Case Studies in Dementia

Common and Uncommon Presentations

Case Studies in Dementia

Common and Uncommon Presentations

Edited by

Serge Gauthier and Pedro Rosa-Neto

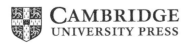

CAMBRIDGE
UNIVERSITY PRESS

CAMBRIDGE
UNIVERSITY PRESS

University Printing House, Cambridge CB2 8BS, United Kingdom

Published in the United States of America by Cambridge University Press, New York

Cambridge University Press is part of the University of Cambridge.

It furthers the University's mission by disseminating knowledge in the pursuit of education, learning and research at the highest international levels of excellence.

www.cambridge.org
Information on this title: www.cambridge.org/9780521188302

© Cambridge University Press 2011

First published 2011

A catalogue record for this publication is available from the British Library

Library of Congress Cataloguing in Publication data
Case studies in dementia : common and uncommon presentations / edited by Serge Gauthier, Pedro Rosa-Neto.
p. ; cm.
Includes bibliographical references and index.
ISBN 978-0-521-18830-2 (pbk.)
1. Dementia–Case studies. I. Gauthier, Serge, 1950- II. Rosa-Neto, Pedro.
[DNLM: 1. Dementia–diagnosis–Case Reports. 2. Diagnostic Techniques and Procedures–Case Reports. WM 220]
RC521.C37 2011
616.8′3–dc22

2010039408

ISBN 978-0-521-18830-2 Paperback

Contents

Contributors

Dag Aarsland
Psychiatric Clinic, Stavanger University Hospital, Stavanger, and AHUS University Hospital, University of Oslo, Oslo, Norway

Adrià Arboix
Cerebrovascular Division, Department of Neurology, Hospital Universitari del Sagrat Cor, Universitat de Barcelona, Barcelona, Spain

Carlos Bazán III
Department of Radiology, School of Medicine, University of Texas Health Science Center at San Antonio and the Audie Murphy Veterans Hospital, San Antonio, TX, USA

James T. Becker
Departments of Neurology, Psychiatry, and Psychology, Alzheimer's Disease Research Center, University of Pittsburgh School of Medicine, Pittsburgh, PA, USA

Sylvie Belleville
Institut universitaire de Gériatrie de l'Université de Montréal, Montréal, QC, Canada

Kevin M. Biglan
Department of Neurology University of Rochester, Rochester, NY, USA

Sandra E. Black
Department of Medicine (Neurology), LC Campbell Cognitive Neurology Research Unit, Sunnybrook Health Sciences Centre, University of Toronto, Canada

Mariana Blanco
Division of Neurology and Rotman Research Institute, Baycrest Centre for Geriatric Care, Toronto, Canada

Rémi W. Bouchard
Département des Sciences Neurologiques, Centre Hospitalier Affilié Hôpital de l'Enfant-Jésus and Faculté de Médecine, Université Laval. Quebec City, Province of Quebec, Canada

Bruce J. Brew
Department of Neurology and Centre for Applied Medical Research, St. Vincent's Hospital, Sydney, Australia

David J. Burn
Institute for Ageing and Health, Newcastle University, Newcastle upon Tyne, UK

Leonardo Caixeta
Hospital das Clínicas, Federal University of Goias, Brazil

Richard Camicioli
Divisions of Neurology and Neuropathology, University of Alberta Hospital, Edmonton, Canada

Paulo Caramelli
Federal University of Minas Gerais, Belo Horizonte (MG) and University of São Paulo, Brazil

Neil Cashman
Brain Research Centre, Faculty of Medicine, University of British Columbia, Canada

Nicholas W. S. Davies
Department of Neurology & Centre for Applied Medical Research, St. Vincent's Hospital, Sydney, Australia

Yan Deschaintre
Hôpital Notre-Dame, Centre Hospitalier de l'Université de Montréal (CHUM), Montréal, QC, Canada

Rachel S. Doody
Baylor College of Medicine, Department of Neurology, Alzheimer's Disease and Memory Disorders Center, Houston, TX, USA

Bruno Dubois
Centre des maladies cognitives et comportementales, Hôpital de la Pitié-Salpêtrière, Paris, France

Uwe Ehrt
Psychiatric Clinic, Stavanger University Hospital, Stavanger, Norway

Stephane Epelbaum
Centre des maladies cognitives et comportementales, Hôpital de la Pitié-Salpêtrière, Paris, France

Ryan V. V. Evans
Department of Neurology University of Rochester, Rochester, NY, USA

Joseph M. Ferrara
Department of Neurology, University of Louisville, Louisville, KY, USA

Bruno Franchi
Geriatric Medicine, Royal Adelaide Hospital, Adelaide, Australia

Morris Freedman
Division of Neurology, Dept of Medicine, Mt. Sinai Hospital, University Health Network, and University of Toronto, Canada

Anders Gade
Memory Disorders Research Group, The Neuroscience Centre, Rigshospitalet, Copenhagen University Hospital, Copenhagen, Denmark

Serge Gauthier
Alzheimer's Disease Research Unit, McGill Center for Studies in Aging, Douglas Mental Health University Institute, McGill University, Quebec, Canada

Marta Grau-Olivares
Cerebrovascular Division, Department of Neurology, Hospital Universitari del Sagrat Cor, Universitat de Barcelona, Barcelona, Spain

Matthew E. Growdon
UCSF Memory and Aging Center, San Francisco, CA, USA

Will Guest
Brain Research Centre, Faculty of Medicine, University of British Columbia, Canada

Marie Christie Guiot
Montreal Neurological Institute and Hospital, McGill Center for Studies in Aging, Montréal, QC, Canada

Shahul Hameed
Division of Neurology, Departments of Medicine and Pathology, University of British Columbia, Canada

Mirna Lie Hosogi-Senaha
Federal University of Minas Gerais, Belo Horizonte (MG) and University of São Paulo, Brazil

Ging-Yuek Robin Hsiung
Division of Neurology, Departments of Medicine and Pathology, University of British Columbia, Canada

Masamichi Ikawa
Second Department of Internal Medicine (Neurology), Faculty of Medical Sciences, University of Fukui, Fukui, Japan

Rajive Jassal
Divisions of Neurology and Neuropathology, University of Alberta Hospital, Edmonton, Canada

Vesna Jelic
Department of Geriatric Medicine and Department of Neurology, Karolinska University Hospital-Huddinge, Stockholm, Sweden

Peter Johannsen
Memory Disorders Research Group, The Neuroscience Centre, Rigshospitalet, Copenhagen University Hospital, Copenhagen, Denmark

Edward S. Johnson
Divisions of Neurology and Neuropathology, University of Alberta Hospital, Edmonton, Canada

Mary M. Kenan
Baylor College of Medicine, Department of Neurology, Alzheimer's Disease and Memory Disorders Center, Houston, TX, USA

Bert-Jan Kerklaan
Department of Neurology and Alzheimer Centre, VU University Medical Centre, Amsterdam, the Netherlands

Benjamin Lam
L.C. Campbell Cognitive Neurology Research Unit, Department of Medicine (Neurology), Sunnybrook Health Sciences Centre, University of Toronto, Canada

Gabriel C. Léger
Hôpital Notre-Dame, Centre Hospitalier de l'Université de Montréal (CHUM), Université de Montréal, McGill University, Montréal, QC, Canada

Gabriel Leonard
McGill Center for Studies in Aging, Montreal Neurological Hospital and Institute, Montréal, QC, Canada

Emilie Lepage
Institut universitaire de Gériatrie de l'Université de Montréal, Montréal, QC, Canada

Irene Litvan
Department of Neurology, University of Louisville, Louisville, KY, USA

Oscar L. Lopez
Departments of Neurology and Psychiatry, Alzheimer's Disease Research Center, University of Pittsburgh School of Medicine, Pittsburgh, PA, USA

Ian R. A. Mackenzie
Division of Neurology, Departments of Medicine and Pathology, University of British Columbia, Canada

Mario Masellis
Department of Medicine (Neurology), LC Campbell Cognitive Neurology Research Unit, Sunnybrook Health Sciences Centre, University of Toronto, Canada

Fodi Massoud
Hôpital Notre-Dame, Centre Hospitalier de l'Université de Montréal (CHUM), Montréal, QC, Canada

Paige Moorhouse
Dalhousie University, Halifax, NS, USA

John C. Morris
Alzheimer's Disease Research Center, Washington University School of Medicine, St. Louis, MO, USA

Taim Muayqil
Divisions of Neurology and Neuropathology, University of Alberta Hospital, Edmonton, Canada

Yannick Nadeau
Department of Medicine (Neurology), LC Campbell Cognitive Neurology Research Unit, Sunnybrook Health Sciences Centre, University of Toronto, Canada

Inger Nennesmo
Department of Pathology, Karolinska University Hospital-Huddinge, Sweden

Jørgen E. Nielsen
Memory Disorders Research Group, The Neuroscience Centre, Rigshospitalet, Copenhagen University Hospital, Copenhagen, Denmark

Ricardo Nitrini
Behavioral and Cognitive Neurology Unit of the Department of Neurology, University of São Paulo School of Medicine, São Paulo, Brazil

Sven-Eric Pålhagen
Department of Neurology, Karolinska University Hospital-Huddinge, Stockholm, Sweden

Robert Perry
Department of Neuropathology, Newcastle General Hospital, Newcastle upon Tyne, UK

Gerald Pfeffer
Division of Neurology, University of British Columbia, Canada

Machiel Pleizier
Department of Neurology and Alzheimer Centre, VU University Medical Centre, Amsterdam, the Netherlands

Steffen Plickert
St. Katharinen Hospital, Dept. of Neurology, Frechen, Germany

Gil D. Rabinovici
UCSF Memory and Aging Center, San Francisco, CA, USA

Philippe H. Robert
Centre Mémoire de Ressources et de Recherche, CHU, Université de Nice Sophia–Antipolis, France

Lothar Resch
Divisions of Neurology and Neuropathology, University of Alberta Hospital, Edmonton, Canada

Gustavo C. Román
Department of Neurology, School of Medicine, University of Texas Health Science Center at San Antonio and the Audie Murphy Veterans Hospital, San Antonio, TX, USA

Maxime Ros
Service de Chirurgie, Hôpital Purpan, Toulouse, France

Pedro Rosa-Neto
Alzheimer's Disease Research Unit, McGill Center for Studies in Aging, Verdun, Quebec, Canada

Aiman Sanosi
Division of Neurology, Department of Pathology, Department of Medicine, University of British Columbia, Canada

Philip Scheltens
Department of Neurology and Alzheimer Centre, VU University Medical Centre, Amsterdam, the Netherlands

Christian Schmidt
Georg-August-University Hospital, Dept. of Neurology, German National Reference Center for the Surveillance of Transmissible Spongiform Encephalopathies, Goettingen, Germany

Eric Schmidt
Service de Neurochirurgie, Hôpital Purpan, Toulouse, France

Jean-Paul Soucy
Montreal Neurological Hospital and Institute, Montréal, QC, Canada

Jette Stokholm
Memory Disorders Research Group, The Neuroscience Centre, Rigshospitalet, Copenhagen University Hospital, Copenhagen, Denmark

David Summers
University of Edinburgh, Western General Hospital, Department of Neuroradiology, Edinburgh, UK

Rawan Tarawneh
Alzheimer's Disease Research Center, Washington University School of Medicine, Saint Louis, MO, USA

Louis Verret
Neurologist, Département des Sciences Neurologiques, Centre Hospitalier Affilié Hôpital de l'Enfant-Jésus and Faculté de Médecine, Université Laval. Quebec City, Province of Quebec, Canada

Huali Wang
Dementia Care and Research Center, Peking University Institute of Mental Health, Beijing, China

Bengt Winblad
Department of Neurology, Karolinska University Hospital-Huddinge and Karolinska Institutet, Alzheimer Disease Research Centre, Karolinska University Hospital, Stockholm, Sweden

Makoto Yoneda
Second Department of Internal Medicine (Neurology), Faculty of Medical Sciences, University of Fukui, Fukui, Japan

Xin Yu
Dementia Care and Research Center, Peking University Institute of Mental Health, Beijing, China

Inga Zerr
Georg-August-University Hospital, Dept. of Neurology, German National Reference Center for the Surveillance of Transmissible Spongiform Encephalopathies, Goettingen, Germany

Preface

The main idea behind *Case Studies in Dementia* is to provide an overview of the spectrum of clinical presentations of various diseases, which have dementia as a common denominator. As a rapidly expending field of clinical neurology, the differential diagnosis and clinical assessment of dementia is becoming progressively more sophisticated and complex. We hope that these case studies will prove useful to medical students, family doctors and neurology residents in their understanding of neurology and the care they provide to their patients.

Serge Gauthier and Pedro Rosa Neto

Acknowledgments

We thank the team of contributors for their cases, comments, and clinical insights. Their diligent work made the edition of this book a pleasurable task. We also would like to thank Dorothée Schoemaker (MCSA), Mary Sanders, Nisha Doshi, and Caroline Brown (Cambridge University Press) for their terrific editorial assistance.

Introduction to the diagnosis of dementia

Serge Gauthier and Pedro Rosa-Neto

This chapter will outline general strategies to establish the presence and the differential diagnosis of dementia, and the case studies in this book will allow the reader to explore more in-depth specific causes of dementia across different age groups. We emphasize the diagnosis of dementia in this book, the first step in the management of dementia.

Is dementia present?

A broad interpretation of the current definition of dementia written in the DSM-IV-R is that an intellectual decline involving at least two cognitive domains must be sufficient to interfere with daily life. Thus the clinician must establish through a systematic history with the subject and an informant if there is a decline in memory, language, praxis, gnosis, and/or executive abilities, and if this decline is associated with impairment in activities of daily living (ADL).

Screening questions about changes within the past year in recall for appointments, recent events, or conversations, can be followed immediately and during a follow-up visit with more detailed questions relevant to:

(1) memory: do you look for things in your room; do you need reminders for appointments
(2) language: do you say sometimes "give me the thing there, what do you call it?"
(3) praxis: do you have difficulty using kitchen appliances or tools?
(4) gnosis: do you have difficulties recognizing people?
(5) executive abilities: do you find it harder to plan a meal for the family or friends; do you need help when playing a card game, can you adjust if there is a change of plans?

Case Studies in Dementia: Common and Uncommon Presentations, ed. S. Gauthier and P. Rosa-Neto. Published by Cambridge University Press. © Cambridge University Press 2011.

Testing for cognitive impairment is usually done using the Mini-Mental State Examination (MMSE; Folstein *et al.*, 1975). If the MMSE is above 26/30, the Montreal Cognitive Assessment (MoCA; Nasreddine *et al.*, 2005) is usually performed, also giving a total score of 30, but encompassing some executive tests such as the Trail B and the clock. More detailed neuropsychological tests may be required depending on the level of education of the subject, the nature of his complaints (language for instance), and the severity of his decline. Thus, the Severe Impairment Battery is used if the MMSE is below 15/30 (Panisset *et al.*, 1994).

From population studies (Pérès *et al.*, 2007), four ADLs were found to be particularly altered in early dementia:

(1) use of telephone and other means of communication
(2) planning an outing and completing it efficiently
(3) using medications safely
(4) using money appropriately.

These specific ADLs can be asked about for screening purpose, followed immediately or during a follow-up visit with questions on other instrumental (meal preparation, leisure, and housework) and basic (hygiene, dressing, continence, eating) ADLs.

Although surprisingly missing from the current definition of dementia, neuropsychiatric symptoms can precede the onset of cognitive decline and nearly always accompany them. It is thus important to ask about the following common symptoms in a semi-structured way or using an instrument such as the Neuropsychiatric Inventory (NPI; Cummings J, 1997).

(1) apathy
(2) agitation and aggressivity
(3) anxiety and depression
(4) aberrant motor behaviors
(5) delusions and hallucinations
(6) irritability
(7) night-time behaviors

What is the cause of dementia?

It is surprising how a good history addressing the common cognitive, functional (ADL), and behavioral symptoms encountered in dementia will lead to a short differential diagnosis, since the most common causes of dementia have a typical pattern of presentation:

Alzheimer's disease (AD) may be preceded by a prodrome of anxiety, mild depressive mood, irritability, nearly always starts with impaired recent memory, followed by word-finding difficulties, decreased orientation to time and place. MMSE usually 25/30 or less at time of diagnosis.

Dementia with Lewy Bodies (DLB) nearly always starts with visual hallucinations and fluctuations in cognitive ability. The MMSE may be 22 at times, 26 at other times. Parkinson Disease Dementia (PDD) by definition starts with motoric symptoms of resting tremor, bradykinesia, and/or rigidity, followed at least a year later by visual hallucinations and fluctuations in cognitive ability.

Fronto-temporal dementias (FTD) usually start with language impairment or with social disinhibition. The former can lead to mistakenly low MMSE scores and the latter with mistakenly high MMSE scores. This and other cognitive tests must always be interpreted within the context of cognitive, functional, and behavioral symptoms, and not be used as "a test of dementia."

The common causes of dementia may have atypical presentations, as illustrated in this book. Rare causes of dementia, particular in young subjects (before age 50) require special work-up as demonstrated as well in this book.

What confirmatory tests are required?

Although the history is the cornerstone of the diagnosis of dementia, complementary laboratory tests usually include:

(1) basic blood tests (hematologic, endocrine, hepatic, renal function, screening, B12, VDRL, HIV)
(2) brain imaging using Computer Scanning (CT) or Magnetic Resonance Imaging (MRI) studies

Special tests will depend on the suspected cause of dementia and include:

(1) Special blood tests (coeruloplasmin for Wilson's disease, for example)
(2) Special brain imaging such as Positron Emission Tomography (PET) for glucose metabolism (FDG-PET), amyloid load (PIB, for instance)
(3) Electroencephalography (in Creutzfeldt–Jacob disease)
(4) Lumbar puncture (some protein markers in AD, in neurosyphilis)
(5) Immunology work-up for antibody-mediated dementias (paraneoplastia syndromes, Hashimoto's encephalitis)
(6) Genetic and molecular studies (metabolic and inherited diseases).

General advice in dealing with dementia

• It takes time and patience to obtain key elements of history leading to a diagnosis of dementia and its cause; repeated assessments are sometimes required; additional data may be required from visits at home by occupational therapists or other health professionals.

- Go back to the beginning of the symptoms, since most family members will discuss current problems; the sequence of symptoms is the key to the diagnosis.
- Time tells, e.g. some types of dementia are diagnosed with key physical findings that appear well after the onset of cognitive decline, such as slowing of saccadic eye movements in progressive supra-nuclear palsy.
- There may be more than one cause of dementia, e.g. "mixed-dementia" is more common than a single cause of dementia in elderly subjects (over age 75).
- Psychiatric symptoms may mask a dementia, e.g. depression often co-exists with early AD, and patients with odd personality disorders can have a dementia.
- If the diagnosis is not clear, get advice from colleagues in different disciplines, including neuropsychology, social services, occupational therapy. A consensus approach in difficult cases may be the best way to move forward.

The future

Things will get more complicated as the field in moving towards a diagnosis of common causes of "dementia" in their pre-dementia stages of disease. For instance, an early diagnosis of AD may be possible when only memory is impaired, if at least one biological marker of the disease is found by CSF examination, genetic testing, or neuro-imaging (Dubois *et al.*, 2007). Possibly DLB and PDD will be diagnosed earlier with sleep disturbances such as REM Behavior Disorder associated with an abnormal biological marker (still to be identified). There will be risks (such as a catastrophic reaction), benefits (such as early treatment and arrest or delay of progression), and additional costs (most from neuroimaging procedures) for earlier diagnosis. More to follow on this in the next edition of this book!

REFERENCES AND FURTHER READING

American Psychiatric Association (1994). *Diagnostic and Statistical Manual of Mental Disorders* (DSM IV), 4th edn. Washington, DC: American Psychiatric Association.

Cummings JL (1997). The Neuropsychiatric Inventory: assessing psychopathology in dementia patients. *Neurology*, **48**(5 Suppl 6), S10–16. Review.

Folstein M, Folstein S, McHugh P (1975). Mini-mental state – practical method for grading cognitive state of patients for clinician. *J Psychiat Res*, **12**, 189–98.

Geschwind MD, Shu H, Haman A, Sejvar JJ, Miller BL (2008). Rapidly progressive dementia. *Ann Neurol*, **64**, 97–108.

Nasreddine ZS, Phillips NA, Bedirian V, *et al.* (2005). The Montreal Cognitive Assessment, MoCA: a brief screening tool for mild cognitive impairment. *J Am Geriatr Soc*, **53**, 695–9.

Panisset M, Roudier M, Saxton J, Boller F (1994). Severe impairment battery. A neuropsychological test for severely demented patients. *Arch Neurol*, **51**(1), 41–5.

Pérès K, Helmer C, Amieva H, *et al.* (2008). Natural history of decline in instrumental activities of daily living performance over the 10 years preceding the clinical diagnosis of dementia: a prospective population-based study. *J Am Geriatr Soc*, **56**(1), 37–44. Epub 2007 Nov 20.

Rossor MN, Fox NC, Mummery CJ, Schott JM, Warren JD (2010). The diagnosis of young-onset dementia. *Lancet Neurol*, **9**(8), 793–806.

Subjective cognitive complaint

Stephane Epelbaum and Bruno Dubois

Clinical history – main complaint

A 70-year-old woman consulted for a severe cognitive complaint encompassing numerous domains (i.e. memory, language, calculation...). She described her difficulties as follows:

- "I forget what I did yesterday or even a few hours ago."
- "I am unable to perform mental calculation."
- "I gave an appointment to my daughter and forgot it. When she called me I did not even remember the purpose of this appointment."
- "I did not remember answering my mail."
- "I have trouble finding my words. They are often on the tip of my tongue."
- "I have difficulties remembering my friends' names."
- "I come into a room and do not remember why I entered it."
- "I have trouble finding things in my house."
- "I lose the notion of time so that a recent event feels far gone."
- "I make more and more spelling mistakes."

General history

She is a university educated woman in good general health. She lives with her husband and has two children. She does not have any chronic medical problem and takes no medication. A depression was diagnosed and successfully treated for 6 months with fluoxetine 5 years ago.

Family history

Her father died of myocardial infarct at the age of 75.

Case Studies in Dementia: Common and Uncommon Presentations, ed. S. Gauthier and P. Rosa-Neto.
Published by Cambridge University Press. © Cambridge University Press 2011.

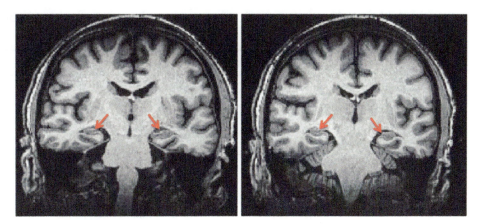

Fig. 1.1.   MRI (T1 coronal slices) showing minimal cerebral atrophy especially in the hippocampal regions (arrows).

Examination

BP: 140/80; pulse: 65 regular. MMSE: 29/30, serial-7s correct but effortful. Five-word test: 10/10. FAB: 17/18. Normal naming, no dysgraphia or dyslexia. Normal neurologic examination. Anxiety and mild depression were also noted (MADRS = 18).

Special studies

MRI showed no focal atrophy especially of the hippocampal regions (see Fig. 1.1).

Neuropsychological tests were normal except for impaired working memory on the digit span test (digit span forward = 6, digit span backward = 3) and a low free recall in the Free and Cued Selective Reminding Test (FCSRT): free recall = 17/48* (significant decrease), total recall = 48/48, delayed total = recall 16/16, no intrusion; Mattis dementia rating scale = 137/144; DO 80 = 78. No apraxia, dyscalculia, Gerstmann syndrome, or visuospatial difficulties.

Diagnosis

The initial diagnostic impression was a subjective cognitive complaint with an attention disorder of probable psychogenic origin.

Follow-up

Fluoxetine was administered. After 6 months, subjective improvement was noted.

Table 1.1. The three mnesic processes one has to assess in case of cognitive complaint

Process	Assessment (with the FCSRT)	Causes
Registration	Immediate recall	Attention deficit due to – Depression – Confusion – Drug therapies
Storage	Retrieval with cue	Hippocampal (or hippocampo–mamillo–thalamic circuit) lesion in – Alzheimer's disease – Korsakoff's syndrome – Limbic encephalitis
Retrieval	Spontaneous retrieval	Executive dysfunction in – Vascular cognitive impairment – Depression – Normal aging – Fronto-temporal dementia

Discussion

Subjective cognitive complaint (SCC) is frequent in normal aging with a prevalence of 50% after 55 years of age (Lowenthal *et al.*, 1967). The problem is that SCC may be the symptomatic expression of several conditions including Alzheimer's disease. To better understand the diagnostic algorithm of SCC, we must have in mind the physiopathology of long-term episodic memory.

Episodic memory is the capacity to recall personal events that can be identified in time or in space. For instance, to recall one's last meal, its taste, smell, the conversation, and state of mind during the meal. To be recalled, the stimulus (whatever it is: a list of words, sentences, stories, images, drawings, smells...) must go through three different and successive stages (See Table 1.1). The three mnesic processes one has to assess in case of cognitive complaint are as follows.

• The first one is registration, which mainly relies on attention resources, which facilitate the capture of information by the perceptual and sensory cortical areas (visual cortex for images, auditory cortex for verbal items...). This stage is impaired in conditions that may interfere with attention processes: depression, anxiety, professional stress, sleep disorders, aging, treatment such as anticholinergic drugs or benzodiazepines... In all these cases, there might be a recall deficit not because of a long-term memory problem, but only because of registration impairment. In all these situations, the information will not be well registered and the recall performance will be decreased in relation to attention disorders.

• The second step is storage, i.e. the transformation of registered perceptual events into memory traces: after the perceptual and identification stages by the sensory cortices and related associative areas, the information is transferred to the hippocampus to be transformed by the hippocampal mamillothalamic circuit into memory traces. In case of hippocampal lesions, such as in Alzheimer's disease, or mamillothalamic lesions, such as in Korsakoff syndrome, the perceived information cannot be stored as memory traces in long-term memory. In such conditions, the information will be lost and cannot be recalled any more: this feature corresponds to a true genuine memory impairment.

• The last stage is retrieval: this stage relies on the ability to activate strategic processes to recollect stored information. This process is directly related to the functioning of the frontal lobes. This is why retrieval abilities are decreased in frontal lesions, fronto-temporal dementias, subcortico-frontal dementias and in functional states such as depression or even normal aging, where the activation of retrieval strategies is decreased and effortful. In these conditions, the recall performance will be decreased in relation with a retrieval deficit.

To summarize, memory disorders in everyday life can result from attention disorders, retrieval difficulties as well as genuine memory deficit due to Alzheimer's disease. The best way to disentangle the diagnostic problem is to assess memory by objective tests that may control for attention and that can facilitate the retrieval. This is the case of the Free and Cued Selected Recall Test (FCSRT) (Grober *et al.*, 1988). The FCSRT has been recommended in the new diagnostic criteria of AD for the assessment of episodic long-term memory (Dubois *et al.*, 2007). Semantic cues are used to control for an effective encoding of the 16 items just after their presentation and to maximize retrieval (in case of a dysexecutive syndrome) after a 30-minute delay. Therefore, low total recall, despite the facilitation procedures, indicates the existence of an amnestic syndrome of the hippocample type, mostly in relation to an Alzheimer's disease.

The FCSRT

Sixteen words have to be learned following a standardized procedure. The 16 items to be learned are presented on four successive cards of four items each. These items are presented in quadrants on a sheet of paper as a word (e.g. grapes) which goes with a unique category cue (e.g. fruit). The subject is asked to point to and name aloud each item (e.g. grapes) after hearing the appropriate cue (e.g. fruit). After all four items were identified correctly, the card is removed, and *immediate cued recall* of the four items is tested by giving the cues again in order to control for encoding.

Once a group of four items had been successfully encoded (evidenced by complete immediate recall), the next set of four items is presented. **This first phase of the test is done to control the *registration* process and provides a score called *immediate recall*.** By this way, the examiner knows that the subject has registered all the items. Unfortunately, only a few memory tests control that the information – used to study long-term memory – has been truly registered. Then, three successive recall trials are performed, each consisting of two parts. First, a free recall of as many items as possible and second, a cued recall in response to orally presented semantic category for those items that were not spontaneously retrieved by the patient. This provides a *free recall score* and a *total recall score*, (the latter being the sum of free and cued recall). As semantic cueing, in normal controls, normalizes the performance of recall by facilitating the retrieval of stored information, the total score is expected to be higher than 44/48.

To evaluate the efficacy of semantic cues used to facilitate retrieval from stored information, an *Index of Sensitivity of Cueing* (*ISC*) was defined, which is determined as: (total recall − free recall)/(48 − free recall). **A low index reflects a *storage* deficit** (because free and cued recalls do not differ to a great extent). **Conversely, a high index, points toward *retrieval* difficulties** (because cues are frequently needed to recall the information). After a 30-minute delay, filled by other non-verbal tests, a delayed recall task is proposed with the same procedure of free and cued recall, providing a score for *delayed free recall* and a score for *delayed total recall* (*DTR = maximal score of 16*). During the test, the number of *intrusions* (i.e. words absent from the list and falsely "recalled") is recorded.

In conclusion, SCC can be observed in many circumstances and has varied causes, the first of which being an attention disorder. This disorder is frequent in anxiety (Craik *et al.*, 1995; Ganguli *et al.*, 2004), depression (McGlone *et al.*, 1990; Tierney *et al.*, 1996; Schmand *et al.*, 1997), and drug therapies (benzodiazepines, anticholinergics...) or even in normal aging. An attention disorder is a handicap in daily life when dual tasks are required or working memory is needed. By contrast, neuropsychological tests are frequently normal in these conditions because the examiner avoids eliciting divided attention.

However, subjective cognitive complaint can also be caused by an organic cerebral affection such as Alzheimer's disease (AD). In this case, the storage of information is impaired and controlling the efficacy of the registration process is no longer enough to allow its normal recall (Hodges, 1998; Dubois and Albert, 2004). This justifies a complete neuropsychological assessment if any doubt about a neurodegenerative process remains after the initial neurological consult. Perceptions of patients' symptoms from an informant or proxy may be more significant as they are more strongly related to objective memory performance (McGlone *et al.*, 1990) and are predictive of conversion to AD (Tierney *et al.*,

1996). Particular attention should be paid to intra-individual decline, which improves the identification of patients with prodromal AD (Storandt *et al.*, 2006). The fact that subjective cognitive complaint is sometimes due to a neuro-degenerative disorder justifies additional exams and paraclinical testing as proposed by the revised NINCDS–ADRDA criteria for the diagnosis of AD. In the case of specific memory impairment (storage deficit) (Dubois *et al.*, 2007) anatomical (MRI) and/or functional (PET or TEMP) cerebral imaging and/or amyloid β, Tau and phospho-Tau biomarkers in the CSF are useful supportive arguments to ascertain the diagnosis of AD.

Take home messages

Subjective cognitive complaint is frequent (50% of the population after 50 years of age) and corresponds to numerous etiologies.

To diagnose the etiology of a SCC, one must refer to the specific cognitive stage impaired (registration, storage, and retrieval) and use specific tests that may resolve the issue.

The possibility of a neurodegenerative disorder as a cause of SCC must lead to caution. Paraclinical and complete neuropsychological testing is required as soon as this etiology is possible after an initial neurological consult.

REFERENCES AND FURTHER READING

Craik FIM, Anderson ND, *et al.* (1995). Memory changes in normal ageing. In Baddeley AD, Wilson BA, Watts FN. *Memory Disorders* Chichester: Wiley, 211–42.

Dubois B, Albert ML (2004). Amnestic MCI or prodromal Alzheimer's disease? *Lancet Neurol*, 3(4), 246–8.

Dubois B, Feldman HH, *et al.* (2007). Research criteria for the diagnosis of Alzheimer's disease: revising the NINCDS-ADRDA criteria. *Lancet Neurol*, 6(8), 734–46.

Ganguli M, Rodriguez E, *et al.* (2004). Detection and management of cognitive impairment in primary care: The Steel Valley Seniors Survey. *J Am Geriatr Soc*, 52(10), 1668–75.

Grober E, Buschke H, *et al.* (1988). Screening for dementia by memory testing. *Neurology*, 38(6), 900–3.

Hodges J (1998). The amnestic prodrome of Alzheimer's disease. *Brain*, 121(9), 1601–2.

Lowenthal PM, Berrman PL, *et al.* (1967). *Aging and Mental Disorders: A Social Psychiatric Study*. San Francisco (CA): Jossey-Bass.

McGlone J, Gupta S, *et al.* (1990). Screening for early dementia using memory complaints from patients and relatives. *Arch Neurol,* **47**(11), 1189–93.

Schmand B, Jonker C, *et al.* (1997). Subjective memory complaints in the elderly: depressive symptoms and future dementia. *Br J Psychiatry,* **171**, 373–6.

Storandt M, Grant EA, *et al.* (2006). Longitudinal course and neuropathologic outcomes in original vs. revised MCI and in pre-MCI. *Neurology,* **67**(3), 467–73.

Tierney MC, Szalai JP, *et al.* (1996). The prediction of Alzheimer disease. The role of patient and informant perceptions of cognitive deficits. *Arch Neurol,* **53**(5), 423–7.

Man with subjective complaints but abnormal CSF

Machiel Pleizier and Philip Scheltens

Clinical history – main complaint

A 65-year-old technical worker with previous management function had been unable to work because of pulmonary problems for 7 years. He visited the memory clinic because of slowly progressive memory complaints over the past year, concerning names of familiar people and recent facts. Things get lost and difficulty with multitasking was observed by others. No interference with daily functioning is reported and he denies depressive symptoms.

His wife and children confirm memory complaints, but they also noticed changes in behavior. In increasingly common conflict situations the patient sometimes uses verbal and physical violence. There are numerous life events, such as the undesired cessation of work and some other private circumstances, but the patient is reported to show no emotion, while a marked character change is denied by the spouse.

General history

This highly educated man had been diagnosed with extrinsic allergic alveolitis 7 years ago. He has used prednisolone in the past and now only uses fluticasone inhaler if necessary. Neurologic evaluation 5 years ago, because of black-outs during car driving, revealed no abnormalities. His electroencephalogram (EEG) and magnetic resonance imaging (MRI) were reported to be normal. He stopped smoking 7 years ago and uses three units alcohol daily. Patient lives with his wife and has two children and three grandchildren.

Family history

The patient's father suffered from dementia in his 70s and died 8 years after onset of symptoms. No specific diagnosis was made.

Case Studies in Dementia: Common and Uncommon Presentations, ed. S. Gauthier and P. Rosa-Neto. Published by Cambridge University Press. © Cambridge University Press 2011.

Examination

His blood pressure was 145/95 mm Hg. Further general physical and neurologic examination revealed no abnormalities. Mini-Mental State Examination (MMSE) was 29/30 and Frontal Assessment Battery (FAB) 18/18. He demonstrated difficulties with clock-drawing by wrong placement of hands. There was intact recollection of recent news items.

Special studies

Routine laboratory investigations showed no abnormalities. Apolipoprotein E (APOE) status was $\varepsilon2/\varepsilon3$. Cerebrospinal fluid (CSF) analysis showed abnormal values for brain-specific proteins: beta-amyloid$_{1-42}$ (Aβ_{1-42}) 387 pg/mL (reference value > 500 pg/mL), total tau 458 pg/mL (reference value < 350 pg/mL) and phosphorylated tau at threonine 181 (p-tau) 78 pg/mL (reference value < 60 pg/mL). EEG showed diffuse mild disturbances with abundance of drowsiness. MRI demonstrates periventricular white matter hyperintensities (WMH) and some atrophy in frontal and parietal regions without temporal or hippocampal atrophy. Neuropsychological assessment showed dysfunction in one episodic memory test with normal performance in other (episodic) memory tests and all other cognitive domains.

Diagnosis

A diagnosis of subjective memory complaints (SMC) was made. The fact that CSF values were abnormal was not taken into account at that time because of lack of a clinical diagnosis of dementia. Referral to a psychiatrist was advised for evaluation of a possible mood disorder and for counseling on how to deal with his behavioral disturbances.

Follow-up

One year later, both the patient and his wife confirmed improvement of his behavior following psychotherapy. However, the patient still exhibited aggressive and impulsive behavior with obsessive thoughts regarding his work as a volunteer. Memory, overview, and initiative were preserved, confirmed by repeated neuropsychological tests. Slight diminished executive functioning and dysfunction in learning abilities were noted, but in comparison with earlier assessment no decline was found. MMSE was 28/30 with loss of two points on recall. FAB showed a diminished score of 14/18. Repeated MRI of the brain showed mild parietal atrophy and the presence of two microbleeds. Patient's history together with abnormal CSF values and MRI made a diagnosis of incipient Alzheimer's disease (AD) with frontal features more likely. Since memory was spared and more frontal features were present, 18-fluorodeoxyglucose positron emission tomography (FDG-PET) was made to differentiate with behavioral variant frontotemporal dementia (bvFTD). No abnormalities were seen in the frontal, parietal, and posterior cingulate cortices. At that time a diagnosis of mild cognitive impairment (MCI) was made.

Six months later, further progression was noted with withdrawal from social interaction, impaired memory, interference with IADL function, together with difficulty driving his car. A diagnosis of AD was made, 1½ years after the initial presentation with memory complaints.

Discussion

SMC or subjective cognitive impairment (SCI) in the absence of MCI or dementia is more and more accepted as a separate clinical entity. In subjects aged 65 years or more, a prevalence was found between 25% and 56% (Jonker *et al.*, 2000). SCI is associated with aging, MCI, dementia, and depression. Depression, anxiety, disturbed sleep, fatigue, and loss of energy were responsible for a conversion from SCI to MCI, but subsequently reverted back to SCI after follow-up (Glodzik-Sobanska *et al.*, 2007). Since SCI is often not systematically investigated with exclusion of MCI, dementia or depression, it is hard to reliably determine its prevalence and outcome. Conflicting data are observed in outcome studies: while a three times greater risk of AD was found in highly educated persons with SCI in comparison with non-SCI subjects, others found no evidence that SCI predicted dementia or MCI (Reisberg and Gauthier, 2008). Furthermore, follow-up series showed progressive decline in about 55%–60% of SCI subjects over 7 to 9 years (Reisberg *et al.*, 2008).

Research into predictive factors for progression to dementia in SCI is extensive.

Increase of theta power in baseline EEG in SCI subjects has been shown to predict decline or conversion to MCI and dementia. In healthy subjects without cognitive complaints, slowing of cognitive speed is correlated with AD-associated changes in both CSF and EEG (Stomrud *et al.*, 2010).

CSF AD profiles (characterized by a abnormal ratio $A\beta_{1-42}$:total tau) in amnestic or non-amnestic MCI patients have been shown to be highly predictive in many studies, a.o. the DESCRIPA study. Although in this study subjects with SCI had a CSF AD profile in 50% of the cases, they did not show cognitive deterioration in the 3-year follow-up period (Visser *et al.*, 2009).

MRI studies have shown structural changes as the presence of WMH and medial temporal lobe atrophy between SCI subjects and persons without cognitive complaints (Van der Flier *et al.*, 2004). Although in MCI patients MTA predicted conversion to AD, this has not been determined yet in SCI.

FDG-PET in SCI subjects demonstrated hypometabolism in the parietotemporal regions and the parahippocampal gyrus with lower metabolic rates in the latter region in APOE ε4 positive subjects. These findings resemble those found in AD (Reisberg and Gauthier, 2008).

When SCI is diagnosed, all possible explanations for cognitive impairment have to be ruled out. Consultation with a psychiatrist or psychologist can be very helpful in case of suspected mood disorder. Also, somatic reasons like thyroid dysfunction and vitamin deficiencies have to be excluded. Follow-up studies are recommended to determine deterioration on neuropsychological tests or changes on imaging findings, especially in subjects in whom slowness in EEG background pattern, pathological CSF findings or APOE ε4 homo- or heterozygosity are demonstrated.

In sum, this patient was initially diagnosed with SCI and subsequently underwent psychiatric evaluation. In spite of subjective improvement, a relative rapid decline was observed in 1½ years and AD was diagnosed. Initial CSF analysis already showed pathological vaues probably reflecting brain amyloid deposition. MRI and FDG PET did not show specific findings to support a diagnosis of AD probably explained by the non-ε4 carrier status. This case illustrates the early changes in biomarkers found in AD.

Take home messages

SCI without depression may reflect the earliest pre-dementia state.

In SCI increased theta power in EEG and AD profile in CSF analysis forecast decline to MCI or dementia despite normal brain imaging.

Follow-up of patients with SCI is necessary to rule out other treatable causes and prediction of further cognitive decline.

REFERENCES AND FURTHER READING

Flier WM van der, Buchem MA van, Weverling-Rijnsburger AWE, *et al.* (2004). Memory complaints in patients with normal cognition are associated with smaller hippocampal volumes. *J Neurol* **251**, 671–5.

Glodzik-Sobanska L, Reisberg B, De Santi S, *et al.* (2007). Subjective memory complaints: presence, severity and future outcome in normal older subjects. *Dement Geriatr Cogn Disord* **24**, 177–84.

Johnson JK, Head E, Kim R, *et al.* (1999). Clinical and pathological evidence for a frontal variant of Alzheimer disease. *Arch Neurol* **56**, 1233–9.

Jonker C, Geerlings MI, Schmand B (2000). Are memory complaints predictive for dementia? A review of clinical and population-based studies. *Int J Geriatr Psychiatry* **15**, 983–91.

Norden AG van, Fick WF, Laat KF de, *et al.* (2008). Subjective cognitive failures and hippocampal volume in elderly with white matter lesions. *Neurology,* **71**, 1152–9.

Reisberg B, Gauthier S (2008). Current evidence for subjective cognitive impairment (SCI) as the pre-mild cognitive impairment (MCI) stage of subsequently manifest Alzheimer's disease. *Int Psychogeriatr* **20**, 1–16.

Reisberg B, Shulman M, Monteiro I, *et al.* (2008). A seven-year prospective study of outcome in older persons with and without subjective cognitive impairment. *Alzheimers Dement* **4**, T529.

Stomrud E, Hansson O, Minthon L, *et al.* (2010). Slowing of EEG correlates with CSF biomarkers and reduced cognitive speed in elderly with normal cognition over 4 years. *Neurobiol Aging,* **31**(2), 215–23.

Visser PJ, Verhey F, Knol DL, *et al.* (2009). Prevalence and prognostic value of CSF markers of Alzheimer's disease pathology in patients with subjective cognitive impairment or mild cognitive impairment in the DESCRIPA study: a prospective cohort study. *Lancet Neurol* **8**, 619–27.

Vlies AE van der, Koedam ELGE, Pijnenburg YAL, *et al.* (2009). Most rapid cognitive decline in APOE epsilon4 negative Alzheimer's disease with early onset. *Psychol Med* **39**, 1907–11.

Case 3

When mild cognitive impairment really is Alzheimer's disease

Rawan Tarawneh and John C. Morris

*This case was published in *Archives of Neurology* during the preparation of this manuscript (Cairns et al., 2009).

Case presentation

An 85-year-old man enrolled in a longitudinal study of healthy aging and Alzheimer disease (AD) at the Washington University Alzheimer Disease Research Center (ADRC) was followed annually over 6 years. He was judged to be cognitively normal (CDR 0) at his initial and next three annual assessments through the age of 88 years. At his fifth annual assessment (age 89), his collateral source (CS) reported a decline from his baseline cognitive performance. He was reported to be more forgetful and had impaired ability to make decisions. His Mini-Mental State Examination (MMSE) score was 26. At his sixth assessment at age 90, his CS reported further decline in cognitive function that mildly interfered with his daily activities. For example, his driving was impaired and he experienced a motor vehicle accident. He was unable to recall recent events in which he had participated. He was diagnosed with dementia of the Alzheimer's type (DAT) and died shortly after his 91st birthday. A post-mortem examination was completed (Cairns *et al.*, 2009).

General history

He had 12 years of education and was a retired civil servant. His medical history was notable for congestive heart failure with an automated implanted cardiac defibrillator (AICD) placement, hypertension, critical aortic stenosis, atrial fibrillation, diabetes mellitus, and peripheral vascular disease. Medications included simvastatin, aspirin, clopidogrel, isosorbide dinitrate, furosemide, ramipril, and carvedilol.

Family history

His father died at the age of 83 and his mother died at the age of 92. There was no family history of Alzheimer's disease. Both his father and mother were hypertensive and his mother was diabetic.

Examination

Vital signs at his last assessment: BP: 130/58, pulse rate 62/min and irregularly irregular. The MMSE score at age 90 was 28 (Folstein *et al.*, 1975).

There were no carotid bruits. Lungs were clear. There was an ejection systolic murmur in the left second intercostal space with minimal radiation to the left sternal edge. There were no heaves or thrills. There was +1 pitting edema in both legs. All peripheral pulses were palpable. Abdomen was soft with no organo-megaly and no ascites.

He was alert and oriented to time, place, and person. Attention span was intact. Language was normal in fluency, comprehension, and repetition, but there was mild hesitancy. There was some difficulty with object naming. Cranial nerves were intact including fundoscopic exam. Visual acuity was 20/30 bilaterally. Power and tone was normal throughout. Deep tendon reflexes were +1 and symmetric. Plantar reflexes were flexor. Sensation was intact to light touch and pinprick. Vibration was slightly decreased at the toes and ankles, but otherwise intact. Gait was slow and cautious, but otherwise normal.

Special studies

A psychometric battery was performed within 2 weeks of each annual clinical assessment. The battery included three measures of episodic memory (Logical Memory and Associate Learning from the Wechsler Memory Scale (Wechsler D and Stone CP, 1973) and the Free and Selective Reminding Test [sum of three free recall trials]) (Grober *et al.*, 1988), two measures of semantic memory: [Information and the Boston Naming Test (Goodglass H and Kaplan E, 1983)], measures of working memory [Mental Control and Digit Span (forward and backward) (Wechsler D and Stone CP, 1973) and word fluency] (Thurstone LL and Thurstone LG, 1949), and measures of visuospatial ability [Block Design (Wechsler D and Stone CP, 1973), Digit Symbol (Wechsler D and Stone CP, 1973) and the Trailmaking Test A (Armitage SG, 1946)]. Scores were converted to z scores using means and standard deviations from the first time of assessment of a reference group of 310 individuals who were enrolled at our ADRC as CDR 0

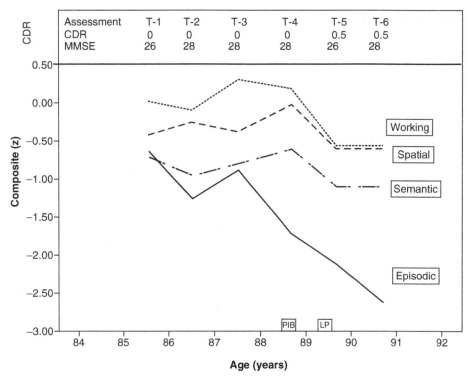

Fig. 3.1.   Clinical and cognitive course of the individual described in this case. CDR, Clinical Dementia Rating; LP, lumbar puncture; MMS, Mini-Mental State Examination; and T-1, first clinical assessment. Composite z scores are given for episodic memory, semantic memory, working memory, and visuospatial ability. At age 89.5 years, he underwent a lumbar puncture for research studies of the cerebrospinal fluid (CSF). The CSF analysis demonstrated increased total tau (575 pg/mL, normally < 500 pg/mL) and $ptau_{181} = 83$ pg/mL (normally < 80 pg/mL). The CSF $A\beta_{42}$ levels were low (303 pg/mL; normally > 500 pg/mL). The $A\beta_{40}$ level (12,943 pg/mL) was within normal range. This CSF profile is consistent with that of Alzheimer's disease (Sunderland et al., 2003, Fagan et al., 2009). Reproduced by permission from Cairns et al. (2009) © 2009 American Medical Association All rights reserved.

and remained at such a rating as long as they were followed (for at least two assessments) (Johnson et al., 2009). The z scores from each cognitive domain then were averaged to form composites (Storandt et al., 2006).

The most striking feature of the longitudinal cognitive performance of this man was a sharp decline, beginning after his third assessment, on the episodic memory composite and eventually totaling two standard deviations (Fig. 3.1). It was accompanied by a less precipitous decline in working memory (totaling half a standard deviation) beginning after his fourth assessment. Semantic memory and visuospatial ability were relatively preserved throughout his six assessments.

Diagnosis

The detection of dementia at our ADRC is based on observations from a collateral source of decline from an individual's previously attained level of cognitive function that is sufficient to interfere with that individual's customary activities (DSM-IV) (The American Psychiatric Association, 1994). Observations obtained from the CS and the individual regarding the possibility of cognitive and functional decline during the clinical assessment are synthesized with the Clinical Dementia Rating (CDR) (Morris, 1993).

The CDR is performed in two components: a semi-structured interview with a collateral source, and an interview with the individual that includes some objective testing. The CDR is determined by rating cognitive, behavioral, and functional changes resulting from dementia in each of six categories: Memory, Orientation, Judgment and Problem Solving, Community Affairs, Home and Hobbies, and Personal Care (Morris, 1993). Each category is scored independently on a five-point scale of impairment (0 = no impairment, 0.5 = questionable or very mild, 1 = mild, 2 = moderate, and 3 = severe impairment); one category, Personal Care, does not have a 0.5 impairment level. The CDR scoring table includes descriptive "anchors" that guide the rater in determining individual domain ratings based on both collateral source report and subject performance.

The CDR determinations and etiologic diagnoses are made independently of the results from the individual's psychometric testing and from results of research diagnostic procedures, including the CSF assays. CDR stage 0.5 denotes very mild dementia and is characterized by relatively mild cognitive decline and subtle functional impairment. The clinician judges the most likely etiology of dementia in accordance with standard criteria. The CDR staging of 0.5 and etiologic diagnosis of very mild DAT are sensitive and accurate for underlying neuropathologic AD (Storandt et al., 2006), although many of these individuals elsewhere would be classified as "mild cognitive impairment" (MCI) (Petersen et al., 2009).

Criteria for amnestic MCI include objective evidence of cognitive impairment as defined by poor performance on a measure of episodic memory by an individual in comparison with normative values from a group of age- and education-matched controls (Petersen et al., 2009). This approach thus represents an inter-individual comparison of psychometric test performance. It does not, however, determine whether the impaired performance represents a decline for that individual. Moreover, individual differences in cognitive ability are too large to permit assessment of very early DAT by comparison with normative values (Storandt et al., 2009). Because putatively normal samples likely are contaminated with individuals with preclinical AD (Sliwinski et al., 1996), the cutpoints are too permissive and fail to capture some persons in the initial symptomatic stages of AD, resulting in an ascertainment bias (Tuokko *et al.*, 2003; Storandt, 2010). Rather than comparing an individual's performance with a normative group to detect early-stage DAT, it is necessary to evaluate the person's longitudinal course.

Although our case met criteria for amnestic MCI at his fifth assessment, it also was possible to diagnose early-stage DAT at the CDR 0.5 level using the principle of intra-individual decline based on collateral source observations. This diagnosis was independently supported by his cognitive decline, CSF results, and post-mortem examination.

Follow-up

The participant died of congestive heart failure shortly after his 91st birthday. His *APOE* genotype was homozygous for ε3. A brain autopsy was performed. External examination showed no cerebral atrophy and an unfixed brain weight of 1310 g (normal range: 1250–1400 g). There was evidence of neuronal loss and gliosis throughout the frontal neocortex on microscopic examination using hematoxylin and eosin staining. Bielschowsky silver staining and immunohistochemistry with anti-Aß and anti-tau antibodies showed focally numerous diffuse plaques throughout the cerebral cortex, but neuritic plaques were relatively infrequent and there were only isolated neurofibrillary tangles. Neurofibrillary tangles, modest granulovacuolar degeneration, and moderate neuronal loss and gliosis were identified in the CA1 subfield of the hippocampus. The parahippocampus showed neuronal loss, gliosis, and a few neurofibrillary tangles with a relative scarcity of neuritic plaques. On biochemical analysis of frozen cerebral cortex, high levels of Aβ_{42} were detected in the frontal, occipital, and precuneus regions.

The neurofibrillary lesions met stage III and amyloid plaques met stage C in the Braak and Braak staging system (Braak and Braak, 1991). The densities of diffuse plaques were sufficient to meet the age-adjusted neuropathological criteria for AD according to Khachaturian criteria (Khachaturian, 1985). The neuritic plaque and tangle densities were consistent with a diagnosis of possible AD by the Consortium to Establish a Registry for Alzheimer's disease (CERAD) criteria (Mirra *et al.*, 1991) and with the "low probability" criteria of the National Institute on Aging-Reagan Institute (NIA-Reagan) criteria (Hyman and Trojanowski, 1997).

Discussion

The diagnosis of very mild DAT in this case was supported independently by his declining longitudinal psychometric performance in the episodic and working memory domains and by an "Alzheimer" CSF profile of elevated tau and decreased Aβ_{42} levels. Although the MMSE scores did not deteriorate, this measure has ceiling effects that make it insensitive to early stages of dementia (Lawrence *et al.*, 2001). Neuropathological assessment supported the clinical diagnosis of very mild DAT, with many diffuse Aβ plaques but relatively few neuritic plaques or neocortical neurofibrillary tangles.

This case illustrates that the accurate diagnosis of DAT can be made in individuals who meet criteria for MCI. The DAT diagnosis was based on inform-ant observations that the individual had declined from previously attained levels of cognitive function (intra-individual decline), rather than comparing his cog-nitive performance to normative values. It is very likely that the diffuse Aβ plaques, which are not considered in CERAD and NIA-Reagan neuropathologic criteria for AD, were indicators of the pathobiological process that caused this individual's clinical and cognitive deterioration, as there was no other pathology that could account for this clinical course.

The diagnosis of DAT in individuals with MCI or earlier degrees of impairment

With the increasing number of older adults, AD is rapidly becoming a major health concern for various regions of the world. The symptomatic onset of AD is insidious and almost always begins with a period of cognitive impairment that interferes only subtly with daily functioning. As novel therapies targeting amyloid and other potentially "disease-modifying" targets become available in the future, the ability to detect early stages of disease may identify individuals who are more likely to benefit from such therapies.

MCI has been proposed as a condition of impairment intermediate between what is considered "normal for aging" and that which is sufficient for a diagnosis of dementia or AD. The utility of MCI to identify individuals as high risk for further cognitive decline and progression to DAT was first suggested in 1999, and was adopted by the American Academy of Neurology practice parameter for early detec-tion of dementia in 2001 (Petersen *et al.*, 2009). The concept of MCI has evolved considerably over the years, as evidenced by revisions of the diagnostic criteria.

The original criteria for MCI focused on memory impairment (Petersen *et al.*, 2001). The criteria for MCI were expanded to recognize impairment in non-memory domains (Winblad *et al.*, 2004). Essentially, two subtypes emerged: amnestic (including memory impairment) and non-amnestic (non-memory cognitive domains impaired). The amnestic subtype is further divided into single domain if only memory is involved and multi-domain if, in addition to memory, one or more domains are involved. Furthermore, the revised criteria allow the presence of some difficulty in performing daily functions in the diagnosis of MCI. However, this should not be to a degree that is sufficient to impair those functions, which would otherwise qualify for a diagnosis of dementia. There are several limitations in this approach. First, the distinction between "some difficulty" versus "impairment" in performing daily functions is arbitrary and depends on the judgment of the clinician, resulting in a non-standard distinction as to who is considered to have MCI rather than dementia. Second, MCI criteria do not require the determination of an etiological basis for the cognitive impairment. Third, some individuals meeting MCI criteria may be below the cutpoint for cognitive performance because of an incipient non-AD dementing disorder, a reversible disorder (e.g. cognitive side effects of medications), or simply because they are at the lower end of normal (but stable) cognitive performance. Thus, there is a considerable degree of heterogeneity in the MCI population; although many individuals characterized as having MCI eventually progress to a diagnosis of DAT, others may not progress or may progress to other forms of dementia and a small proportion may actually improve or revert to normal.

Take home messages

1. It is important to assess an individual's cognitive function compared with their own baseline level of performance in detecting the earliest stages of dementia.
2. This allows the diagnosis of dementia in individuals at earlier stages of symptomatic AD than is common elsewhere, and at a stage where future disease-modifying therapies may have the best chance for success.

REFERENCES AND FURTHER READING

Armitage SG (1946). An analysis of certain psychological tests used in the evaluation of brain injury. *Psych Mono*, 1–48.

Braak H, Braak E (1991). Neuropathological stageing of Alzheimer-related changes. *Acta Neuropathol*, **82**, 239–59.

Cairns NJ, Ikonomovic MD, Benzinger T, *et al.* (2009). Absence of Pittsburgh Compound B detection of cerebral amyloid beta in a patient with clinical, cognitive, and cerebrospinal fluid markers of Alzheimer disease. *Arch Neurol*, **66**, 1557–62.

Fagan AM, Mintun MA, Shah AR, *et al.* (2009). Cerebrospinal fluid tau and ptau(181) increase with cortical amyloid deposition in cognitively normal individuals: implications for future clinical trials of Alzheimer's disease. *EMBO Mol Med* **1**, 371–80.

Folstein MF, Folstein SE, McHugh PR (1975). "Mini-mental state". A practical method for grading the cognitive state of patients for the clinician. *J Psychiatr Res* **12**, 189–98.

Goodglass H, Kaplan E (1983). *Boston Naming Test Scoring Booklet*, Philadelphia, PA: Lea & Febiger.

Grober E, Buschke H, Crystal H, Bang S, Dresner R (1988). Screening for dementia by memory testing. *Neurology*, **38**, 900–3.

Hyman BT, Trojanowski JQ (1997). Consensus recommendations for the postmortem diagnosis of Alzheimer disease from the National Institute on Aging and the Reagan Institute Working Group on diagnostic criteria for the neuropathological assessment of Alzheimer disease. *J Neuropathol Exp Neurol* **56**, 1095–7.

Johnson DK, Storandt M, Morris JC, Galvin JE (2009). Longitudinal study of the transition from healthy aging to Alzheimer disease. *Arch Neurol* **66**, 1254–9.

Khachaturian ZS (1985). Diagnosis of Alzheimer's disease. *Arch Neurol* **42**, 1097–105.

Lawrence J, Davidoff D, Katt-Lloyd D, Auerbach M, Hennen J (2001). A pilot program of improved methods for community-based screening for dementia. *Am J Geriatr Psychiatry*, **9**, 205–11.

Mirra SS, Heyman A, Mckeel D, *et al.* (1991). The Consortium to Establish a Registry for Alzheimer's Disease (CERAD). Part II. Standardization of the neuropathologic assessment of Alzheimer's disease. *Neurology* **41**, 479–86.

Morris JC (1993). The Clinical Dementia Rating (CDR): current version and scoring rules. *Neurology* **43**, 2412–14.

Petersen RC, Doody R, Kurz A, *et al.* (2001). Current concepts in mild cognitive impairment. *Arch Neurol*, **58**, 1985–92.

Petersen RC, Roberts RO, Knopman DS, *et al.* (2009). Mild cognitive impairment: ten years later. *Arch Neurol* **66**, 1447–55.

Sliwinski M, Lipton RB, Buschke H, Stewart W (1996). The effects of preclinical dementia on estimates of normal cognitive functioning in aging. *J Gerontol B Psychol Sci Soc Sci*, **51**, P217–25.

Storandt M, Grant EA, Miller JP, Morris JC (2006). Longitudinal course and neuropathologic outcomes in original vs revised MCI and in pre-MCI. *Neurology* **67**, 467–73.

Storandt M, Mintun, MA, Head D, Morris JC (2009). Cognitive decline and brain volume loss as signatures of cerebral amyloid-beta peptide deposition identified with Pittsburgh compound B: cognitive decline associated with Abeta deposition. *Arch Neurol* **66**, 1476–81.

Storandt M, Morris JC (2010). Ascertainment bias in the clinical diagnosis of Alzheimer's disease. *Arch Neurol*, **67**, 1364–9.

Sunderland T, Linker G, Mirza N, *et al.* (2003). Decreased beta-amyloid1–42 and increased tau levels in cerebrospinal fluid of patients with Alzheimer disease. *JAMA* **289**, 2094–103.

The American Psychiatric Association (1994). *Diagnostic and Statistical Manual of Mental Disorders (DSM)*.

Thurstone LL, Thurstone LG (1949). *Examiner Manual for the SRA Primary Mental Abilities Test*. Chicago, IL, Science Research Associates.

Tuokko H, Garrett DD, Mcdowell I, Silverberg N, Kristjansson B (2003). Cognitive decline in high-functioning older adults: reserve or ascertainment bias? *Aging Ment Health*, **7**, 259–70.

Wechsler D, Stone CP (1973). *Manual: Wechsler Memory Scale*, New York.

Winblad B, Palmer K, Kivipelto M, *et al.* (2004). Mild cognitive impairment – beyond controversies, towards a consensus: report of the International Working Group on Mild Cognitive Impairment. *J Intern Med* **256**, 240–6.

Case 4

Lost for words

Paige Moorhouse

Clinical history – main complaint

A 67-year-old right-handed woman with a history of a 3 cm mid left parietal lobe intra-cerebral hemorrhage (ICH) of uncertain etiology 5 years before was admitted to the inpatient neurology service after an acute episode of witnessed productive aphasia and inability to obey commands during an outpatient neurology assessment. The episode lasted 20 minutes and was not associated with other focal neurologic signs or change in level of consciousness. The reason for referral to the outpatient clinic was concern on the part of her family about her ability to function independently at home over the past several months.

General history

The patient is a high school educated, retired home care worker who lives alone with her son living close by. She has five grown children. Her hemorrhagic stroke 5 years ago was associated with transient right hemiplegia. She made a complete functional recovery, but her course was complicated by a post-stroke seizure disorder occurring 1 year after her stroke. She experienced a generalized tonic clonic seizure (preceded by right visual field aura and a feeling of apprehension) and required ICU admission. Her presentation was further complicated by post-ictal delirium. Her seizure disorder was initially treated with dilantin, but she was unable to tolerate a dose escalation and was therefore switched to valproic acid. There have been no recorded seizures for the past 4 years.

Cognitive history indicates that she has noticed minor deficits of short-term memory and word finding since her stroke, but denied any functional deficits associated with her cognition. Her son has described a 3-year history of decreased attention to personal care, laundry, nutrition, and housekeeping. Her anticonvulsant levels have been lower than expected on several occasions suggesting

Case Studies in Dementia: Common and Uncommon Presentations, ed. S. Gauthier and P. Rosa-Neto.
Published by Cambridge University Press. © Cambridge University Press 2011.

medication non-compliance. After reviewing of her bank statements, her family suspects she may have gambled away her monthly food budget at a video lottery terminal. There is no history of depressive symptoms, but she has been less socially active and has not been calling out on the telephone in the past year.

Past medical history includes atrial fibrillation, and mitral valve regurgitation confirmed on echocardiography. She has a history of hyperlipidemia and hypertension, a 20 pack-year history of smoking (quit 10 years ago) and does not consume alcohol. There are no other vascular risk factors. Medications include ECASA 81 mg daily, clonazepam 0.5 mg QHS, bisoprolol 10 mg daily, atorvastatin 20 mg daily, irbesartan 150 mg daily, valproic acid 250 mg twice daily.

Family history

There is no family history of stroke, acute coronary syndrome, or dementia.

Examination

Alert, co-operative, and slightly disheveled in appearance with a flat affect. She was not emotionally labile during the assessment. BP 120/78; pulse 60 irregularly irregular. She had difficulty following complex instructions during the neurologic examination, however had 5/5 strength globally, symmetric brisk reflexes, down-going toes, and paratonia in the upper extremities. Her sensory, cranial nerve, and cerebellar examinations were within normal limits.

Cognitive assessment: MMSE 27/30 (1/3 delayed recall, 2/3 on 3-step command), Frontal Assessment Battery (FAB) 8/18 (abnormal) with points lost for abstraction (0/3), verbal fluency, and conflicting instructions tasks. She was initially not able to provide any words belonging to a semantic (four-legged animals) or phonemic (words beginning with F) category; however, when this task was repeated, she was able to give six words in a phonemic category as part of the FAB. She was able to place the numbers correctly on when asked to draw a clock; however, she placed the hands at ten and eleven when asked to place them at "ten after eleven." She was able to name high frequency words such as "pen," "watch" but could not name a "shin," "thigh" or "sole." She was unable to interpret the saying "a stitch in time saves nine."

Special studies

Unenhanced CT head: no new lesions. Volume loss measuring 3.5 cm in mid left temporal lobe and gliosis in the left temporal fossa and mild to moderate cerebral and cerebellar atrophy (Fig. 4.1).

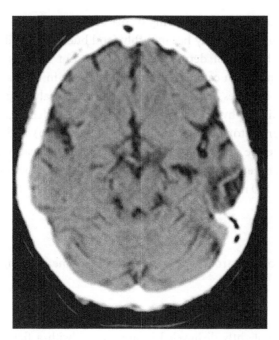

Fig. 4.1.   Unenhanced CT scan showing gliosis and atrophy in the left temporal lobe and generalized cerebral and cerebellar atrophy.

Carotid ultrasound (bilateral): no stenosis
EEG: Focal slowing in left mid temporal and posterior temporal regions. No evidence of focal or generalized epileptiform activity.

Neuropsychological testing performed 3 months after her ICH indicated mild difficulties with problem solving and fine psychomotor co-ordination and subtle language difficulties with word finding, verbal fluency, and verbal memory.

Neuropsychological testing performed during current admission indicates that, compared with prior testing, her present cognitive deficits have a more global pattern with a prominent dysexecutive syndrome. Generally, she was co-operative, but often vague in her responses, and required repetition of instructions for several tasks. She had significant word retrieval problems on confrontational naming as well as on letter and semantic fluency tasks. She had difficulty with several visuospatial tasks including the copying of a complex geometric figure. She had significant difficulty on tests of working memory. Although her recall of verbal information was very poor, visual memory was average to superior. She had severe impairment of novel problem solving, hypothesis testing, and mental flexibility with severe perseveration. She demonstrated difficulty in the acquisition of new material, but adequate retention of information once learned. Hand–eye co-ordination and fine motor movements were moderately impaired in the dominant hand and severely impaired in the non-dominant hand. There was no apraxia. Her score on a measure of overall knowledge and everyday judgment was average, but insight into her cognitive deficits was limited.

Diagnosis

Vascular cognitive impairment: post-stroke dementia with dysexecutive syndrome.

Follow-up

The patient was started on citalopram with the goal of improving her initiative and a cholinesterase inhibitor for her VCI. Her family was provided with strategies to compensate for her impaired verbal learning and executive dysfunction including automating her bills, having meals delivered, and supervision of medications. They were encouraged to break down complex instructions into simple steps and provide such instructions in several formats (written, verbal, pictures). She was discharged home to live independently with a referral for further home care services.

Over the next 3 months, the patient experienced a vast improvement in her initiative for activities of daily living and social outings. She refused home care services, but her family felt reasonably confident in her ability to function with informal assistance.

Over the next 6 months, she experienced three brief witnessed periods of expressive aphasia lasting up to 15 minutes, which were not associated with any other focal neurological deficits or loss of consciousness. These episodes were attributed to focal seizures, although transient ischemic attack (TIA) cannot be ruled out. Her anticonvulsant medication was changed to lamotrigine and titrated.

Discussion

Vascular cognitive impairment (VCI) refers to a heterogeneous group of cognitive disorders related to small and large cerebral vessel disease. VCI encompasses several syndromes, including: vascular dementia (including post-stroke and multi-infarct dementia), mixed primary neurodegenerative disease and vascular dementia, and cognitive impairment of vascular origin that does not meet dementia criteria (VCI-ND). Although post-stroke dementia (the clinical archetype of dementia associated with large vessel disease) is often the result of embolic stroke, primary cerebral hemorrhage is a less common cause of post-stroke dementia. The prevalence of dementia after stroke ranges from 14%–32%, with 5-year incidence of post-stroke dementia of 33% (Barba *et al.*, 2000; Henon *et al.*, 2001).

The pattern of cognitive deficits in VCI varies considerably. Single strategic large vessel infarcts can have specific cognitive profiles, while subcortical lesions are often associated with a cluster of features known as "subcortical syndrome" or "dysexecutive syndrome" characterized by slowed information processing speed, emotional lability, and executive dysfunction (impairment of the ability to plan, organize, initiate, and shift between tasks). As is the case with this patient, standard cognitive assessments such as the Mini-Mental State Examination (Folstein *et al.*, 1975) are often insensitive to these abnormalities (Royall *et al.*, 1998); however, dysexecutive syndrome is often readily apparent on measures that assess the dorsolateral prefrontal cortex such as the Frontal Assessment Battery (FAB) (Dubois *et al.*, 2000).

The clinical course of post-stroke dementia is difficult to predict with up to one-third of people having a change in their diagnostic category (NCI, CIND, dementia) within 1 year after stroke (Tham *et al.*, 2002). Risk factors for progression and functional decline include age, pre-existing cognitive impairment, polypharmacy, hypotension during acute stroke (del Ser *et al.*, 2005), and depression (Brodaty *et al.*, 2007). Neuroimaging findings such as medial temporal atrophy tend to be more important in predicting future cognitive decline than infarct location or the presence of white matter hyperintensities (Firbank *et al.*, 2006; Stephens *et al.*, 2004).

Therapy in this case should focus on minimizing the risk of future strokes (Srikanth *et al.*, 2006), control of current symptoms and minimization of other contributing causes of cognitive impairment. Here, the issue of secondary prevention is complicated by the absence of diffusion-weighted MRI images at the time of her original stroke, which may have helped to differentiate primary intracerebral hemorrhage from an embolic stroke with secondary hemorrhage. In the absence of such information, secondary preventative strategies for the control vascular risk factors and anticoagulation remain appropriate. Treatment of hypertension with perindopril and indapemide has been shown to reduce dementia and cognitive decline associated with recurrent stroke (Tzourio *et al.*, 2003). Similarly, a recent study found a reduction in recurrent stroke for those with a history of stroke or transient ischemic attack, treated with atorvastatin (Amarenco *et al.*, 2006). The decision of whether to give warfarin for atrial fibrillation requires careful consideration and balancing of the risk of recurring hemorrhage vs the risk of thromboembolism (Estol and Kase, 2003). Such decisions should be revisited as the patient ages, and if comorbidities such as congestive heart failure and diabetes arise.

Given that this patient lives alone, without formal supports, maximizing her function is particularly important. Although there is a biochemical basis for use of cholinesterase inhibitors in VCI (Roman and Kalaria, 2006; Sato *et al.*, 2001), metanalyses suggest that the benefits of cholinesterase inhibitors and memantine in mild to moderate VCI are small (Kavirajan *et al.*, 2007). However, a trial of a cholinesterase inhibitor with measurable outcomes (in the form of target symptoms) identified at the outset is reasonable, particularly since a neurodegenerative process (such as Alzheimer's disease) cannot be ruled out as a contributing factor. This is suggested by the evident expansion of cognitive domains affected from the first neuropsychiatric assessment to the second to include visuospatial function. Further, although executive dysfunction is common in VCI, it is not unique to VCI (Reed *et al.*, 2007). Selective serontonin reuptake inhibitors have been shown to be helpful for executive dysfunction in VCI and depressive symptoms in AD, particularly apathy (Opler *et al.*, 1994; Rao *et al.*, 2006; Lyketsos *et al.*, 2004).

Finally, ongoing partial seizures may contribute to cognitive impairment (Tatum *et al.*, 1989). This patient's lamotrigine should be titrated to minimize future seizures.

REFERENCES AND FURTHER READING

Amarenco P, Bogousslavsky J, Callahan AR, *et al.* (2006). High-dose atorvastatin after stroke or transient ischemic attack. *N Engl J Med* **6**, 549–59.

Barba R, Martinez-Espinosa S, Rodriguez-Garcia E, Pondal M, Vivancos J, Del Ser T (2000). Poststroke dementia: clinical features and risk factors. *Stroke* **7**, 1494–501.

Brodaty H, Withall A, Altendorf A, Sachdev PS (2007). Rates of depression at 3 and 15 months poststroke and their relationship with cognitive decline: the Sydney Stroke Study. *Am J Geriatr Psychiatry* **6**, 477–86.

del Ser T, Barba R, Morin MM, *et al.* (2005). Evolution of cognitive impairment after stroke and risk factors for delayed progression. *Stroke* **12**, 2670–5.

Dubois B, Slachevsky A, Litvan I, Pillon B (2000). The FAB: a Frontal Assessment Battery at bedside. *Neurology* **11**, 1621–6.

Estol CJ, Kase CS (2003). Need for continued use of anticoagulants after intracerebral hemorrhage. *Curr Treat Options Cardiovasc Med* **3**, 201–9.

Firbank MJ, Burton EJ, Barber R, *et al.* (2006). Medial temporal atrophy rather than white matter hyperintensities predict cognitive decline in stroke survivors. *Neurobiol Aging*, **28**(11), 1664–9.

Folstein MF, Folstein SE, McHugh PR (1975). "Mini-mental state". A practical method for grading the cognitive state of patients for the clinician. *J Psychiatr Res*, **3**, 189–98.

Henon H Durieu I, Guerouaou D, Lebert F, Pasquier F, Leys D (2001). Poststroke dementia: incidence and relationship to prestroke cognitive decline. *Neurology* **7**, 1216–22.

Kavirajan H, Schneider LS (2007). Efficacy and adverse effects of cholinesterase inhibitors and memantine in vascular dementia: a meta-analysis of randomised controlled trials. *Lancet Neurol* **9**, 782–92.

Lyketsos CG, Rosenblatt A, Rabins P (2004). Forgotten frontal lobe syndrome or "Executive Dysfunction Syndrome." *Psychosomatics* **3**, 247–55.

Opler LA, Ramirez PM, Lee SK (1994). Serotonergic agents and frontal lobe syndrome. *J Clin Psychiatry* **8**, 362–3.

Rao V, Spiro JR, Rosenberg PB, Lee HB, Rosenblatt A, Lyketsos CG (2006). An open-label study of escitalopram (Lexapro) for the treatment of 'Depression of Alzheimer's disease' (dAD). *Int J Geriatr Psychiatry* **3**, 273–4.

Reed BR, Mungas DM, Kramer JH, *et al.* (2007). Profiles of neuropsychological impairment in autopsy-defined Alzheimer's disease and cerebrovascular disease. *Brain,* **3**, 731–9.

Roman GC Kalaria RN (2006). Vascular determinants of cholinergic deficits in Alzheimer disease and vascular dementia. *Neurobiol Aging* **12**, 1769–85.

Royall DR, Polk M (1998). Dementias that present with and without posterior cortical features: an important clinical distinction. *J Am Geriatr Soc,* **1**, 98–105.

Sato A, Sato Y, Uchida S (2001). Regulation of regional cerebral blood flow by cholinergic fibers originating in the basal forebrain. *Int J Dev Neurosci,* **3**, 327–37.

Srikanth VK, Quinn SJ, Donnan GA, Saling MM, Thrift AG (2006). Long-term cognitive transitions, rates of cognitive change, and predictors of incident dementia in a population-based first-ever stroke cohort. *Stroke* **10**, 2479–83.

Stephens S, Kenny RA, Rowan E, *et al.* (2004). Neuropsychological characteristics of mild vascular cognitive impairment and dementia after stroke. *Int J Geriatr Psychiatry* **11**, 1053–7.

Tatum WOT, Ross J, Cole AJ (1998). Epileptic pseudodementia. *Neurology,* **5**, 1472–5.

Tham W, Auchus AP, Thong M, *et al.* (2002). Progression of cognitive impairment after stroke: one year results from a longitudinal study of Singaporean stroke patients. *J Neurol Sci* **204**, 49–52.

Tzourio C, Anderson C, Chapman N, *et al.* (2003). Effects of blood pressure lowering with perindopril and indapamide therapy on dementia and cognitive decline in patients with cerebrovascular disease. *Arch Intern Med* **9**, 1069–75.

Woman with right-sided numbness

Adrià Arboix and Marta Grau-Olivares

Clinical history – main complaint

An 82-year-old woman (right-handed and autonomous) had a former history of hypertension, type 2 diabetes treated with oral hypoglycemic agents, rheumatoid arthritis, dysthymic disorder, and left dorsal herpes zoster with residual post-herpetic neuralgia.

General history

The patient was admitted to the emergency department because of sudden onset of a sensory disorder in the right hemibody associated with mild frontal head-ache. Physical examination revealed a right faciobrachiocrural superficial and deep hemihypoesthesia, which was compatible with a right pure sensory lacunar syndrome. Results of a standard battery of laboratory tests were within normal ranges or negative; the only abnormalities were a serum cholesterol concentration of 6.5 mmol/L (normal < 6.2 mmol/L) and serum triglycerides of 2.4 mmol/L (normal < 1.7 mmol/L). The chest roentgenogram was normal. The ECG showed occasional ventricular extrasystoles and right bundle-branch block. The brain computed tomography (CT) scan revealed mild diffuse cortical atrophy. A left thalamic lacunar infarction was visualized on the magnetic resonance imaging (MRI) scan (Fig. 5.1). MR angiography of the brain and supraaortic vessels did not show occlusive lesions consistent with atherosclerosis. The transthoracic echocar-diogram disclosed a mild hypertensive cardiopathy with preserved left ventricular ejection fraction and normal left atrial size. Mitral ring calcification was observed.

The neuropsychological assessment did not show any evidence of dementia. The Mini-Mental State Examination (MMSE) score was 25/30 (normal). The patient was fully alert and oriented (self, time, space). Language and fluency were normal as well as immediate and delayed memory. The patient showed only a

Case Studies in Dementia: Common and Uncommon Presentations, ed. S. Gauthier and P. Rosa-Neto. Published by Cambridge University Press. © Cambridge University Press 2011.

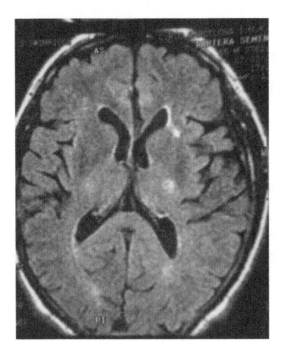

Fig. 5.1.   **MRI FLAIR** shows hypersignal on the left thalamus suggesting lacunar infarction.

slow performance in a psychomotor task and certain difficulty in executive tasks, such as attention and concentration, and planning.

At the time of hospital discharge, partial recovery of sensory deficit was achieved (Rankin score 2, National Institutes of Health Stroke Scale [NIHSS] score 3). Treatment consisted of platelet antiaggregants and strict control of vascular risk factors.

The clinical course was uneventful, but 7 months later she presented with an episode of language disorder, altered consciousness, and motor deficit in the right hemibody, which developed suddenly upon awakening. At the emergency department, a brain CT did not reveal intraparenchymatous intracranial bleeding.

Family history

Father died at the age of 78 of acute stroke.

Examination

The physical examination showed a conscious patient with moderate motor aphasia, right homonymous hemianopsia, and balanced faciobrachiocrural hemiparesis in association with hemihypoesthesia of the right hemibody. Cardiac

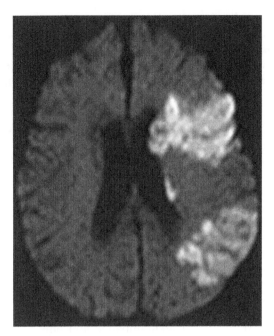

Fig. 5.2. Diffusion brain MRI shows acute cerebral ischemia in the territory of the left middle cerebral artery.

arrhythmia without signs of heart failure was noted. The NIHSS score was 21. The patient showed a non-fluent language and was unable to repeat syllables or words, but the comprehension was quite preserved. She was also disoriented (self, time, space) and showed important memory impairment (immediate and delayed recall). The MMSE score was 3 as she had severe motor aphasia and furthermore she was illiterate.

Special studies

The brain MRI scan showed acute cerebral ischemia in the territory of the left middle cerebral artery (Fig. 5.2). The 24-h Holter ECG monitoring disclosed paroxysmal atrial fibrillation. A diagnosis of cerebral infarction of cardioembolic origin was made. Treatment with platelet antiaggregants was discontinued and oral anticoagulation with warfarin at therapeutic doses was started.

Diagnosis

A final tentative diagnosis of vascular cognitive impairment that fulfilled criteria of multi-infarct dementia was established.

Table 5.1. DSM-IV-TR criteria for vascular dementia

1 Focal neurological signs and symptoms (e.g. exaggerated deep muscular reflexes, Babinskin's sign, semiology of pseudobulbar palsy, gait abnormalities, motor limb weakness, etc.) or Evidence of focal neurological impairment on radiological studies (e.g. multiple cortical infarcts with involvement of the underlying white matter substance).
2 The cognitive deficits in the above criteria cause significant impairment in day-to-day functioning, social or occupational functioning and represent a significant decline from the previous level of functioning.
3 Focal neurologic signs and symptoms or radiologic evidence indicative of cerebrovascular disease are present that are judged to be etiologically related to the dementia.
4 The deficits do not occur exclusively during the course of delirium.
5 The course of deficits is characterized by sustained periods of clinical stability interrupted by a sudden and significant loss of cognitive functions and functioning activities.

Follow-up

Living performance after stroke was severely impaired and home assistance for daily living activities was needed. Treatment included speech therapy and physical rehabilitation.

Discussion

Multi-infarct dementia is a vascular-type cognitive impairment due to recurrent cerebral infarcts. Vascular cognitive impairment has been recently recognized, despite the clinical relevance of this condition. The estimated incidence of post-stroke dementia at 3 months varies between 25% and 41% (Erkinjuntii and Pantoni, 2000). In general, one-fourth of acute stroke patients meet criteria of vascular dementia (Leys *et al.*, 2005). On the other hand, 50% of patients with first-ever lacunar infarct – a stroke subtype characterized by favorable short-term outcome and absence of neuropsychological impairment – will also suffer from mild vascular cognitive impairment at the end of the acute phase of the disease (Arboix and Martí-Vilalta, 2009). Additionally, all patients with ischemic or hemorrhagic stroke will present some type of neuropsychological impairment, the clinical symptoms and severity of which are related to the cerebral topography involved, the affected hemisphere, the volume of the lesion, and the concomitant presence of previous vascular lesions, either silent or symptomatic, visible on neuroimaging studies.

Several specific diagnostic criteria can be used to diagnose vascular dementia but the DSM-IV-TR criteria are the most extensively used (Table 5.1).

Subtypes of vascular cognitive impairment

Many subtypes of vascular dementia have been described to date. The spectrum includes multi-infarct dementia, post-stroke dementia, dementia due to hemorrhagic lesions, and dementia due to ischemic cerebral small-vessel disease. Ischemic cerebral small-vessel disease includes strategic infarct dementia, Alzheimer's disease with cerebrovascular disease, and subcortical vascular dementia (Erkinjuntii and Pantoni, 2000; Roman, 2003).

Multi-infarct dementia

Multi-infarct dementia reflects the traditional view that multiple and recurrent large cortical infarcts are required for dementia to develop. Co-existing subcortical infarcts, lacunes, and white matter changes may be found (Hachinski *et al.*, 1974). Multi-infarct dementia is related to atherothrombotic stroke, cardiac embolic stroke, and major hemodynamic events. Typical clinical features of this condition include focal neurological signs, such as hemiparesis, lateralized sensory changes, and stepwise deterioration with cognitive impairment and aphasia. Multi-infarct dementia, however, is not the most common type of vascular dementia in elderly people, who are more likely to have mixed Alzheimer's disease and vascular dementia.

Post-stroke dementia

Post-stroke dementia that occurs in close temporal relationship with a thromboembolic or hemorrhagic stroke includes multi-infarct dementia and hemorrhage-associated dementia. The prognosis for recovery of cognitive symptoms after stroke is generally favorable, although persistent or progressive cognitive decline may occur in some patients. Post-stroke dementia develops in up to one-third of patients within the first year after the acute cerebrovascular event (Lenzi and Altieri, 2007). In fact, post-stroke dementia has long been considered the prototypical subtype of vascular dementia, and it might therefore be expected that all patients with post-stroke dementia would meet the criteria for vascular dementia. The most important demographic predictor of post-stroke dementia is age. The association with stroke risk factors is less robust. Evidence suggests heterogeneity of the underlying pathology, with many cases resulting from different vascular causes and changes in the brain, as well as from degenerative pathology. Degree of pre-existing subcortical white matter disease, infarct volume, and global and medial temporal lobe atrophy have been identified as some of the relevant imaging determinants of post-stroke dementia (Roman, 2003). A greater degree of severity of cognitive impairment after stroke has been associated with increased risk of post-stroke dementia (Erkinjuntti and Pantoni, 2000).

Intracerebral hemorrhage

Intracerebral hemorrhage, usually multiple, might cause widespread brain injury leading to dementia. Chronic hypertension is the most common underlying disease. The clinical syndrome usually comprises headache, nausea, reduced consciousness and, depending on the site of the hemorrhage, different neurological symptoms, such as contralateral hemiparesis and sensory loss, cranial nerve palsies, eye movement abnormalities, or weakness. In some cases, subarachnoid hemorrhage leads to normal pressure hydrocephalus, which is a potentially treatable secondary dementia disorder. Another pathogenetic basis of post-hemorrhagic dementia is amyloid angiopathy (Erkinjuntti, 1996), which makes the vessel wall liable to recurrent rupture and hemorrhage.

Vascular dementia due to ischemic cerebral small-vessel disease

Ischemic cerebral small-vessel disease includes strategic infarct dementia, Alzheimer's disease with cerebrovascular disease, and subcortical vascular dementia.

Strategic infarct dementia

Smaller infarcts in particular regions, for example, in the deep central gray matter, may have an important role in causing dementia (Arboix and Martí-Vilalta, 2009). Lacunar infarcts involving the thalamus, internal capsule, and basal ganglia are sometimes associated with widespread cognitive effects, including confusion and memory impairment (Arboix and Martí-Vilalta, 2009). Infarcts involving the dorsomedial and anterior thalamus might also produce significant executive symptoms and profound amnesia, which can persist in some cases. Cognitive symptoms associated with strategic infarcts are often reversible by 12 months, and they are therefore not a common cause of persistent dementia. In some unusual cases, strategic infarct dementia may also be caused by non-small-vessel disease (e.g. cortical infarcts of the angular gyrus or the hippocampus).

Alzheimer's disease with cerebrovascular disease

Evidence is accumulating that Alzheimer's disease is commonly associated with cerebrovascular risk factors, including diabetes, hypertension, and smoking. Vascular and degenerative diseases interact in terms of clinical expression of cognitive impairment, and vascular dementia and Alzheimer's disease share common pathogenetic mechanisms (Snowdon et al., 1997). Many individuals with Alzheimer's disease, especially those beyond 85 years of age, show significant vascular co-morbidity to the extent that they are more accurately characterized as having mixed vascular–Alzheimer's dementia. Although in older patients, a mixed etiology is likely to be more common than either pure

Alzheimer's disease or vascular dementia, clinical criteria for ante-mortem diagnosis of mixed dementia are currently lacking (Erkinjuntti and Pantoni, 2000; Lenzi *et al.*, 2007).

Subcortical vascular dementia

In clinical studies, the proportion of vascular dementia caused by small-vessel disease or subcortical vascular dementia ranges from 36% to 67% (Erkinjuntti and Pantoni, 2000; Grau-Olivares and Arboix, 2009). In subcortical vascular dementia, the primary types of brain lesions are lacunar infarcts and ischemic white matter lesions, with demyelination and loss of axons, a decreased number of oligodendrocytes, reactive astrocytosis, and the primary lesion site is the subcortical region (Grau-Olivares and Arboix, 2009). This type of vascular dementia includes the old entities "lacunar state" and "Binswanger's disease." These entities are related to a pseudobulbar syndrome, defined by the triad of Thurel of dysarthria, dysphagia (mainly to liquids), and mimic disturbances (laugh or spasmodic cry). Lacunar state and Binswanger's disease are the two main pathophysiological pathways involved in subcortical vascular dementia, and often co-exist in the same patient (Arboix and Martí-Vilalta, 2009). In the first case, occlusion of the arteriolar lumen due to arteriolosclerosis leads to the formation of lacunes, which results in a lacunar state (état lacunaire). In the second case, critical stenosis and hypoperfusion of multiple medullary arterioles causes widespread incomplete infarction of deep white matter, with a clinical picture of Binswanger's disease.

Patients with subcortical vascular dementia often have a history of multiple cerebrovascular risk factors, including hypertension, diabetes, and ischemic heart disease. The onset of dementia is insidious in over half of the patients and the course is usually continuous and slowly progressive. The clinical symptoms are usually low mental speed, extrapyramidal symptoms (rigidity, hypokinesia), bilateral pyramidal symptoms (short steps, vivid reflex activity in the legs), and positive masseter reflex. Other neurological signs are imbalance and falls, urinary frequency and incontinence, dysarthria, and dysphagia. Behavioral and psychiatric symptoms include depression, personality change, emotional lability, emotional bluntness, and mental slowness. This syndrome is also called "the subcortical syndrome" or "frontosubcortical syndrome" (Leys *et al.*, 2005).

The typical cognitive syndrome in patients with subcortical vascular dementia is the dysexecutive syndrome. It includes slowed information processing, memory deficits, behavioral and psychiatric symptoms, as well as impairment in goal formulation, initiation, planning, organizing, executing, and abstracting. The essential neuroimaging changes in subcortical vascular dementia include extensive ischemic white matter lesions and multiple lacunar infarcts in the deep gray and white matter structures. These manifestations probably result from ischemic interruption of parallel circuits from the prefrontal cortex to the basal ganglia and corresponding thalamocortical connections (Leys *et al.*, 2005).

Identification of early and mild stages of subcortical vascular dementia is an important area for research, because this form of vascular dementia is one of the most common causes of cognitive decline in elderly people. Subcortical vascular dementia is commonly not recognized and remains undiagnosed, but it accounts for a significant number of cases of dementia and results in many admissions to nursing homes. Better recognition of the disease is necessary for maximum benefit to be derived from treatments that are currently available to delay disease progression, as well as the introduction of primary and secondary therapeutic prevention measures.

Take home messages

Multi-infarct dementia is a subtype of vascular dementia caused by recurrent cerebral infarcts.

Adequate secondary prevention of cerebral ischemia is mandatory to prevent multi-infarct dementia.

REFERENCES AND FURTHER READING

Arboix A, Martí-Vilalta JL (2009). Lacunar stroke. *Exp Rev Neurotherapeutics*, **9**, 179–96.

Erkinjuntti T, Pantoni L (2000). Subcortical vascular dementia. In Gauthier S, Cummings JL, eds. *Yearbook of Alzheimer's Disease and Related Disorders*. London: Martin Dunitz; 101–33.

Erkinjuntti, T (1996). Clinicopathological study of vascular dementia. In Prohovnik I, Wade J, Knezevic T, *et al.*, eds. *Vascular Dementia: Current Concepts*. London: Wiley & Sons.

Grau-Olivares M, Arboix A (2009). Mild cognitive impairment in stroke patients with ischemic cerebral small-vessel disease: a forerunner of vascular dementia? *Exp Rev Neurotherapeutics*, **9**, 1201–17.

Hachinski VC, Lassen NA, Marshall J (1974). Multi-infarct dementia: a cause of mental deterioration in the elderly. *Lancet* **2**, 207–10.

Lenzi GL, Altieri M (2007). Short term evolution as a marker of vascular dementia versus Alzheimer's disease. *J Neurol Sci*, **257**, 182–4.

Leys D, Hénon H, Mackowick-Cordiolani MA, Pasquier F (2005). Postroke dementia. *Lancet Neurol*, **4**, 752–9.

Roman G, Sachdev P, Royall DR, Bullock RA, Orgogozo JM, López-Pousa S, Arizaga R, Wallin A (2004). Vascular cognitive disorder: a new diagnostic category updating vascular cognitive impairment and vascular dementia. *J Neurol Sci*, **226**, 81–7.

Roman GC (2003). Stroke, cognitive decline and vascular dementia: the silent epidemic of the 21st century. *Neuroepidem* **22**, 161–4.

Snowdon DA, Greiner LH, Mortimer JA, Riley KP, Greiner PA, Markersberg WR (1997). Brain infarction and the clinical expression of Alzheimer disease. The Nun Study. *JAMA* **277**, 813–17.

Case 6

Don't be fooled by a misleadingly high MMSE score

David J. Burn

Clinical history – main complaint

A 72-year-old man with a 10-year history of Parkinson's disease had experienced visual hallucinations with preserved insight 2 years previously, subsiding on withdrawal of selegiline. At the most recent consultation, his wife described him as having periods of being "absent" and "confused," more withdrawn and with recurring visual hallucinations associated with some paranoid ideation.

General history

University educated man who worked until retirement as an engineer. Long-standing hypertension. Lives with his wife; two children living in UK. His medication comprised co-careldopa 25/100, two tablets three times daily, bendroflumethiazide 2.5 mg daily, atenolol 50 mg daily and senna two tablets nocte.

Family history

Both parents deceased (father aged 67 of myocardial infarction and mother aged 79 of bowel cancer). No family history of neurodegenerative disease known.

Examination

BP 160/90 lying, falling to 135/82 on standing after 2 minutes; pulse 78 regular. MMSE 27/30, Addenbrooke's Cognitive Examination (ACE-R) score 78/100. He had particular problems on the verbal fluency, clock drawing, and visuoperceptual abilities (dot counting and fragmented letters) sections of the ACE-R. Recall was

Case Studies in Dementia: Common and Uncommon Presentations, ed. S. Gauthier and P. Rosa-Neto. Published by Cambridge University Press. © Cambridge University Press 2011.

well preserved. Physical examination revealed a fairly symmetric and moderately severe parkinsonian syndrome, with akinetic-rigid features dominant and little in the way of rest tremor. Postural reflexes were mildly impaired.

Special studies

CT brain scan showed some patchy white matter changes consistent with diffuse small vessel disease in both cerebral hemispheres, although this was not marked.

His Neuropsychiatric Inventory score (NPI-4, comprising the items hallucinations, delusions, depression, and apathy) was 24 out of a maximum of 48, with his wife registering positive responses for all four stem questions. She also positively endorsed three out of four of the items on the Mayo Fluctuations Questionnaire (flow of ideas seeming disorganized, unclear or not logical at times, staring into space for long periods of time and excessively drowsy or lethargic, but not sleeping for more than 2 hours during the day).

Diagnosis

The initial diagnostic impression was of a dementia syndrome relating to his Parkinson's disease, although the doctor was initially uncomfortable with what he regarded as a "normal" MMSE score of 27 out of 30.

Follow-up

After 3 and 6 months, repeat MMSE scores were 23 and 25, respectively. Despite some initial diagnostic uncertainty, the patient was commenced on a cholinesterase inhibitor with considerable improvement in his psychotic features and lessening of his periods of confusion.

Discussion

Dementia affects up to 80% of people with Parkinson's disease. Current age is the biggest risk factor for the development of dementia. Other clinical predictors include a so-called postural instability–gait difficulty motor phenotype (that is, a rather symmetric akinetic-rigid syndrome with little or no rest tremor) and early impairments on semantic fluency and drawing of overlapping pentagons (Burn *et al.*, 2006, Williams-Gray *et al.*, 2007). Unlike Alzheimer's disease, memory loss may not be prominent in PD-associated dementia (PD-D), particularly in the early stages (Emre *et al.*, 2007). The MMSE, which is biased towards mnemonic deficits, is therefore insensitive to the diagnosis, and this has been confirmed in two recent studies (Riedel *et al.*, 2008 Mamikonyan *et al.*, 2009). Instruments that include measures of executive function (including verbal fluency and clock drawing) and visuoperceptual abilities, such as the ACE-R, are better suited to detecting the characteristic cognitive dysfunction of early PD-D.

In common with dementia with Lewy bodies (DLB), PD-D is also characterized by fluctuating cognition, manifest clinically as periods of absence or confusion and which may wax and wane over very short periods of time. Fluctuating cognition has a major impact upon the ability of the person to manage their activities of daily living (Bronnick *et al.*, 2006). Although not strictly validated for use in PD-D, the Mayo Fluctuations Questionnaire is a quick and easy to administer instrument, which provides some indication of this problem. Carer endorsement of three out of four of the questions (as in the example presented here) is highly suggestive of fluctuating cognition (Ferman *et al.*, 2004).

People with PD-D frequently have a considerable neuropsychiatric burden, with high levels of depression and apathy, together with psychotic features (notably visual hallucinations with or without delusional misinterpretation and paranoid ideation) (Aarsland *et al.*, 2007). The four item NPI (NPI-4) is both sensitive and feasible to use routinely in the clinic to detect key symptoms. This instrument captures the frequency and severity of each symptom. Recently devised diagnostic criteria for PD-D take the clinical phenomenology into account and are to be recommended when making the diagnosis (Emre *et al.*, 2007).

Rationalization of anti-parkinsonian and other medications is an important first step in the management of PD-D. A graded withdrawal of anticholinergic drugs, monoamine oxidase type B inhibitors, and dopamine agonists can lead to at least a temporary improvement or resolution of psychotic symptoms, as in the example presented here. Nocturia, urinary frequency, and urgency are common problems in the person with PD, but conventional non-specific muscarinic receptor antagonists (e.g. oxybutynin, probantheline) should be avoided as these drugs may cross the blood–brain barrier and worsen cognitive and neuropsychiatric problems.

PD-D is characterized by a profound cholinergic deficiency, in addition to the dopaminergic deficit, which underpins the movement disorder. Consequently, cholinesterase inhibitors are a logical therapeutic choice. These agents may improve cognition, particularly fluctuating attention, and can also benefit neuropsychiatric symptoms (Emre *et al.*, 2003). Figure 6.1 illustrates a typical objective improvement that may be seen from the use of cholinesterase inhibitors in PD-D.

(a)   (b)

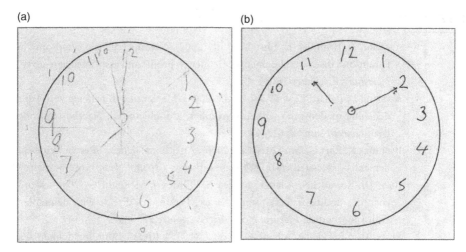

Fig. 6.1. (a) A patient with PD-D is asked to put the numbers on the face of a clock and to draw the clock hands showing the time "10 to 2." The attempt illustrates the profound visuospatial impairment typical of PD-D. Global cognition at the time of this assessment, according to the Mattis Dementia Rating Scale (DRS-2), was 112 (out of a maximum score of 144). A DRS-2 score of less than 123 has 93% sensitivity and 91% specificity for discriminating PD-D from non-demented PD using the *Diagnostic and Statistical Manual* Dementia criteria as a "gold standard." (b) The same patient has been treated with the cholinesterase inhibitor rivastigmine, and is asked 3 months later to attempt the same task. The illustration shows a significant improvement in the number placement and hand drawing. The DRS-2 score at this time on treatment has also improved to 131.

A recent trial has suggested that the N-methyl-D-aspartate receptor antagonist memantine may have modest benefits in PD-D (Aarsland *et al.*, 2009). Further studies are necessary to determine the long-term clinical effectiveness and cost–benefit of these drugs in managing PD-D.

Take home messages

The MMSE is insensitive to the diagnosis of dementia associated with Parkinson's disease

Assessment should include some attempt to measure fluctuating cognition and neuropsychiatric burden since both may be relatively clinically "silent," yet these symptoms can have a major impact upon the patient and their carer.

REFERENCES AND FURTHER READING

Aarsland D, Brønnick K, Ehrt U, *et al.* (2007). Neuropsychiatric symptoms in patients with Parkinson's disease and dementia: frequency, profile and associated care giver stress. *J Neurol Neurosurg Psychiatry* **78**, 36–42.

Aarsland D, Ballard C, Walker Z, *et al.* (2009). Memantine in patients with Parkinson's disease dementia or dementia with Lewy bodies: a double-blind, placebo-controlled, multicentre trial. *Lancet Neurol* **8**, 613–18.

Bronnick K, Ehrt U, Emre M, *et al.* (2006). Attentional deficits affect activities of daily living in dementia-associated with Parkinson's disease. *J Neurol Neurosurg Psychiatry* **77**, 1136–42.

Burn DJ, Rowan EN, Allan L, Molloy S, O'Brien J, McKeith IG (2006). Motor subtype and cognitive decline in Parkinson's disease, Parkinson's disease with dementia, and dementia with Lewy bodies. *J Neurol Neurosurg Psychiatry* **77**, 585–9.

Emre M, Aarsland D, Albanese A, *et al.* (2003). Rivastigmine for dementia associated with Parkinson's disease. *N Engl J Med* **351**, 2509–18.

Emre M, Aarsland D, Brown R, *et al.* (2007). Clinical diagnostic criteria for dementia associated with Parkinson disease. *Mov Disord* **22**, 1689–707.

Ferman TJ, Smith GE, Boeve BF, *et al.* (2004). DLB fluctuations: specific features that reliably differentiate DLB from AD and normal aging. *Neurology* **62**, 181–7.

Mamikonyan E, Moberg PJ, Siderowf A, *et al.* (2009). Mild cognitive impairment is common in Parkinson's disease patients with normal Mini-Mental State Examination (MMSE) scores. *Parkinsonism Relat Disord* **15**, 226–31.

Riedel O, Klotsche J, Spottke A, *et al.* (2008). Cognitive impairment in 873 patients with idiopathic Parkinson's disease. Results from the German Study on Epidemiology of Parkinson's Disease with Dementia (GEPAD). *J Neurol* **255**, 255–64.

Williams-Gray CH, Foltynie T, Brayne CEG, Robbins TW, Barker RA (2007). Evolution of cognitive dysfunction in an incident Parkinson's disease cohort. *Brain* **130**, 1787–98.

Case 7

Hemiparesis followed by dementia

Yan Deschaintre, Fadi Massoud, and Gabriel C. Léger

Clinical history – main complaint

A 73-year-old woman presented to the emergency room with mild left hemi-paresis since awakening the day before. History was difficult to obtain from the patient. Her husband mentioned memory decline with functional limitations in the last few months. For example, he reported that she misplaced money and that he no longer let her go to the supermarket by herself.

General history

She was a right-handed, retired real estate agent living with her husband. They had no children. She led a sedentary lifestyle, smoked actively, and consumed two drinks of alcohol daily.

Past medical history included diffuse atherosclerosis with renovascular hyper-tension diagnosed at age 58, high blood cholesterol, and a right parieto-temporal ischemic stroke at age 71 with no apparent sequelae. There was no history of coronary heart disease.

Past surgical history included both right carotid endarterectomy and iliac angio-plasty at age 58, and hysterectomy with bilateral salpingo-oophorectomy at age 35.

Medications on admission included aspirin 80 mg daily, cilazapril (Inhibace) 5 mg daily, irbesartan (Avapro) 150 mg daily, amlodipine (Norvasc) 10 mg daily, metoprolol (Lopresor) 100 mg am + 50 mg pm, terazosin (Hytrin) 2 mg daily, simvastatin (Zocor) 10 mg daily, ezetimibe (Ezetrol) 10 mg daily, and venlafaxine (Effexor XR) 300 mg daily.

Family history

Parents and siblings (ten sisters and seven brothers) had no particular medical history regarding vascular disease or dementia.

Case Studies in Dementia: Common and Uncommon Presentations, ed. S. Gauthier and P. Rosa-Neto. Published by Cambridge University Press. © Cambridge University Press 2011.

Examination

Awake and alert, looked well, and collaborated, but made inappropriate jokes (disinhibited).

BP 162/72; pulse 64 regular; temperature 36.9 C; capillary glucose 6.2.

Normal speech. MMSE 23/30: lost two points on calculation, three on delayed recall, one on reading, and one on copying (slight disorientation in time and place was noted the following days). Clock-drawing was deficient: numbers initially written in words, with some repetition and misplacement, and time (9h45) indicated by writing "10–1/4" rather than drawing hands. "Five words test" (Dubois *et al.*, 2002) 9/10 (on immediate recall: two words recalled spontaneously and three with cueing; on delayed recall: three spontaneously, one with cueing and one still missed). MoCA done 3 months later was 16/30; points lost on trail making test, cube copying, clock-drawing (only contour was correct), calculation, fluency (eight words in 1 minute), abstraction, delayed recall (one word recalled spontaneously, one with cueing, two with multiple choice), and orientation.

Normal heart, lung, and abdominal examinations. No carotid bruits, normal pulses throughout. Normal cranial nerves. Slight left hemiparesis with slowed rapid alternating movements, but no drift on extended arms (rapidly normalized in the following days). No sensory loss. Symmetric deep tendon reflexes.

Special studies

CT scan showed a known old right parieto-temporal infarct and a right caudate nucleus lacune. MRI done within 3 days of presentation showed the same ischemic lesions without diffusion restriction, with mild leukoaraiosis and atrophy for age. SPECT showed diffuse bilateral cortical hypoperfusion, with severe deficit in the right parieto-temporal region compatible with the known old infarct (see Fig. 7.1).

Carotid ultrasound and angioCT showed bilateral 50%–60% internal carotid stenosis, with no intracranial stenosis.

Trans-thoracic cardiac ultrasound was normal apart from a moderate left ventricular hypertrophy with mild diastolic dysfunction. 24 h-Holter showed normal sinus rhythm.

Two electroencephalograms, awake and with sleep deprivation, showed only a mild, diffuse, intermittent slowing, possibly attributable to somnolence, with no epileptic activity.

Neuropsychological tests showed severe executive functions deficits (sensitivity to interference, altered inhibition, mental rigidity, organization/planning difficulties, etc.), moderate to severe memory deficits (affecting encoding, retrieving, and

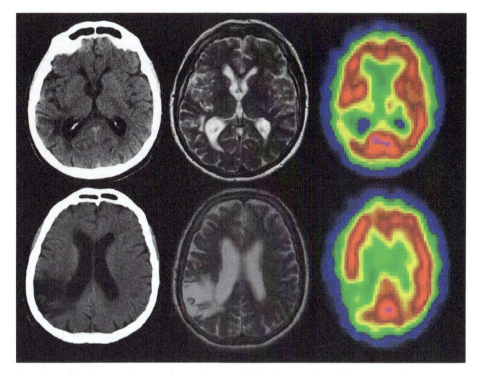

Fig. 7.1.   Right caudate lacune and parieto-temporal infarction with mild leukoaraiosis
and atrophy as shown respectively on CT scan, MRI (T2 weighted images),
and SPECT.

consolidation), and mild visuoconstructive and ideomotor apraxia. Further
questioning of the husband revealed that these deficits had been noted for more
that a year and appeared to be progressive.

Routine blood tests were normal, including: TSH, calcium, vitamin B12, and
VDRL.

Diagnosis

The initial diagnostic impression was mixed dementia, although a purely vascular
dementia could not be ruled out.

Follow-up

Repeated MMSE showed decline over time, despite temporary improvement after
initiation of a cholinesterase inhibitor, galantamine (Reminyl ER), 3 months after

Table 7.1. Follow-up of MMSE and BP over time

Time	Presentation	3 months	7 months	17 months
MMSE	23	20 (ChEI initiated)	22	18
BP	162/72 (Rx adjusted)	155/75 (Rx adjusted)	144/90 (Rx adjusted)	111/48

Notes: BP: Blood pressure.
ChEI: Cholinesterase inhibitor.
Rx: Anti-hypertensive medication.

presentation. Blood pressure remained high during initial follow-up, requiring several anti-hypertensive medication adjustments (see Table 7.1).

CT scan at 19 months was unchanged, without new vascular lesion.

Discussion

Vascular dementia, mixed dementia, and Alzheimer's disease can be seen as a continuum. Typically, vascular dementia is characterized by a very slow or stepwise decline, particularly in executive functions (Moorhouse and Rockwood, 2008). This stepwise decline is thought to be caused by new vascular lesions. In non-demented individuals with silent brain infarcts, further cognitive decline is only seen with new additional vascular lesions on MRI (Vermeer *et al.*, 2003). In contrast, Alzheimer's disease is characterized by a progressive decline, mainly in episodic memory, and is associated with hippocampal atrophy (Dubois *et al.*, 2007). Mixed dementia shares features of both.

Conceptually, mixed dementia is a dementia where both vascular lesions and Alzheimer's pathology co-exist to produce cognitive impairment sufficient to interfere with functioning. In recent autopsy series, the majority of demented patients showed both vascular lesions and Alzheimer's pathology. These seem to interact synergistically (or at least additively): given a similar degree of Alzheimer's pathology, patients with additional vascular lesions had poorer cognitive function, or, with similar clinical severity of dementia, they had less Alzheimer's pathology (Zekry *et al.*, 2002). Each pathology also appears to promote the other: demented patients have a greater incidence of stroke and stroke patients have a greater incidence of dementia (Leys *et al.*, 2005).

There are no widely accepted criteria to define mixed dementia (Zekry *et al.*, 2002; Langa *et al.*, 2004). As for vascular dementia criteria, one of the main difficulties is establishing a causal relationship between vascular lesions and cognitive impairment (Chui *et al.*, 2000). Strategic lesions usually associated with cognitive impairment, such as large cortical or bilateral thalamic infarcts, are found as often in patients with and without post-stroke dementia (Ballard *et al.*, 2004). Subcortical white matter ischemia or leukoaraiosis is associated with a decrease in cognitive functions (Vermeer *et al.*, 2003; van der Flier *et al.*, 2005), but with advances in neuroimaging, white matter changes are now observed in the majority of elderly, only 10% of which are demented. Thus, vascular lesions may not be sufficient to cause dementia, but they likely contribute to cognitive impairment when present. Even when scarce, their presence indicates a higher risk of developing future vascular lesions, which could eventually lead to dementia (Vermeer *et al.*, 2003).

Mixed dementia also requires a neurodegenerative, or, more specifically, an Alzheimer's disease component. Alzheimer's disease criteria emphasize memory impairment, progressive decline, and hippocampal atrophy (Dubois *et al.*, 2007). However, memory impairment can also be caused by vascular lesions. For example, in the medial temporal lobe; progressive decline can be seen with increasing silent subcortical vascular lesions; hippocampal atrophy has been associated with vascular lesions (Zekry *et al.*, 2002; Moorhouse and Rockwood, 2008). Other evidence of Alzheimer's pathology can be sought with PET scan and CSF biomarkers, but interpretation of these results is still controversial. Definite diagnosis of Alzheimer's disease still requires histopathological evidence.

Irrespective of the underlying cause, occurrence of dementia after stroke can be described as post-stroke dementia. It affects about 30% of stroke survivors, depending on the follow-up duration, and is most often a vascular dementia (Leys *et al.*, 2005). In this case study, although a temporal relationship between cognitive impairment and stroke was not clear, the significant vascular burden coupled with executive dysfunction suggested a vascular component. Specific visuoconstructive and ideomotor apraxia could stem from the stroke involving the right parietal region. Severe executive dysfunction would be atypical in early Alzheimer's disease, but the memory complaint with specific storage deficit (Budson and Price, 2005), as evidenced by the five words test (Dubois *et al.*, 2002), the delayed recall of the MoCA, and the neuropsychological assessment, as well as the progressive decline reported by the husband and observed during follow-up in the absence of new vascular lesion, is suggestive of an Alzheimer's component.

A strictly vascular dementia was less likely but could not be excluded. Brain imaging did not show hippocampal atrophy nor specific hypoperfusion suggestive of Alzheimer's disease. Because follow-up imaging was done by CT scan rather than MRI, vascular burden progression could have been missed. Newer imaging techniques such as tensor diffusion imaging can show changes in the normal

Table 7.2. Treatment effects on cognition and global functioning according to type of dementia

		Alzheimer's	Mixed dementia	Vascular dementia
Donepezil (Aricept)	Cognition	+		+
	Global functioning	+		+
Rivastigmine (Exelon)	Cognition	+	(+)	+
	Global functioning	+	(ns)	ns
Galantamine (Reminyl)	Cognition	+	+	+
	Global functioning	+	+	ns
Memantine (Ebixa)	Cognition	+		+
	Global functioning	+		ns

Notes: ChEI: Cholinesterase inhibitor.
+: Showed statistically significant improvement.
ns: Did not show statistically significant improvement.

appearing white matter which correlate better with cognitive impairment than the usual T2 or FLAIR sequences (Moorhouse and Rockwood, 2008).

Vascular dementia and Alzheimer's disease share the same risk factors (de la Torre, 2004). In this case, in addition to well-known vascular risk factors, estrogen deficiency secondary to bilateral oophorectomy at age 35 might have increased both her risk of vascular disease and Alzheimer's disease. Replacement hormonotherapy to prevent dementia is controversial, but vascular risk factor prevention is thought to delay cognitive decline, especially when there is a vascular component (Deschaintre *et al.*, 2009). In randomized controlled trials, only anti-hypertensive medications have been shown to prevent dementia (Peters *et al.*, 2008). Special attention was given for controlling blood pressure in this case.

Cholinesterase inhibitors and the NMDA partial antagonist memantine (Ebixa) have all been shown to improve both cognition and global functioning in Alzheimer's disease. In vascular dementia, donepezil (Aricept) improved both cognition and global functioning, but galantamine (Reminyl), rivastigmine (Exelon), and memantine (Exelon) significantly improved only cognition. In mixed dementia defined as Alzheimer's disease with significant cerebrovascular disease, only galantamine (Reminyl) has been specifically studied: it improved both cognition and global functioning (Erkinjuntti *et al.*, 2002). In an exploratory analysis of patients presumed to have mixed dementia rather than vascular dementia because of their age ($\geq$75 years old), rivastigmine (Exelon) tended to improve cognition but not global functioning (Ballard *et al.*, 2008). A summary of these data is shown in Table 7.2.

Other medications have been studied for the treatment of mixed or vascular dementia but failed to demonstrate a significant positive effect.

Take home messages

Vascular lesions and Alzheimer's pathology:

* Share the same risk factors
* Promote each other
* Often co-exist
* Interact synergistically

Mixed dementia is now recognized as the most frequent dementia.
    Treatment includes vascular risk factors prevention, especially high blood pressure.

REFERENCES AND FURTHER READING

Ballard C, Burton E, Barber R, *et al.* (2004). NINDS AIREN neuroimaging criteria do not distinguish stroke patients with and without dementia. *Neurology*, **63**(6), 983–8.

Ballard C, Sauter M, Scheltens P, *et al.* (2008). Efficacy, safety and tolerability of rivastigmine capsules in patients with probable vascular dementia: the VantagE study. *Curr Med Res Opin*, **24**(9), 2561–74.

Budson AE, Price BH (2005). Memory dysfunction. *N Engl J Med*, **352**(7), 692–9.

Chui HC, Mack W, Jackson JE, *et al.* (2000). Clinical criteria for the diagnosis of vascular dementia: a multicenter study of comparability and interrater reliability. *Arch Neurol*, **57**(2), 191–6.

de la Torre JC (2004). Is Alzheimer's disease a neurodegenerative or a vascular disorder? Data, dogma, and dialectics. *Lancet Neurol*, **3**(3), 184–90.

Deschaintre Y, Richard F, Ley SD, Pasquier F (2009). Treatment of vascular risk factors is associated with slower decline in Alzheimer's disease. *Neurology*, **73**(9), 674–80.

Dubois B, Feldman HH, Jacova C, *et al.* (2007). Research criteria for the diagnosis of Alzheimer's disease: revising the NINCDS-ADRDA criteria. *Lancet Neurol* **6**(8): 734–46.

Dubois B, Touchon J, Portet F, Ousset PJ, Vellas B, Michel B (2002). ["The 5 words": a simple and sensitive test for the diagnosis of Alzheimer's disease]. *Presse Med*, **31**(36), 1696–9.

Erkinjuntti T, Kurz A, Gauthier S, Bullock R, Lilienfeld S, Damaraju CV (2002). Efficacy of galantamine in probable vascular dementia and Alzheimer's disease combined with cerebro-vascular disease: a randomised trial. *Lancet*, **359**(9314), 1283–90.

Langa KM, Foster NL, Lawson EBJ (2004). Mixed dementia: emerging concepts and thera-peutic implications. *JAMA*, **292**(23), 2901–8.

Leys D, Hénon H, Mackowiak-Cordoliani MA, Pasquier F (2005). Poststroke dementia. *Lancet Neurol*, **4**(11), 752–9.

Moorhouse P, Rockwood K (2008). Vascular cognitive impairment: current concepts and clinical developments. *Lancet Neurol*, **7**(3), 246–55.

Peters R, Beckett N, Forette F, *et al.* (2008). Incident dementia and blood pressure lowering in the Hypertension in the Very Elderly Trial cognitive function assessment (HYVET-COG): a double-blind, placebo controlled trial. *Lancet Neurol* **7**(8), 683–9.

van der Flier WM, van Straaten EC, Barkhof F, *et al.* (2005). Small vessel disease and general cognitive function in nondisabled elderly: the LADIS study. *Stroke*, **36**(10), 2116–20.

Vermeer SE, Prins ND, den Heijer T, *et al.* (2003). Silent brain infarcts and the risk of dementia and cognitive decline. *N Engl J Med*, **348**(13), 1215–22.

Zekry D, Hauw JJ, Gold G (2002). Mixed dementia: epidemiology, diagnosis, and treatment. *J Am Geriatr Soc*, **50**(8), 1431–8.

Case 8

Young man with behavioral symptoms

Philippe H. Robert

Clinical history – main complaint

At the age of 54, Mr. H came in consultation to the psychiatric department for his wife: "My wife has a bipolar disorder and I would like to have information in order to help her more." The psychiatric interview mentioned that Mr. H presents some neurotic personality features associated with some impulsivity.

Ten years later at the age of 64, Mr. H went to the Memory consultation: "I have some memory problem and would like to be tested." His wife added "He changed a lot in 1 year. He is now terribly irritable particularly with me."

General history

Mr. H. has a high level of education. He was Director of an informatic department in an important company. He retired at the age of 63. Past medical history includes only coronary disease (chirurgical treatment at age 57).

Family history

No familial history of dementia.

Examination

First assessment age 64

- Mini-Mental Score Examination (MMSE): 30/30
- Kaplan Baycrest Neuropsychological Assessment (KBNA):
  - Attention task, flexibility, verbal fluency: normal performances
  - Episodic and immediate memories: performances < normal

Case Studies in Dementia: Common and Uncommon Presentations, ed. S. Gauthier and P. Rosa-Neto.
Published by Cambridge University Press. © Cambridge University Press 2011.

- Behavioral assessment:
  - NPI (wife interview); irritability, anxiety, apathy
  - Patient interview: Mr. H is aware of his memory problem and explains that irritability and anxiety are related to the perception of his memory difficulties. He is aware of these difficulties but does not accept them. He also explains that he is losing interest in his usual hobbies (tennis, bridge, art)

Age 67

- Mini-Mental Score Examination (MMSE): 21/30
- Grober & Buschke Selective and cue reminding test: quantitative and qualitative pathological performance
- Ray figure: pathological performances
- Trail making test A& B: pathological performance (slower than normal without errors)
- Behavioral assessment:
  - NPI (wife interview); irritability, aggressiveness, and delusion ("he is very jealous and does not accept that I can have activity without him"), apathy
  - Patient interview: Mr. H denies the information provided by his wife ("this is exaggerated, I am not like this"). He is aware of the memory difficulties, but denies that this could have an effect in his daily living activities. He feels as active as in the past
  - Clinician point of view: loss of spontaneous ideas during the discussion and during the test; loss of interest but able to be curious when stimulated

Age 68

- Mini-Mental Score Examination (MMSE): 18/30
- Apraxo-aphasic syndrome
- Behavioral assessment:
  - NPI (wife interview): apathy is predominant. Verbal aggressively (only with his wife) delusion.
  - Patient interview: Mr. H has accepted to go once a week to a day-care unit. He explains that this is good place. He even remembers that he visited a museum last week. Finally, looking at his wife, he said that sometimes it is good to be without her.
  - Clinician point of view: during the testing and interview Mr. H had some difficulties in finding words. He worries about this and seems irritable about himself on this point. Loss of interest and loss of initiative are important, but Mr. H is always emotionally responsive during the discussion when the interviewer or the psychologist makes a joke, or focuses on Mr. H's past topic of interest.

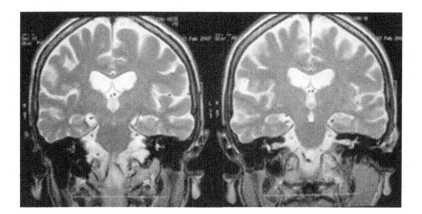

Fig. 8.1. Coronal T2 weighted MRI (2 consecutive slices) showing declines and hippocampal volume (right > left) and no significant signal changes in the white matter.

Special studies

There was evidence of hippocampal atrophy predominantly in the right side on the MRI (Fig. 8.1).

Diagnosis

Alzheimer's disease

Follow-up

Today Mr. H is still living at home. He comes 2 days a week to the day-care hospital.

He takes a cholinergic treatment and pushes to be enrolled in a disease-modifying treatment clinical trial. His wife participates in a caregiver-training program.

Discussion

Medical history is a cornerstone of medical practice. In addition, recording history serves to gather information about the personality of the patient.

A majority of patients develop neuropsychiatric symptoms, also called behavioral and psychological symptoms of dementia (BPSD) during the course of their illnesses.

Several neuropsychiatric symptoms are present very early in the disease process. Apathy and depressive symptoms are the most frequently observed neuropsychiatric symptoms in mild cognitive impairment. Neuropsychiatric symptoms are primary manifestations of the disease process, but other psychological and social factors also play a role in determining which patients will manifest behavioral symptoms.

A very important point is that very different BPSD such as delusion, irritability, or apathy can occur at the same time in the same patient. However, the cause of each symptom may differ.

For Mr. H, irritability, anxiety, and delusion are related both to the personal history of the patient and his wife. They are also the consequences of the cognitive deficit and the patient psychological reaction to the perception of his memory loss.

Apathy is related to the disease process. It is important to clarify the characteristics of the behavioral symptom. Mr. H. has a major loss of self-initiated behavior and interest. However, he is able to respond to external cognitive and emotional stimulation. This will help in choosing the best non-pharmacological strategies.

Take home messages

Taking clinical history and behavioral assessment are cornerstones for the diagnosis but also for defining the therapeutic strategies.

Different behavioral symptoms coming from multiple causes can occur at the same time.

FURTHER READING

Gauthier S, Cummings J, Ballard C, *et al.* (2010). Management of behavioral problems in Alzheimer's disease. *Int Psycho-Geriatrics*: in press.

Robert PH, Onyike CU, Leentjens AFG, *et al.* (2009). Proposed diagnostic criteria for apathy in Alzheimer's disease and other neuropsychiatric disorders. *Eur Psychiatry*, **24**: 98–104.

Waldemar G, Burns A (2009). *Alzheimer's Disease*. Oxford: Oxford University Press.

Case 9

Woman with visual complaints

Serge Gauthier, Sylvie Belleville, Emilie Lepage,
and Jean-Paul Soucy

Clinical history

A 53-year-old woman reports difficulties over the past 6 months in handling her
work as a specialized clothes cutter in a garment factory. She has the impression
of seeing superimposed images while reading, watching television, and walking,
to the point that she fell off the sidewalk. She has difficulties writing her name,
reading, and writing numbers such as "3700" and in setting time on her alarm
clock, but she could use her banking card with a PIN number. She described
occasional difficulties putting on a nightgown or a sweater. She has forgotten
birthdays and has been calling her mother repeatedly to check on dates of
upcoming events. She has hesitation in explaining verbally how to get somewhere,
but she can orient herself well using public transportation.

General history

Grade 9 educated right-handed woman in good general health. Lives with her
husband, no children. About to end Arimidex treatment post-breast cancer
surgery 5 years previously. Mild arterial hypertension controlled with Avapro
(irbesartan) and Norvasc (amiodipine besylate).

Family history

No family history of Alzheimer's disease.

Examination

Eleven months after onset of symptoms: BP 120/85; pulse 72 regular. MMSE 20/30,
Boston Naming 10/15. Difficulties with serial-7s. Unable to complete Trail B or

Case Studies in Dementia: Common and Uncommon Presentations, ed. S. Gauthier and P. Rosa-Neto.
Published by Cambridge University Press. © Cambridge University Press 2011.

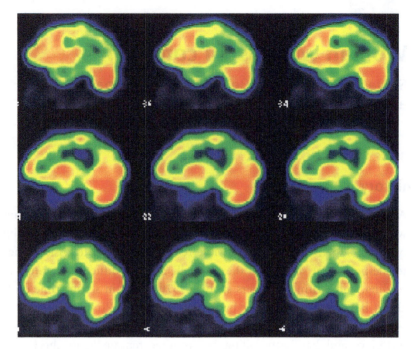

Fig. 9.1.   ECD SPECT showing hypoperfusion in the posterior temporo-parietal regions sparing the frontal cortex.

to draw a clock. No sign of peripheral arterial disease. No carotid bruits. Normal general neurologic examination, including visual fields by confrontation.

Special studies

MRI with and without enhancement 1 month after onset of symptoms showed no focal atrophy.

EEG 6 months after onset of symptoms showed intermittent theta 5 to 7 Hz low voltage in the anterior and mid-temporal regions bilaterally.

A quantified regional perfusion study using 99mTc SPECT eleven months after onset of symptoms showed significant hypoperfusion of the left parieto-temporal regions and very slight of the right parietal region. This was unchanged on repeat examination eight months later (Fig. 9.1).

Neuropsychological testing was done 1 and 2 years after onset of symptoms (Table 9.1) and demonstrated predominantly an apraxia (ideomotor, melokinetic, constructive) and spatial deficits, with some memory impairment, but intact recognition of objects and speech. The follow-up assessment showed worsening of the apraxia.

Table 9.1. Patient's results on neuropsychological tests

	One year after onset		Two years after onset	
	C.G.	z score	C.G.	z score
Global cognition				
Mattis dementia rating scale (MDRS) (/144)	98	−8.9*	90	−10.6*
Executive functions				
Stroop Victoria				
Time (sec)	92.61	8.4*	95.56	8.7*
Errors	2	2.1*	6	7.2*
Verbal memory				
Free and cued recall (RL/RI) (/16)				
Free recall (first trial)	5	−2*	5	−2*
Cued recall (first trial)	12	−1.6*	7	−4.6*
Free recall (20 minutes delay)	8	−2.1*	8	−2.1*
Cued recall (20 minutes delay)	14	−2.1*	12	−4.6*
Visuo-perceptual functions				
Benton judgment of line orientations (/30)	1	−5.9*	NA**	
Boston naming test (/15)	10	−1.5*	9	−2.1*
Constructional functions				
Copy of Rey Figure (score) (/36)	1	−23*	NA**	
Construction subtest from MDRS (/3)	0		1	
Limb praxis				
Ideomotor praxis (/7)	6		4	
Imitation praxis (/2)	2		2	
Melokinetic praxis (/3)	0		1	

Notes: *Indicates that C.G. is impaired.
**Indicates that C.G. is unable to do the task.

Diagnosis

The initial diagnostic impression was a focal cognitive deficit related to early Alzheimer's disease, non-familial.

Follow-up

Donepezil was given and well tolerated up to 10 mg a day. There was no evident clinical change over 1 year, whereas the MMSE improved from 19/30 to 22/30. She had to stop working and obtained full medical disability.

Discussion

Alzheimer's disease can present with focal symptoms and neuropsychological findings, particularly in highly educated persons (Joanette *et al.*, 2000). Evolution over time reveals a more widespread cortical impairment, supporting the diagnosis of a neurodegenerative process such as Alzheimer's disease (Neary *et al.*, 1986).

SPECT is a relatively simple technique available world-wide, and if read by a competent radiologist, can be very useful in early diagnosis of Alzheimer's disease (Habert *et al.*, 2009). This may require serial examinations 6 months apart.

There is an ongoing debate about the diagnosis of Alzheimer's disease when memory impairment is minimal ("possible AD" according to the NINCDS-ADRDA criteria; McKahnn *et al.*, 1984), or when there is little functional impairment (pre-dementia stage; Dubois *et al.*, 2007). It is possible but not yet fully established that the combination of impaired working memory and one or a combination of: reduced metabolism on FDG-PET, reduced perfusion on SPECT, hippocampal atrophy on MRI, amyloid deposition on PIB-PET, elevated tau and reduced aß in CSF would be diagnostic of early Alzheimer's disease (see case from Dr. Bruno Dubois *et al*).

These criteria would not have helped in this case, since memory was relatively intact at presentation. Atypical presentations of Alzheimer's disease account for about 15% of cases. This case falls under the umbrella of "posterior cortical atrophy," first described by Benson *et al.* in 1988, usually presenting with visuo-spatial difficulties including visual fields defects. Such patients are often seen by opthalmologists before being referred to neurologists. Other common symptoms include alexia, agraphia, acalculia, anomia, digital agnosia, apraxia. Onset of symptoms is usually around 55 to 60, and progression is faster than usual in Alzheimer's disease. Memory appears largely preserved over a long period of time. Pathologically there are a large number of neurofibrillary tangles in the primary and associative visual cortices and in the inferior parietal lobes, and much less so in the hippocampus (Renner *et al.*, 2004).

Take home messages

Not all cases of dementia have memory impairment at onset.
SPECT can be useful in atypical presentations of dementia.

REFERENCES AND FURTHER READING

Benson DF, Davis RJ, Snyder BD (1988). Posterior cortical atrophy. *Arch Neurol* **45**, 789–93.

Dubois B, Feldman H, Jacova C, *et al.* (2007). Research criteria for the diagnosis of Alzheimer's disease: revisiting of the NINCDS-ADRDA criteria. *Lancet Neurol*, **6**, 734–46.

Habert MO, Horn JF, Sarazin M *et al.* (2009). Brain perfusion SPECT with an automated quatitative tool can identify prodromal Alzheimer's disease among patients with mild cognitive impairment. *Neurobiol Aging*, doi:10.1016/j.neurobiolaging.2009.01.013.

Joanette Y, Belleville S, Gely-Nargeot, Ska B, Valdois S (2000). Plurality of patterns of cognitive impairment in normal aging and in dementia. *Rev Neurol (Paris)*, **156**, 759–66.

McKhann G, Drachman D, Folstein M *et al.* (1984). Clinical diagnosis of Alzheimer's disease: report of the NINCDS-ADRDA Work Group under the auspices of Department of Health and Human Services Task Force on Alzheimer's Disease. *Neurology*, **34**, 939–44.

Neary D, Snowden JS, Bowen DM *et al.* (1986). Neuropsychological syndromes in presenile dementia due to cerebral atrophy. *J Neurol Neurosurg Psychiatry*, **49**, 163–74.

Renner JA, Burns JM, Hou CE *et al.* (2004). Progressive posterior cortical dysfunction: a clinicopathologic series. *Neurology*, **63**, 1175–80.

Case 10

Difficulty playing tennis

Matthew E. Growdon and Gil D. Rabinovici

Clinical history – main complaint

A 77-year-old right-handed woman presented to clinic with a 7-year history of slowly progressive difficulty with visuospatial processing followed by language and memory dysfunction. The patient first noticed problems with visuospatial function while playing tennis 7 years ago. She experienced difficulty directing the ball and would at times miss the ball entirely when swinging her racquet. She subsequently developed problems with depth perception resulting in a series of car accidents and ultimately necessitating revoking her driver's license. Four years after the onset of her visual symptoms she began to have difficulty manipulating objects. She also reported difficulty reading. In the year prior to her clinic visit the patient noticed problems with short-term memory; she developed trouble recalling recent events, and she began misplacing objects and asking questions repeatedly. She also reported mild word-finding difficulties and occasional mispronunciation of words.

General history

The patient received an associate's degree and worked as an accountant until the age of 50. She lives with her husband and maintains an active social life. Her past medical history is significant for hypertension, arthritis, and hypothyroidism. Her medications are levothyroxine, ramipril, hydrochlorothiazide, and a multivitamin.

Family history

Her mother died at age 88 and was diagnosed with Parkinson's disease in late life. A paternal aunt was diagnosed with Alzheimer's disease at age 80 and died 8 years later.

Case Studies in Dementia: Common and Uncommon Presentations, ed. S. Gauthier and P. Rosa-Neto. Published by Cambridge University Press. © Cambridge University Press 2011.

Examination

The general physical examination was normal. On mental status examination, the patient was alert and fully oriented. Her speech was fluent with occasional word finding pauses. She made one phonemic paraphasic error. On short-term memory testing she registered three items and recalled all three after a short delay. She was able to recite months of the year backwards without difficulty. There was subtle apraxia of the bilateral upper extremities on transitive and intransitive tasks, left greater than right. She had great difficulty mimicking hand positions and drawing a cube and pyramid. She showed mild ocular apraxia (though not ocular ataxia) and had difficulty integrating a complex visual scene, instead focusing on individual elements (simultanagnosia). She had preserved insight into her deficits.

The patient demonstrated left-sided extinction to simultaneous bilateral visual stimulation, but there was no hemispatial neglect and visual fields were full. There was saccadic breakdown of smooth pursuit. Extraocular movements were full with normal velocity. The remainder of the cranial nerve examination was normal. On motor examination there was mild paratonia of the left arm without rigidity; power was full throughout. Sensory examination revealed agraphesthesia in both hands, left greater than right, with intact primary sensation. Deep tendon reflexes were normal and symmetric and plantar responses were flexor bilaterally. There were no tremors, co-ordination was intact throughout, and gait was normal except for mildly diminished left arm swing.

Special studies

A neuropsychological testing battery was performed. Mini-Mental State Examination (MMSE) score was 26/30; she lost 3 points for orientation and 1 point for poor copy of overlapping pentagons. Her episodic memory was relatively spared. She scored 3, 5, 6, and 7 across learning trials of the 9-item California Verbal Learning Test, recalling six items after delays of 30 seconds and 10-minutes. She recognized 7 items with 1 false positive. Visual memory was more impacted than verbal memory, as evidenced by a score of 2/17 on delayed recall of the Rey-Osterreith figure. She was able to correctly select this figure from four options. She scored 3/17 when asked to copy the Rey-Osterreith figure. On a subset of the Visual Object and Space Perception Battery, she scored 5/10, further underscoring her deficits in visuospatial ability. She was only able to complete 3/5 simple calculations. On language testing, she scored 9/15 on the 15-item Boston Naming Test. She scored 3/5 on a test of syntax comprehension, but it is important to note that she had difficulty visualizing the stimuli. She generated 10 D words and

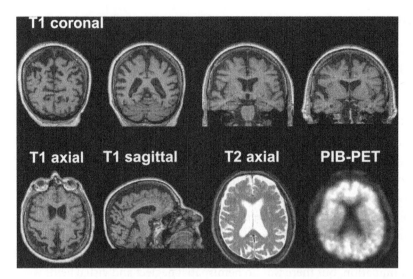

Fig. 10.1.   Coronal T1-weighted MRI images presented posterior (left) to anterior (right) demonstrate prominent biparietal atrophy and sparing of hippocampi (top row). The posterior-predominant atrophy pattern can be better appreciated on axial and sagittal images (bottom left). T2-weighted imaging shows absence of significant vascular disease. PIB-PET (bottom right) demonstrates increased cortical signal consistent with the presence of amyloid-beta plaques. All images are presented in radiological orientation.

12 animals in 1 minute. Executive function proved hard to evaluate with traditional tests due to the patient's deficits in visuospatial processing.

Electrolytes, liver, and renal function tests, thyroid function tests, rapid plasmin reagin and vitamin B12 levels were normal. Cerebrospinal fluid showed 1 white blood cell per mm^3, 0 red blood cells per mm^3, glucose of 60 mg/dl (reference range 40–70), and protein of 36 mg/dl (range 15–45). VDRL of the cerebrospinal fluid was non-reactive, and a test for Lyme antibodies was negative. Apolipoprotein E genotype was ε2/ε3.

Brain MRI showed marked atrophy of the bilateral medial and lateral parietal lobes, right slightly greater than left, in the setting of mild generalized cortical atrophy (Fig. 10.1).

Hippocampal volumes were preserved for age, and there were minimal periventricular white matter changes on T2-weighted images.

Diagnosis

Based on the patient's history of slowly progressive visuospatial dysfunction followed by mild deficits in language and memory, physical and cognitive examination findings suggestive of biparietal dysfunction and marked parietal atrophy on brain imaging, the patient was diagnosed with posterior cortical atrophy (PCA). The most likely underlying histopathology was felt to be Alzheimer's disease (AD), based on the strong relationship between the PCA clinical syndrome and underlying AD (Renner *et al.*, 2004; Tang-Wai *et al.*, 2004). Corticobasal degeneration was also considered, but was felt to be less likely given the paucity of movement abnormalities and parkinsonian features seven years after symptom onset. Dementia with Lewy bodies was considered unlikely, given the absence of parkinsonism, neuropsychiatric symptoms, or fluctuations. A vascular etiology was dismissed, given the absence of cortical vascular lesions on brain imaging, and Creutzfeldt–Jakob disease was felt to be highly unlikely given the long disease course. Treatment with a cholinesterase inhibitor was recommended.

Follow-up

The patient returned for a follow-up visit 2 years later. In the interim, she experienced worsening visuospatial symptoms. She occasionally walked into glass doors and developed trouble seeing steps, such that her family placed brightly colored tape along the edges of the stairs in her house in order to guide her. She developed a dressing apraxia. Language problems, primarily in the form of word-finding difficulties, became more pronounced. She reported that her left hand was harder to control, and she could not use it to manipulate buttons while dressing. Despite worsening symptoms, her neuropsychological testing profile remained relatively constant. Positron emission tomography (PET) with the β-amyloid imaging tracer [^{11}C] Pittsburgh Compound-B (PIB) conducted as part of a research study showed increased tracer uptake throughout cortex suggesting the presence of fibrillar β-amyloid plaques (Fig. 10.1) and supporting the impression of underlying AD (Fig. 10.1).

Discussion

Frank Benson first described a series of patients with progressive and relatively restricted deficits of higher-order visual function associated with pronounced parieto-occipital atrophy, a syndrome he coined posterior cortical atrophy (PCA) (Benson *et al.*, 1988). PCA has since gained recognition as a distinct clinical entity. The presenting symptoms are most often referable to the parietal lobes and include variable combinations of Balint syndrome (ocular apraxia, ocular ataxia, and simultanagnosia), Gerstmann syndrome (acalculia, agraphia, finger agnosia, and left-right disorientation), environmental agnosia and sensory transcortical aphasia (Renner *et al.*, 2004; Tang-Wai *et al.*, 2004). The dorsal visual stream is most often disrupted leading to difficulty judging spatial relationships, locating objects, and navigating. Trouble with driving is common, and patients are at risk for motor vehicle accidents (as demonstrated in this case). Presentations referable to the ventral visual stream (e.g. visual agnosia, pure alexia) and disturbances of primary visual processing are less common (Tang-Wai *et al.*, 2004). Episodic memory, insight, and executive functions are relatively spared (McMonagle *et al.*, 2006). Given their severe problems with visuospatial processing, patients with PCA often present to an optometrist or ophthalmologist, and it is not unusual for patients to be fitted for new glasses or even to undergo cataract removal before presenting to the neurologist.

Structural or functional brain imaging usually reveals marked posterior cortical atrophy, hypometabolism, or hypoperfusion involving parietal and posterior temporal lobes but extending into association and even primary visual cortex, a more posterior atrophy pattern than that seen in clinically "typical" (i.e. amnestic) AD (Migliaccio *et al.*, 2009; Nestor *et al.*, 2003; Whitwell *et al.*, 2007). In contrast, hippocampus and medial temporal cortex are relatively preserved, mirroring the clinical sparing of episodic memory. Cortical atrophy is often asymmetric, with greater involvement of the right hemisphere (Whitwell *et al.*, 2007). At autopsy, most patients are found to have underlying Alzheimer's disease (AD), though the syndrome has also been associated with post-mortem diagnoses of dementia with Lewy bodies (DLB), corticobasal degeneration (CBD), and prion disease (Renner *et al.*, 2004). The presence of parkinsonism early in the disease course should raise the suspicion for underlying DLB or CBD (Tang-Wai *et al.*, 2004). The distribution of AD pathology in PCA is atypical, with a very high burden of neurofibrillary tangles (NFT) found in primary and association visual cortex and relatively decreased numbers of NFT seen in medial temporal and prefrontal cortex compared to patients with an amnestic clinical phenotype. Some studies have also reported an atypical distribution of senile plaques compared to amnestic AD, but this finding appears less robust and consistent than the differences in NFTs (Tang-Wai *et al.*, 2004). Interestingly, our patient showed a diffuse pattern of PIB binding equally involving anterior and posterior cortex (Fig. 10.1).

Most series of PCA demonstrate a female preponderance and an early age-at-onset in the sixth or early seventh decade (McMonagle *et al.*, 2006; Migliaccio *et al.*, 2009; Tang-Wai *et al.*, 2004). However, the present case demonstrates that the syndrome can present later in life. The biological mechanisms that lead to differential degeneration of visuospatial networks in PCA are unknown. One study reported a lower incidence of the apolipoprotein ε4 allele in PCA compared to AD (Schott *et al.*, 2006), but this result has not been reproduced in other cohorts (Migliaccio *et al.*, 2009; Tang-Wai *et al.*, 2004). Some have speculated that patients with developmental cognitive disability may be particularly vulnerable to focal neurodegeneration (Rogalski *et al.*, 2008), but this remains an unproven hypothesis.

As this case demonstrates, AD can present with focal symptoms and neuropsychological profiles that are distinct from the typical amnestic presentation. A multimodal approach (including a thorough clinical history, neurological examination, a comprehensive neuropsychological evaluation, and neuroimaging) is particularly important for accurate diagnosis in such atypical clinical syndromes. In the future, cerebrospinal fluid biomarkers or amyloid imaging, currently used primarily for research purposes, may supplement the clinical evaluation and assist in molecular diagnosis of underlying AD in patients with pathologically heterogeneous cortical syndromes such as PCA.

Early recognition of PCA can be helpful, since patients often retain insight and executive functions and are thus likely to respond to rehabilitation efforts to adapt to visual loss such as changes to the living environment and referrals to services for the blind (Mendez *et al.*, 2002). An accurate diagnosis of cortical visual dysfunction can spare patients from unnecessary ophthalmologic procedures. Given the preservation of insight, clinicians should be particularly vigilant for depressive symptoms that may respond to treatment. Finally, given the strong association between PCA and underlying AD, patients presenting with PCA should be considered for current and future AD pharmacologic therapies.

Take home messages

Posterior cortical atrophy (PCA) is a clinical syndrome of visuospatial dysfunction in the setting of neurodegeneration in visual association cortex.

PCA represents a diagnostic challenge and is often mistaken for primary ocular disease.

PCA is strongly associated with underlying Alzheimer's disease (AD), though the clinical presentation, cognitive and anatomic profiles are distinct from those seen in amnestic presentations of AD.

Molecular imaging and CSF biomarkers may in the future supplement the clinical evaluation and improve in vivo prediction of pathology in PCA and other focal cortical syndromes.

PCA patients have unique safety and rehabilitation needs that must be recognized and addressed by the clinician.

REFERENCES AND FURTHER READING

Benson DF, Davis RJ, Snyder BD (1988). Posterior cortical atrophy. *Arch Neurol*, **45**, 789–93.

McMonagle P, Deering F, Berliner Y, Kertesz A (2006). The cognitive profile of posterior cortical atrophy. *Neurology*, **66**, 331–8.

Mendez M, Ghajarania M, Perryman K (2002). Posterior Cortical Atrophy: Clinical Characteristics and Differences Compared to Alzheimer's Disease. *Dement Geriatr Cogn Disord*, **14**, 33–40.

Migliaccio R, Agosta F, Rascovsky K, *et al.* (2009). Clinical syndromes associated with posterior atrophy: early age at onset AD spectrum. *Neurology*, **73**, 1571–8.

Nestor PJ, Caine D, Fryer TD, *et al.* (2003). The topography of metabolic deficits in posterior cortical atrophy with FDG-PET. *J Neurol Neurosurg Psychiatry*, **74**, 1521–9.

Renner JA, Burns JM, Hou CE, *et al.* (2004). Progressive posterior cortical dysfunction: a clinicopathologic series. *Neurology*, **63**, 1175–80.

Rogalski E, Johnson N, Weintraub S, Mesulam M (2008). Increased frequency of learning disability in patients with primary progressive aphasia and their first-degree relatives. *Arch Neurol*, **65**, 244–8.

Schott JM, Ridha BH, Crutch SJ, *et al.* (2006). Apolipoprotein e genotype modifies the phenotype of Alzheimer disease. *Arch Neurol*, **63**, 155–6.

Tang-Wai DF, Graff-Radford NR, Boeve BF, *et al.* (2004). Clinical, genetic, and neuropathologic characteristics of posterior cortical atrophy. *Neurology*, **63**, 1168–74.

Whitwell JL, Jack CR, Jr., Kantarci K, *et al.* (2007). Imaging correlates of posterior cortical atrophy. *Neurobiol Aging*, **28**, 1051–61.

Progressive aphasia complicated by intracerebral bleeding

Gabriel C. Léger

Clinical history – chief complaint

A 63-year-old right-handed woman was referred for language difficulties. Her husband and daughter (a physician) describe a 4-year gradual decline in her ability to express herself and, more recently, difficulties carrying out complex tasks. There was reduced interest (if not ability) in completing both basic and instrumental activities of daily living. The family had also noted a new tendency to gamble, in particular, through the use of video lottery and poker machines.

General history

Completed high school. Worked in a cigarette factory before starting her family at age 35. Had four daughters. Formerly, a 40-pack–year smoker. No known drug allergies. Tubal ligation at age 37. Recovered from a severe weight-loss associated depression 3 years ago, leaving residual of general anxiety and agoraphobia. There was post-menopausal osteoporosis and smoking-related emphysema. No history of cerebral, cardiac, or peripheral vascular disease. No hypertension, diabetes, hypercholesterolemia, thyroid, or autoimmune disease. Medications: hormone replacements, bisphosphonates with calcium and vitamin D, venlafaxine 75, ASA 325, clonidine 0.1, and lorazepam PRN. She had not tolerated paroxetine, which caused increased confusion.

Family history

There was a strong family history of early-onset cognitive problems. Mother, who died at age 45 from colon cancer, had history of progressive memory and praxis difficulties. Sister had behavioral changes and also died at age 45 from a mild head injury. Brother with behavior, language, and memory problems aged 52. Sister sustained hemorrhagic stroke at age 51.

Case Studies in Dementia: Common and Uncommon Presentations, ed. S. Gauthier and P. Rosa-Neto. Published by Cambridge University Press. © Cambridge University Press 2011.

Examination

Unremarkable general physical and neurological examinations, specifically no evidence of peripheral vascular or cardiac disease, and no primitive release signs.

MMSE was 26/30 (backwards spelling) or 22/30 (serial-7's), MoCA 11/30. There was full orientation to time and place. Short-term memory was reasonable. Significant deficits were present in executive and visuospatial functions, as well as language. Language was fluent, characterized by frequent semantic (more than lexical) paraphasias, jargonophasia, occasional word finding difficulties, and decreased understanding. There was reduction in confrontational naming. Both semantic and lexical fluency were severely reduced. Serial-7's and calculations were difficult. Copying of pentagons and transparent cube was impossible. Clock drawing showed poor organization and loss of abstraction.

Special studies

Brain MRI without gadolinium demonstrated mild diffuse atrophy, slightly more prominent than expected for age, and severe extensive near-confluent white matter hyperintensities on T2 and FLAIR sequences (Fig. 11.1(a)). Gradient-echo sequences were not done. There was otherwise no evidence of cortical or subcortical strokes. Radiological differential diagnosis included ischemic, hypertensive, or toxic leukoencephalopathy, vasculitis, and demyelinating diseases such as multiple sclerosis or the sequelae of a previously undiagnosed post-viral acute demyelinating encephalomyelitis (ADEM).

Lumbar puncture was normal, including inflammatory indices and oligoclonal bands. Studies for CSF amyloid and tau were not available. Studies for rare late onset leukodystrophies, a full autoimmune and inflammatory work-up in addition to a paraneoplastic antibody panel (drawn because of her history of heavy smoking, weight loss, and emphysema), were entirely negative.

Brain SPECT revealed mild diffuse hypoperfusion with further focal blood flow reductions in left posterior peri-sylvian areas (Fig. 11.1(b)).

Doppler studies of the neck and large intracranial arteries were unremarkable. EEG showed mild slowing in left temporal leads.

Genetic testing for mutations in genes coding for Amyloid Precursor Protein (APP), Presenilin-1 and 2 (PS-1 and 2), *Tau*, and Progranulin (PRG), completed because of the strong family history and presenile onset, were negative.

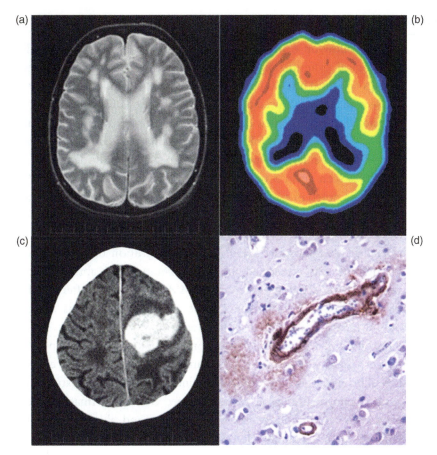

Fig. 11.1.   (a) T2 weighted MRI showing absence of cortical strokes, but extensive white matter changes; (b) blood flow SPECT showing isolated hypoperfusion in posterior language (left posterior perisylvian) areas; (c) left frontal lobar hemorrhage days prior to death; (d) amyloid staining showing presence of diffuse plaques and vessel involvement, including capillaries. Magnification × 400.

Initial diagnostic impression

The initial clinical diagnostic impression was that of a progressive but primarily focal cognitive disorder involving predominantly language, at least in its early course: primary progressive aphasia (PPA). Progression to involve other cognitive domains was obvious at time of work-up, 4 years after symptom onset. The presence of severe white matter changes in the absence of other evidence of vascular disease or risk factors was atypical, and its clinical relevance unclear.

Follow-up

At early follow-up 6 months after presentation, the MMSE had fallen to 16/30. Neurological examination remained otherwise non-focal. There were no new findings on repeat brain CT or blood investigations. Donepezil therapy was initiated.

A second SPECT showed progression of the previously demonstrated left sylvian perfusion deficits and a new deficit involving the right superior parietal area. A third SPECT study immediately following acetazolamide injection demonstrated improvement of the left-sided hypoperfusion, but no change of the deficits on the right.

She was seen again 3 months later. MMSE had increased to 23/30. Improvements were noted in executive and visuospatial function, memory, and language, and attributed to the effect of the cholinesterase inhibitor, although clinical fluctuations could not be ruled out. When seen again six months later, MMSE had fallen once more to 17/30. A trial substitution of the donepezil with oral rivastigmine was attempted, but not tolerated and abruptly stopped in the context of an acute pyelonephritis. MMSE 1 month after resolution of her infection was 3/10. Galantamine was introduced and was associated with a 7-point MMSE increase 3 months later.

Despite a family reported functional stability on follow-up after another 6 months, there was further loss of language abilities with severe understanding difficulties and speech production reduced to a few contextually inappropriate words. Again, neurological exam remained non-focal. Imaging and blood-work revealed no new findings. Memantine was added and, although clinically unchanged 6 months later, the family rejoiced in a mildly improved functional status at home (unaided dressing, showering, and personal hygiene, helping with the dishes, and absence of incontinence or behavioral changes, for a FAST of approximately 5).

There were no significant changes in her status until she sustained a hip fracture from a fall 1 year later, for which she underwent an uneventful hip replacement. Two months later, she suffered a large left frontal lobar hemorrhage (Fig. 11.1(c)). After a family discussion, palliative care was instituted and she passed away peacefully 6 days later, at 68 years of age. Autopsy was performed.

Clinical summary

With apparent disease onset at age 59, this patient presented with slowly progressive language difficulties and personality changes. In the 4 years prior to medical consultation, other cognitive domains became affected, including visuospatial and executive deficits, leading to a formal diagnosis of dementia. Although there was no relevant past medical history, a strong family history of presenile cognitive disorders was present. During the ensuing 5 years, she demonstrated occasional precipitous worsening, very good response to cholinesterase inhibition, but ultimately progressed to near complete dependence. Language remained the most prominent and severely affected cognitive domain. She died, 9 years after symptom onset, from a large left frontal lobar hemorrhage.

Positive tests included only brain MRI, which showed mild atrophy and severe white matter disease, and cerebral blood flow imaging, which revealed global hypoperfusion with marked focal blood flow reductions in eloquent areas, well correlated to her salient cognitive deficits. Etiological investigations including a search for causes of vascular and white matter diseases, as well as genetic, paraneoplastic, inflammatory, autoimmune, nutritional and, infectious disorders were entirely negative.

Autopsy

Autopsy confirmed the presence of a large left frontal hematoma with intraventricular spillage. There was associated diffuse cerebral edema and uncal herniation, ruled as the cause of death.

The brain weighed 1320 grams and was diffusely atrophic, with ventricular dilatation. More focal atrophy was noted in amygdalar and hippocampal regions, as well as temporal neocortex, left greater than right. A special note was made of the presence of a persistent left fetal circulation involving a hypoplastic proximal left posterior cerebral artery and a very prominent left posterior communicating artery (implying that the entire left hemisphere was dependent on the carotid circulation). No macroscopic strokes could be identified.

Microscopy was performed after standard staining with luxol fast blue, HE, and Gallyas, as well as immunohistochemical stains for β-amyloid, tau, and alpha-synuclein. Findings included extracellular neuritic plaques and intracellular neurofibrillary tangles involving medial temporal areas as well as frontal, temporal, tempo-occipital, and parietal neocortex, corresponding to a Braak & Braak stage 5 and, given the clinical history, consistent with a pathological diagnosis of Alzheimer's disease. Diffuse staining for β-amyloid was also found in meningeal and cortical arteries, consistent with severe cerebral amyloid angiopathy (CAA – Fig. 11.1(d)), and the likely etiology of the lobar bleed.

Discussion

Throughout the clinical course, the exact diagnosis in this complicated case remained undetermined. The early onset, with a fairly well-isolated language disorder and later progression to a full-blown dementia was highly suggestive of PPA. The differential diagnosis for PPA includes variants of frontotemporal dementia (FTD – Mesulam *et al.*, 2008, Neary *et al.*, 1998) and atypical Alzheimer's disease (AD – Mesulam *et al.*, 2008). In this case the exact etiology of her disorder was unclear. Certainly, the clinical profile, with the early onset, strong family history, absence of severe memory complaints on history and amnestic deficits on testing, behavioral changes (gambling), and a predominance of executive dysfunction, swayed the diagnosis towards FTD. On the other hand, the significant MRI white matter abnormalities, even if not obviously attributable to vascular disease (because of the absence of both risk factors and evidence of demonstrable vascular disease elsewhere), with the presence of focal cortical hypoperfusion deficits on blood flow imaging seemed to raise the possibility of the existence of at least two pathological processes.

Although difficult to fully appreciate during her life, the clinical progression of our patient's disorder is fully consistent with the ultimate pathological diagnosis. Certain additional tests during life (brain biopsy, but also including less invasive tests) could have betrayed this process.

Early age of onset

AD is more often thought of as a disorder of the aged. Its most important risk factor is aging, with a probability of developing the disorder doubling every 5 years after age 65. The risk increases further with a positive family history. But even in the presenium (before age 65), AD still accounts for as many as 50% of cases of dementia (Knopman *et al.*, 2004). Age of onset in AD is also reduced when a secondary pathology is also present. This is particularly the case for so-called *mixed dementia*, where the accompanying pathology is that of vascular disease (Snowdon *et al.*, 1997). Although CAA can occur in isolation, most cases are found in association with AD (Maia *et al.*, 2007), here also reducing the age of onset.

Contribution from cerebral amyloid angiopathy

CAA results from the deposition of *amyloid* within leptomeningeal and cortical arteries and arterioles. It can frequently also involve capillaries, and occasionally veins. *Amyloid* here refers to non-specific material whose presence can be demonstrated through its ability, after staining with Congo red, to produce apple-green birefringence under polarized light. This property is a result of the protein's deposition to form β-pleated sheets. Although a number of different proteins can undergo such deposition, β-amyloid peptide is the most frequent culprit, and the cause of CAA when associated with AD. The composition of β-amyloid in vessels is not identical to that in the hallmark parenchymal extracellular plaques (which contains a greater proportion of the β-amyloid 1–42 peptides). The processes of β-amyloid deposition in parenchyma in AD and in vessels in CAA thus appear to be independent, the latter probably a result of a failure of clearance (Weller *et al.*, 2009). The topography of β-amyloid deposition in CAA also appears to be different, with a predilection for involvement of occipital structures (Attems *et al.*, 2007). A number of familial forms exist with associated gene mutations, including one involving APP (Levy *et al.*, 1990), which was negative in our patient.

CAA, in the absence of AD, can present in a number of ways. Classically, and best understood, is as spontaneous lobar hemorrhage in the elderly. Thus, the recent Boston criteria for the pre-mortem diagnosis of even *possible* CAA requires the presence of hemorrhage in patients older than 55 years, and in the absence of other possible cause (Knudsen *et al.*, 2001). Rarely, hemorrhage can be subarachnoid in nature (Ohshima *et al.*, 1990) or result in superficial siderosis, especially in association with AD (Feldman *et al.*, 2008). Using such criteria, diagnosis before such a catastrophic event (as in our patient) is not possible. Spontaneous lobar hemorrhage in an otherwise asymptomatic patient placed on anticoagulation for medically unrelated indications is probably frequently the result of an underlying undiagnosed CAA (Hart, 2000).

Less catastrophic *ischemic* strokes in otherwise risk-free individuals have also been attributed to CAA. Strokes tend to be cortical and may be minor, or even completely transient in nature (such as TIAs) (Greenberg *et al.*, 1993). The occasional precipitous worsening and apparent dramatic response to cholinesterase inhibition in our patient could have, at least in part, been the consequence of, and recovery from, such potentially minor events.

Extensive white matter changes have been described in CAA (Caulo *et al.*, 2001), and are very likely to contribute to the clinical manifestation of any associated dementia (Pantoni and Garcia, 1997). These changes can be chronic in nature, or more subacute and potentially pharmacologically (Kinnecom *et al.*, 2007) or even spontaneously reversible (Oh *et al.*, 2004). When acute, the clinical course is often rapidly progressive and is likely the consequence of a rare amyloid-angiopathy related inflammation that may respond to corticosteroids (there was no evidence of acute inflammation in the pathological analysis of our patient). When white matter changes are more chronic, CAA is more likely to be associated with AD, be the consequence of β-amyloid deposition in capillaries (as seen pathologically in our patient – Fig. 11.1), and is more frequently seen in so-called "type-1" CAA (Thal *et al.*, 2008). As with AD, type 1 CAA is also more frequently associated with ApoE ε4 status (Thal *et al.*, 2008). ApoE status in our patient was not known.

Detecting CAA before lobar hemorrhage?

Is it possible to detect the presence of CAA prior to catastrophic events such as a lobar hemorrhage? Is such a question even worth considering – what could be done if a diagnosis of CAA was available pre-morbidly?

The presence of severe white matter changes in the absence of a clear etiology (leukodystrophy, MS, otherwise established vascular disease, ADEM, etc.) with an associated dementia should elicit inclusion of CAA in the differential diagnosis, even before the event of a bleed. Knowledge of such a diagnosis is useful, especially since the occasional precipitous worsening in our patient could have been attributed to strokes, and the absence of stabilization with aspirin led to more aggressive anti-platelet and even anti-thrombotic therapy, which, in the presence of CAA, could be catastrophic. Moreover, some suggest that patients with CAA may be at higher risk of vascular inflammatory complications if treated with β-amyloid immunization (Eng *et al.*, 2004).

Other than brain biopsy, and increased clinical suspicion from evidence such as available in this case, it is possible to elicit a diagnosis of CAA through the detection of microbleeds. These appear as susceptibility artefacts on particular MRI sequences such as gradient-echo and susceptibility weighted imaging (Greenberg *et al.*, 1996, Haacke *et al.*, 2007), which can be routinely available for clinical use. Positron emission tomography (PET) with Pittsburgh Compound B (PiB), currently being investigated as a technique for the detection of parenchymal β-amyloid deposition in AD, is sensitive to accumulation in vessels, and produces a distinct pattern in keeping with the known predominantly posterior vascular involvement (Johnson *et al.*, 2007).

Focal cortical presentation of AD?

AD is not an uncommon cause of focally progressive syndromes leading to dementia. Alladi *et al.* (2007) found that AD accounted for a large proportion of cases of focal syndromes, in particular, PPA (45 to 70%), Posterior Cortical Atrophy (PCA – 100%), and Corticobasal syndrome (CBS – 50%). In PPA, Mesulam himself described AD as an underlying pathology in some cases with the disorder (Mesulam *et al.*, 2008). In their analysis of the progressive aphasias, Gorno-Tempini *et al.* (2004, 2008) have characterized and isolated the clinical characteristics of patients with PPA that eventually progress to AD – the so-called *Logopenic Progressive Aphasia* (LPA). They have also shown that PiB imaging in these patients reveals patterns typical of patients with AD (Rabinovici *et al.*, 2008). Further, on clinical and imaging grounds, LPA patients show considerable overlap with PCA patients (Migliaccio *et al.*, 2009), described elsewhere in this book. By the time our patient sought medical advice, she had already developed additional significant difficulties with visuospatial tasks, in keeping with this diagnosis.

More evidence of AD

Cholinergic deficits and a positive response to AChEIs are present in a number of disorders other than AD, including Lewy body and vascular dementia. Nonetheless, a clear positive response as seen in our patient is often taken as evidence that AD may be the underlying diagnosis.

Acetazolamine challenge SPECT and vascular disease

Cerebral blood flow acetazolamide response reflects preserved vascular autoregulation, the absence of which is usually attributed to vascular disease (Vagal *et al.*, 2009). It can be used to determine the relative contributions of vascular and degenerative disease to the overall cerebral blood flow pattern. In our patient, the pattern of blood flow activation was suggestive of preserved cerebral autoregulation on the left (implying a degenerative etiology to the deficits on that side) and abolished autoregulation on the right (invoking a vascular etiology for the right-sided deficits). The presence of focally reduced autoregulation in the absence of vascular risk factors or evidence of atherosclerosis elsewhere should also raise suspicion that CAA may be present.

Relevance of the persistent fetal circulation

Persistent fetal circulation is a normal variant of the circle of Willis. Dependence of a posterior cerebral artery on the anterior circulation occurs in 16% of normals, but 25% of patients with stroke (Battacharji *et al.*, 1967). It is interesting to speculate whether the presence of such a variant of the left circulation in our patient led to early language deficits, and ultimately the left lobar hemorrhage. Was there chronic hypoperfusion (de la Torre, 2004), particularly in watershed areas (dependent on blood flow from both the middle and posterior cerebral arteries) that led to early neurodegeneration and language involvement?

Take home messages

The exact etiological diagnosis of our patient's illness remained elusive throughout its progression, although in retrospect, there was enough evidence to elicit a diagnosis of AD with CAA. Additional tests, including gradient-echo MRI or SWI, PiB-PET, and lumbar puncture for β-amyloid/tau ratios could have increased our diagnostic confidence dramatically.

This case is interesting because, while complex and atypical, the entire evolution of the illness, and all of the clinical and imaging findings can be explained by the ultimate pathological diagnosis.

Acknowledgments

Special thanks to Drs. Yan Deschaîntres and Sarah Banks for the help with the text, to Dr. France Berthelet for the pathological analysis and slide, and to Jean-Maxime Leroux for the cerebral imaging data.

REFERENCES AND FURTHER READING

Alladi S, Xuereb J, Bak T, *et al.* (2007). Focal cortical presentations of Alzheimer's disease. *Brain*, **130**, 2636–45.

Attems J Quass M, Jellinger KA, Lintner F (2007). Topographical distribution of cerebral amyloid angiopathy and its effect on cognitive decline are influenced by Alzheimer disease pathology. *J Neurol Sci*, **257**, 49–55.

Battacharji SK, Hutchinson EC, Mccall AJ (1967). The Circle of Willis – the incidence of developmental abnormalities in normal and infarcted brains. *Brain*, **90**, 747–58.

Caulo M, Tampieri D, Brassard R, Guiot CM, Melanson D (2001). Cerebral amyloid angiopathy presenting as nonhemorrhagic diffuse encephalopathy: neuropathologic and neuroradiologic manifestations in one case. *Am J Neuroradiol*, **22**, 1072–6.

De La Torre JC (2004). Is Alzheimer's disease a neurodegenerative or a vascular disorder? Data, dogma, and dialectics. *Lancet Neurol*, **3**, 184–90.

Eng JA, Frosch MP, Choi K, Rebeck GW, Greenberg SM (2004). Clinical manifestations of cerebral amyloid angiopathy-related inflammation. *Ann Neurol*, **55**, 250–6.

Feldman HH, Maia LF, Mackenzie IR, Forster BB, Martzke J, Woolfenden A (2008). Superficial siderosis: a potential diagnostic marker of cerebral amyloid angiopathy in Alzheimer disease. *Stroke*, **39**, 2894–7.

Gorno-Tempini ML, Brambati SM, Ginex V, *et al.* (2008). The logopenic/phonological variant of primary progressive aphasia. *Neurology*, **71**, 1227–34.

Gorno-Tempini ML, Dronkers NF, Rankin KP, *et al.* (2004). Cognition and anatomy in three variants of primary progressive aphasia. *Ann Neurol*, **55**, 335–46.

Greenberg SM, Finklestein SP, Schaefer PW (1996). Petechial hemorrhages accompanying lobar hemorrhage: detection by gradient-echo MRI. *Neurology*, **46**, 1751–4.

Greenberg SM, Vonsattel JP, Stakes JW, Gruber M, Finklestein SP (1993). The clinical spectrum of cerebral amyloid angiopathy: presentations without lobar hemorrhage. *Neurology*, **43**, 2073–9.

Haacke EM, Delproposto ZS, Chaturvedi S, *et al.* (2007). Imaging cerebral amyloid angiopathy with susceptibility-weighted imaging. *Am J Neuroradiol*, **28**, 316–17.

Hart RG (2000). What causes intracerebral hemorrhage during warfarin therapy? *Neurology*, **55**, 907–8.

Johnson KA, Gregas M, Becker JA, *et al.* (2007). Imaging of amyloid burden and distribution in cerebral amyloid angiopathy. *Ann Neurol*, **62**, 229–34.

Kinnecom C, Lev MH, Wendell L, *et al.* (2007). Course of cerebral amyloid angiopathy-related inflammation. *Neurology*, **68**, 1411–16.

Knopman DS, Petersen RC, Edland SD, Cha RH, Rocca WA (2004). The incidence of frontotemporal lobar degeneration in Rochester, Minnesota, 1990 through 1994. *Neurology*, **62**, 506–8.

Knudsen KA, Rosand J, Karluk D, Greenberg SM (2001). Clinical diagnosis of cerebral amyloid angiopathy: validation of the Boston criteria. *Neurology*, **56**, 537–9.

Levy E, Carman MD, Fernandez-Madrid IJ, *et al.* (1990). Mutation of the Alzheimer's disease amyloid gene in hereditary cerebral hemorrhage, Dutch type. *Science*, **248**, 1124–6.

Maia LF, Mackenzie IR, Feldman HH (2007). Clinical phenotypes of Cerebral Amyloid Angiopathy. *J Neurol Sci*, **257**, 23–30.

Mesulam M, Wicklund A, Johnson N, *et al*. (2008). Alzheimer and frontotemporal pathology in subsets of primary progressive aphasia. *Ann Neurol*, **63**, 709–19.

Migliaccio R, Agosta F, Rascovsky K, *et al*. (2009). Clinical syndromes associated with posterior atrophy: early age at onset AD spectrum. *Neurology*, **73**, 1571–8.

Neary D, Snowden JS, Gustafson L, *et al*. (1998). Frontotemporal lobar degeneration: a consensus on clinical diagnostic criteria. *Neurology*, **51**, 1546–54.

Oh U, Gupta R, Krakauer JW, *et al*. (2004). Reversible leukoencephalopathy associated with cerebral amyloid angiopathy. *Neurology*, **62**, 494–7.

Ohshima T, Endo T, Nukui H, Ikeda S, Allsop D, Onaya T (1990). Cerebral amyloid angiopathy as a cause of subarachnoid hemorrhage. *Stroke*, **21**, 480–3.

Pantoni L, Garcia JH (1997). Cognitive impairment and cellular/vascular changes in the cerebral white matter. *Ann NY Acad Sci*, **826**, 92–102.

Rabinovici GD, Jagust WJ, Furst AJ, *et al*. (2008). Abeta amyloid and glucose metabolism in three variants of primary progressive aphasia. *Ann Neurol*, **64**, 388–401.

Snowdon DA, Greiner LH, Mortimer JA, Riley KP, Greiner PA, Markesbery WR (1997). Brain infarction and the clinical expression of Alzheimer disease. The Nun Study. *J Am Med Assoc.*, **277**, 813–17.

Thal DR, Griffin WS, De Vos RA, Ghebremedhin E (2008). Cerebral amyloid angiopathy and its relationship to Alzheimer's disease. *Acta Neuropathol*, **115**, 599–609.

Vagal AS, Leach JL, Fernandez-Ulloa M, Zuccarello M (2009). The acetazolamide challenge: techniques and applications in the evaluation of chronic cerebral ischemia. *Am J Neuroradiol*, **30**, 876–84.

Weller RO, Boche D, Nicoll JA (2009). Microvasculature changes and cerebral amyloid angiopathy in Alzheimer's disease and their potential impact on therapy. *Acta Neuropathol*, **118**, 87–102.

Progressive difficulty with naming and object identification

Mariana Blanco and Morris Freedman

Clinical history – main complaint

T.E. presented as a 61-year-old woman with a 5-year history of difficulty finding words and slowly progressive memory decline. Her main symptoms were that she forgot names, needed to make notes, and had problems with written spelling. In addition, she read more slowly than others at her book club and had poor recall of information. In contrast, she was independent in all activities of daily living.

Examination

At initial presentation, mood was good. General neurological exam was unremarkable.

Language examination showed that spontaneous speech was fluent. Prosody, phonology, and syntax were intact. Picture description showed some word-finding difficulties, semantic paraphasias (e.g., knife for scissors) and circumlocutions. Naming was impaired for low frequency items. Repetition and auditory comprehension were intact. Reading was slow with only one error on an irregularly spelled word (colonel). Writing to dictation was good except for irregular words, showing regularization-type errors consistent with surface dysgraphia (debrie for debris). Grammar was intact. World list generation was good for words beginning with the letters F, A, and S but not for words within a semantic category. There was perseveration. Semantic knowledge of words was preserved.

Mini-Mental State Examination (MMSE) was 30/30. On frontal lobe testing, she had difficulty with planning and set shifting, but attention and concentration were not impaired. Memory and visuospatial function were intact.

Special studies

Magnetic Resonance Imaging (MRI) scans are shown in Fig. 12.1. Single photon emission computed tomography (SPECT) revealed mildly reduced cortical perfusion in the left frontal, parietal, and temporal lobes compared to the right.

Case Studies in Dementia: Common and Uncommon Presentations, ed. S. Gauthier and P. Rosa-Neto. Published by Cambridge University Press. © Cambridge University Press 2011.

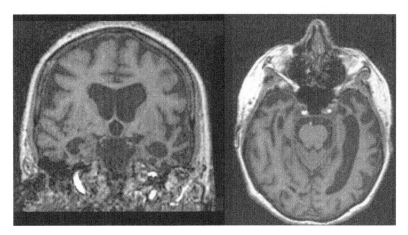

Fig. 12.1. Coronal and axial MRI, five years post-onset, shows bilateral temporal lobe atrophy. The atrophy on the left involves medial and lateral temporal regions, and the temporal pole. The atrophy on the right involves primarily the inferior temporal pole. The temporal horns are enlarged bilaterally, most marked on the left. There is asymmetrical enlargement of the bodies of the lateral ventricles, as well as the third ventricle.

Diagnosis

The initial clinical impression was semantic dementia (SD). However, Alzheimer's disease (AD) could not be ruled out.

Follow-up

She showed progressive deterioration in speech and some aspects of cognition. When asked about her difficulties, she responded: "My difficulty is that I am not able to remember words that I should be able to, that I used to know very well." Semantic paraphasias became more frequent. Comprehension of complex commands, as well as verbal abstract and mathematical reasoning became impoverished. She could not understand the meaning of words that she heard and read. There were frequent neologisms (e.g., koz for calls) and grammar was impaired (e.g., she referred to her daughter as "the girl that we got born"). When she was informed that her "understanding" was going to be tested with a few questions, she said: "See, understanding is even the word that's the pits for me. . ." When she was asked to point to the source of illumination, she said: ". . .the source of illuuumination . . . what's illumination? I don't know. . ." When she was instructed to pretend to hammer a nail on testing for ideomotor apraxia, she said: ". . .hammer a nail, a nail, a nail. See I can't remember what a nail is." She had difficulty recognizing familiar faces and objects.

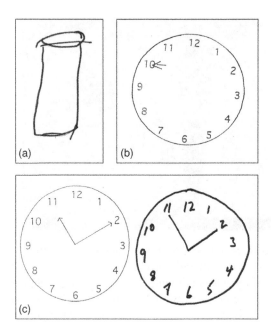

Fig. 12.2.   Clock drawing, 10 years post-onset (MMSE 6/30). (a) Impaired free-drawn clock showing loss of object meaning. (b) Examiner's clock showing a "stimulus pull" toward the number "ten." (c) Clock copy was intact except for proportion of hands. This shows relative preservation of posterior visuospatial function.

For the free-drawn clock, the patient drew a completely different figure from a clock face, suggesting that there was loss of meaning for the word "clock." When asked to set the hands at ten after eleven on the examiner's clock (i.e., a clock with a contour and the numbers but no hands) she drew a short hand pointing to the ten. This indicated a "stimulus pull" toward the number "ten" and suggested frontal system dysfunction. In contrast, copy of a clock was good except for a proportion error on drawing the hands, suggesting that posterior visuospatial function was relatively well preserved (Fig. 12.2).

She subsequently developed behavioral problems affecting her social function. Examples included loss of social graces, playing with feces, refusing daily showers, and aggression. She was admitted to a nursing home 9 years following the initial visit. She eventually developed significant swallowing difficulties and became mute.

Discussion

T.E.'s final clinical diagnosis was Senile dementia (SD). This syndrome comprises one of the three clinical presentations of Primary Progressive Aphasia (PPA). The other two are Progressive Non-Fluent Aphasia (PNFA) and logopenic progressive aphasia. PPA has been recognized under several different labels and concepts over the last century (Mesulam, 2007).

The term SD was coined in 1989 to describe three patients with fluent aphasia, impaired word comprehension and visual comprehension deficits (Snowden *et al.*, 1989). Hodges and Patterson (2007) noted that SD was associated with anterior, bilateral, temporal lobe atrophy that was usually asymmetrical. In 1998, consensus criteria for the diagnosis of SD (see Table 12.1) with this disorder being part of the spectrum of Frontotemporal Lobar Degeneration (FLTD) i.e., frontotemporal dementia (FTD), PNFA, and SD (Neary *et al.*, 1998).

Although little has been published about the epidemiology of SD, the literature suggests that this disorder comprises 18.7% of FTLD cases, and is the least common syndrome produced by FTLD (Johnson et al., 2005). Snowden *et al.* (2007) reported a mean age of onset at 59 years, similar to the mean age of FTD, i.e., the behavioral syndrome of FTLD, but much younger than for patients with PNFA. Hodges *et al.* (2009) reported that the mean age at onset of symptoms was 60.3 (+7.1) years. There was a slight male predominance (60%) and the mean age at diagnosis was 64.2 (+7.1) years, indicating an average lag of 4 years between symptom onset and diagnosis. In this series, the prevalence of family history in a first-degree relative was between 2% and 7%; whereas others have suggested a higher prevalence (22%). Nevertheless, SD is the least familial disorder compared to FTD and PNFA (Rohrer *et al.*, 2009).

SD shows insidious onset and gradual progression that is characterized by impaired understanding of word meaning and/or object identity. Other aspects of cognition, including autobiographical memory for day-to-events and visuospatial abilities are intact or relatively well preserved (Neary *et al.*, 1998). There is controversy about whether a disorder of object identity, i.e., a perceptual disorder, is always present.

As illustrated by the case of T.E., the most prominent early feature of SD is word-finding difficulty. Correspondingly, anomia is one of the main presenting complaints, observed on both spontaneous speech and naming to confrontation. For example, patients may name a "zebra" as "an animal," as specific words may be substituted by a more general term. There is increased use of broad terms as "thing." This word-retrieval failure is caused mainly by poor semantic knowledge about the object or concept to be named. Usually, cueing does not help. At the bedside, a semantic deficit may be suspected when a patient keeps asking for the meaning of words that he or she hears. For example, when asked to point to his or her watch, the patient may say "I don't know what a watch is." In this example, the patient is able to say the word "watch" but has lost its meaning. Speech production is fluent, effortless, and empty. Semantically related words may replace the correct terms leading to what is called semantic paraphasias.

Table 12.1. The clinical diagnostic features of progressive semantic aphasia and associative agnosia (SD)

Clinical profile: Semantic disorder (impaired understanding of word meaning and/or object identity) is the dominant feature initially and throughout the disease course. Other aspects of cognition, including autobiographic memory, are intact or relatively well preserved.

Core diagnostic features	**Supportive diagnostic features**

A. Insidious onset and gradual progression	A. Speech and language
	  1. Press of speech
	  2. Idiosyncratic word usage
	  3. Absence of phonemic paraphasias
	  4. Surface dyslexia and dysgraphia
	  5. Preserved calculation

B. Language disorder characterized by:
  1. Progressive, fluent, empty spontaneous speech
  2. Loss of word meaning, manifest by impaired naming and comprehension
  3. Semantic paraphasias
	B. Behavior
	  1. Loss of sympathy and empathy
	  2. Narrowed preoccupations
	  3. Parsimony
	C. Physical signs
	  1. Absent or late primitive reflexes
	  2. Akinesia, rigidity, and tremor
	D. Investigations:

and/or
C. Perceptual disorder characterized by:
  1. Prosopagnosia: impaired recognition of identity of familiar faces
and/or
  2. Associative agnosia: impaired recognition of object identity
D. Preserved perceptual matching and drawing reproduction
E. Preserved single-word repetition
F. Preserved ability to read aloud and write to dictation orthographically regular words
	1. Neuropsychology:
	    • Profound semantic loss, manifest in failure of word comprehension and naming and/or face and object recognition
	    • Preserved phonology and syntax, and elementary perceptual processing, spatial skills, and day-to-day memorizing
	  2. Electroencephalography (EEG): normal
	  3. Brain imaging (structural and/or functional): predominant anterior temporal abnormality (symmetric or asymmetric)

Source: Copyright © 1998 by AAN Enterprise, Inc. Modified with permission from Lippincott, Williams and Wilkins (Neary *et al.*, 1998).

An important feature of SD is that deterioration of receptive vocabulary is initially more evident for "single word" comprehension rather than comprehension for sentences. The reason is that patients with SD are able to benefit by extracting information from the context of the conversation. This contrasts with Alzheimer's disease in which comprehension tends to be worse with increasing phrase length.

T.E.'s speech–language assessment revealed a key feature of SD, i.e., fairly intact repetition of words or short phrases. Reading aloud and writing to dictation are preserved for orthographically regular words, although not for irregular words. Regularization errors are common, where words are pronounced or written following letter-to-sound rules, referred to as surface dysgraphia (e.g., writing debrie for debris) or surface dyslexia (e.g., reading pint to rhyme with mint).

As in the case of T.E., patients may develop a visual perceptual disorder manifested as prosopagnosia, i.e., inability to recognize familiar faces; and/or associative agnosia, which refers to impaired recognition of objects. However, matching and copy of figures are preserved.

Behavior and personality changes are common, though these should not dominate the early clinical picture. Patients may show a loss of social functioning that results from a combination of emotional withdrawal, depression, apathy, disinhibition, and irritability. Other behavioral features include loss of sympathy and empathy, parsimony, hoarding, narrowed preoccupations, e.g., doing word puzzles all day and constant clock watching (Neary et al., 1998). Changes in eating behaviors are common and patients may develop a sweet tooth (Hodges et al., 2009).

Left and right temporal variants of SD, based on the predominance of atrophy, have distinctive symptom profiles, although they share the main core features of the syndrome. Anomia and impaired comprehension at presentation are more common when there is a left-sided predominance. Patients with right-sided predominance have a higher prevalence of facial recognition problems, social awkwardness, and poor insight (Thompson et al., 2003).

SD is associated with focal atrophy of the anterior temporal lobes bilaterally on MRI. However, left-sided atrophy is more prominent than right. Changes are best seen on coronal MRI cuts and usually correlate well with changes on fluorodeoxyglucose positron emission tomography (PET) imaging and SPECT. Diagnosis of SD should be made with caution when neuroimaging studies are unremarkable.

In SD there may be some involvement of the medial temporal lobes, with atrophy in the amygdala and hippocampus, but this is not as severe as in AD. Therefore, episodic memory is quite good. Other areas of atrophy may include entorhinal cortex, parahippocampal gyrus, fusiform gyrus, and inferior temporal gyrus. Progression may involve disease extension caudally to the posterior temporal lobes and rostrally into the posterior, inferior frontal lobes.

There is no known definitive neuropathology associated with SD. Small series have shown ubiquitin-positive tau-negative pathology as the most frequent finding (Hodges and Patterson, 2007; Snowden et al., 2007). More recently, Hodges and colleagues, in a series of 100 SD patients, reported pathological confirmation in 24 cases: 18 had FTLD with ubiquitin-positive tau-negative inclusions, three had classic tau-positive Pick bodies and three had AD pathology. Of the 18 with ubiquitin-positive inclusions, 13 showed TDP-43 inclusions (Hodges et al., 2009). These findings need to be confirmed in larger samples. The fact that some SD cases showed neuropathology compatible with AD highlights the point that AD can present with a phenotype suggestive of SD and should be considered within the initial differential diagnosis of SD, especially if memory impairment is part of the initial presentation (Snowden et al., 2007). No genetic mutations have been identified, to date, for SD.

The median survival reported for SD is 12.8 years, but there is considerable variability in the speed of progression (Hodges et al., 2009). Moreover, independence in activities of daily living tends to be preserved longer in SD than in AD.

There is no treatment to stop progression or modify the course of SD. Therapy should be targeted toward the provision of support to the patient, family, and care-giver through an interdisciplinary approach, e.g., speech-language pathology, occupational therapy, physiotherapy, social work, and nursing. Early detection of swallowing problems, prevention of falls, adequate education regarding the disease, and assessment of caregiver burden are all important in the care of patients with SD.

Pharmacological management of behavioral problems in SD is similar to that in FTD. Medications such as serotonin reuptake inhibitors, trazodone, and memantine may be considered but further evidence is needed to better support these treatment options. For language symptoms, bromocriptine and galantamine have been tried in small studies of mixed groups of patients with PPA. Results showed a mild slowing of progression of language symptoms but additional evidence is needed to support these findings.

Due to the progressive nature of SD, speech therapy becomes a challenging option. While some speech pathologists focus therapy on rebuilding lost concepts, others try to maintain a structured set of core vocabulary that will produce a better functional outcome. Both of these approaches have shown promising results. A case report by Jokel and colleagues (2006) illustrated that a patient with SD and anomia improved from a personalized program that focused on re-learning names and concepts for objects that were lost. In addition, items that were preserved for naming and understanding were also included in the program. Results indicated that practice delayed the loss of these preserved names and concepts. Thus a trial of speech therapy should be considered for patients with SD.

Take home messages

Core features of SD include fluent, empty speech with loss of word meaning. The latter is manifested by impaired naming and comprehension. Single word repetition is preserved.

SD is a clinical subtype of FTLD with insidious onset and gradual progression. It is one of the three clinical presentations of Primary Progressive Aphasia.

REFERENCES AND FURTHER READING

Hodges JR, Mitchell J, Dawson K, *et al.* (2009). Semantic dementia: demography, familial factors and survival in a consecutive series of 100 cases. *Brain*, **132**, 2734–46.

Hodges JR, Patterson K (2007). Semantic dementia: a unique clinicopathological syndrome. *Lancet Neurol*, **6**, 1004–14.

Johnson JK, Diehl J, Mendez MF, *et al.* (2005). Frontotemporal lobar degeneration: demographic characteristics of 353 patients. *Arch Neurol*, **62**, 925–30.

Jokel R, Rochon E, Leonard C (2006). Treating anomia in semantic dementia: improvement, maintenance, or both? *Neuropsychol Rehabil*, **16**, 241–56.

Mesulam MM (2007). Primary progressive aphasia: a 25-year retrospective. *Alzheimer Dis Assoc Disord*, **21**, S8–S11.

Neary D, Snowden JS, Gustafson L, *et al.* (1998). Frontotemporal lobar degeneration: a consensus on clinical diagnostic criteria. *Neurology*, **51**, 1546–54.

Rohrer JD, Guerreiro R, Vandrovcova J, *et al.* (2009). The heritability and genetics of frontotemporal lobar degeneration. *Neurology*, **73**, 1451–6.

Snowden J, Goulding PJ, Neary D (1989). Semantic Dementia: a form of circumscribed cerebral atrophy. *Behav Neurol*, **2**, 167–82.

Snowden J, Neary D, Mann D (2007). Frontotemporal lobar degeneration: clinical and pathological relationships. *Acta Neuropathol*, **114**, 31–8.

Thompson SA, Patterson K, Hodges JR (2003). Left/right asymmetry of atrophy in semantic dementia: behavioral-cognitive implications. *Neurology*, **61**, 1196–203.

A lady with weakness, fasciculations, and failing memory

Shahul Hameed, Ian R. A. Mackenzie, and Ging-Yuek Robin Hsiung

Clinical history – main complaint

A 73-year-old right-handed woman presented at initial consultation with 6 to 8 months history of progressive weakness in her arms bilaterally.

General history

She described difficulty with manipulating objects with her hand, such as doing up buttons or opening a jar. She was unable to put on her brassiere. She also mentioned difficulty elevating her, making her unable to reach for objects above her head. Sometimes utensils would fall out of her hand when she was cooking. These problems came on insidiously. Initially, she was not paying much attention, thinking that she was just getting older. She had no pain or numbness. Three months prior to presentation, she started to notice slurring of speech, and food started to leak from her mouth. In addition, she started noticing episodic twitching in her muscles and cramping in arms and legs. She also complained of an increased sense of fatigue.

In addition to these motor complaints, she also noticed difficulties with word finding and naming. She was sometimes embarrassed because, when she met up with acquaintances, she could recognize them but was unable to come up with their names. However, she did not pay much attention because she didn't feel that this was out of the ordinary compared with other friends of her age. Functionally she admitted that she was having difficulties with dressing herself. She was still preparing her own cooking and she had been driving herself to go grocery shopping. She denied ever getting lost or having any trouble finding her way around. She was still handling all her own finances and remembered to take her medications.

Her past medical history was notable for osteoarthritis and hypercholesterolemia, but she was not on any prescription medication. She was on a herbal natural medicine for her joint pain, and controlled her cholesterol by dietary restrictions.

Case Studies in Dementia: Common and Uncommon Presentations, ed. S. Gauthier and P. Rosa-Neto. Published by Cambridge University Press. © Cambridge University Press 2011.

She only had an elementary school education, and worked as a sales associate. She lived alone, and at the time of presentation she was independent with all her activities of living. She was twice divorced and had no children.

She was a former smoker but had discontinued smoking more than 20 years previously. She never drank alcohol, and was not aware of any exposure to toxins.

Family history

Her father and mother had died at the age of 82 and 70, respectively, and neither of them had any memory or other neurological concerns at the time of death. Her brother had died at the age of 76, was said to be suffering from diabetes and Alzheimer's disease, but documentation of these diagnoses was not available as he lived in another country.

Examination

On her initial assessment, she was pleasant, co-operative and not in any distress. During conversations, when she could not remember the answers, she tended to use humor and laughter to cover up her deficiency. Her general medical examination was normal.

On cognitive screening tests, she scored 26/30 on the MMSE, and 81/100 on the 3MS. She lost one point with mental reversal, missing a letter when she spelled the word "world" backwards. With delayed recall, she could not remember two out of three words spontaneously, but was able to remember one with categorical cueing and another one with multiple choice cueing. She lost one point with orientation to date. She also lost a point in naming of body parts. With verbal fluency, she only came up with three four-legged animals after 30 seconds, and she also had significant difficulties describing abstraction and similarities, scoring only one out of six points.

On the Montreal Cognitive Assessment, she scored 19/30. She had some trouble understanding the trail making test and she called a rhinoceros a buffalo. She had trouble with the backward digit span, and made two mistakes in serial sevens. With phonemic verbal fluency, she only came up with five words after 1 minute. She lost a point with describing abstract similarities. In the delayed recall task, she scored 2/5 but was able to remember two extra words after categorical and multiple choice cueing.

On cranial nerve examination there was obvious tongue atrophy with fasciculations. The strength of the tongue muscles was decreased bilaterally. All the other cranial nerves were otherwise within normal limits. She was able to whistle and puff up her cheeks fully.

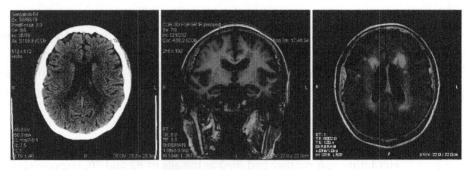

Fig. 13.1.   The CT (left) head demonstrated some mild deep white matter disease, but no other structural abnormalities. The MRI head coronal T1 images (center) demonstrated significant atrophy of the frontal and temporal lobes, as well as hippocampal atrophy much greater than expected for age. The FLAIR MRI images (right) confirmed the presence of white matter disease.

On motor examination, she had clear, albeit mild, atrophy in the interossei and abductor pollicis brevis bilaterally, which was more pronounced on the right than the left. Power testing revealed weakness in her arms bilaterally, more on the right than the left. Her abductor pollicis brevis on the left was 3+/5, whereas on the right was 3/5. The strength of the interossei was 4+/5 on the right and 4−/5 on the left. The strength of biceps and triceps was reasonably good 5/5, but she had clear weakness in shoulder abduction bilaterally 4/5. In the leg muscles, bulk was reasonably good. Her deep tendon reflexes were brisk, 3+ on the right and 2+ on the left. Plantar responses were extensor on the right and equivocal on the left. The power in he leg muscles was fairly good. She walked well on her heels and toes. Fasciculations were visible in her thighs and calves bilaterally. Sensory examination was unremarkable bilaterally. Her gait was reasonably stable and she was able to turn around a corner within two steps without any difficulty. Romberg was negative, and she was able to maintain her stance with the pull-back test.

Special studies

Nerve conduction and EMG studies were obtained and showed evidence of denervation changes consistent of Amyotrophic Lateral Sclerosis. Cervical Spine MRI showed no abnormal signal in the cord. Brain MRI showed: (1) Extensive frontotemporal atrophy, (2) bilateral hippocampal atrophy, and (3) periventricular deep white matter T2 hyperintense changes (Fig. 13.1).

Diagnosis

The diagnostic impression was Frontotemporal dementia with amyotrophic lateral sclerosis (FTD-ALS).

Follow-up

Nine months after her initial review, she showed progressive decline in terms of her weakness leading to a couple of falls, and her cognition also declined considerably. She was hospitalized after her last fall, in which she sustained significant bruising of her right eye and forehead. A repeat MRI brain examination after her recent fall showed a focal intra-axial hemorrhage in the inferior aspect of the right frontal lobe in the gyrus rectus with associated surrounding edema. According to her friend and informant, the patient was a rather stoic and stubborn person, and did not like to be helped by others. Despite the clinical recommendation of not ambulating independently, and having a home care visiting nurse arranged to come to her apartment twice a day, she often tried to do things herself without the nurse's presence. Apparently, she liked to go to bed at around 5–6 pm in the evening, which is when her nurse was scheduled to come and make sure that she has her meals and her medications, but she often had already eaten and got herself ready for bed. Then she tended to wake up at around 4 in the morning, and by the time the nurse came in around 9–10 in the morning, she was already up and had cleaned herself and done all her toileting. Therefore, the nurse had not been able to provide the help that she needed, and could not prevent her falls and eventual head injury.

On the follow-up cognitive examination, she scored 13/30 on MMSE and 47/100 on the MS, which was a significant decline from her previous assessment. Her Frontal Assessment Battery (FAB) score was 5/18. She scored 0 in Similarities, 0 in Lexical fluency, 0 in both Inhibitory Control and in Conflicting Instructions. She scored 2/3 in Luria hand sequence and normal in prehension behavior. Her concentration, orientation, and memory have significantly declined and a formal psychiatric assessment found that she was not competent to make her own decisions. A legal guardian was appointed to manage her medical and financial planning.

She continued to deteriorate and needed PEG tube feeding and home care hospice. She exhibited abnormal behaviors such as inappropriate smiling and laughing during her later follow-up assessments.

An autopsy was performed when she expired 2 years after her initial visit. The neuropathology examination revealed neurons containing Ubiquitin and TDP-43 positive cytoplasmic inclusions, which were numerous within the dentate granule cells (Fig. 13.2 center). Sections of spinal cord showed mild decrease in myelin staining of the corticospinal tracts. (Fig. 13.2 top) There is loss of lower motor neurons in the anterior horn, and some of the remaining cells contain ubiquitin/TDP-43-positive cytoplasmic inclusions (Fig. 13.2, bottom). Sections of mesial temporal lobe also showed tau-positive neurofibrillary tangles and neutrophil threads

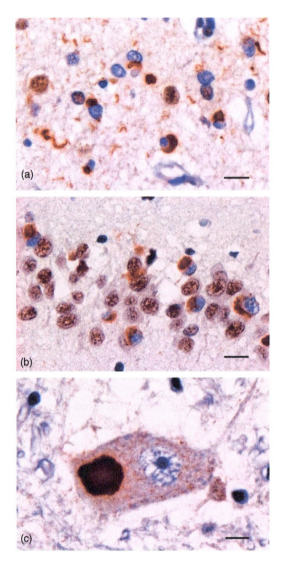

Fig. 13.2. Frontal neocortex micrograph (top) demonstrating TDP-43-immunoreactive neuronal cytoplasmic inclusions and dystrophic neurites. Abundant TDP-43-immunoreactive neuronal cytoplasmic inclusions are found in the hippocampal dentate granule cells (center). TDP-43-immunoreactive compact Lewy body-like cytoplasmic inclusion in a spinal cord lower motor neuron (bottom). [scale bar = 15 microns in Fig. 13.2(a) and (b), and = 5 microns].

restricted to the hippocampus, entorhinal, and transentorhinal cortex. The final neuropathological diagnosis: (1) Amyotrophic lateral sclerosis, (2) frontotemporal lobar degeneration with TDP-43 positive pathology (FTLD-TDP43), and (3) neuro-fibrillary tangles and neutrophil threads, limbic structures (Braak stage 3/6).

Discussion

Amyotrophic Lateral Sclerosis (ALS), the most common adult onset motor neuron disease, is a complex neurodegenerative disease involving both upper motor neuron and lower motor neuron characterized by progressive muscle weakness, muscle wasting, and spasticity. ALS has been traditionally considered to be a disorder affecting only motor systems; however, recent developments show that ALS is a multi-system disorder in which motor system deficits are the most prominent manifestations, but non-motor manifestations can also be observed (Strong, 2008). The El Escorial criteria (revised) form the core of any diagnosis of ALS (Brooks, 1994; Brooks et al., 2000). The sensitivity and specificity of the El Escorial criteria as diagnostic criteria for ALS have been validated in neuropathological studies (Chaudhuri et al., 1995). The prevalence of dementia in ALS ranges from 15% to 40%) (Lomen-Hoerth et al., 2003; Ringholz et al., 2005). The cognitive deficits in ALS ranges from mild frontal lobe dysfunction to full blown Frontotemporal Dementia (FTD) (Lomen-Hoerth, 2004; Strong, 2008). FTD is the second most common cause of dementia in those under the age of 65. It is characterized by the degeneration of frontal and temporal lobes of brain. (Neary et al., 2005) With recent advances in this field, the diagnostic criteria for FTD are also evolving (Neary et al., 1998; Cairns et al., 2007). Recent studies have shown that Transactive Response DNA-binding protein 43 (TDP-43), encoded by the TARDBP gene, has been identified as the major pathological protein of FTLD with ubiquitin-immunoreactive (ub-ir) inclusions (FTLD-U) with or without amyotrophic lateral sclerosis (ALS) as well as sporadic ALS (Neumann et al., 2006; Mackenzie et al., 2007). TDP-43 is a 43 kDa protein abundant in most tissues and well conserved among mammals and invertebrates (Wang et al., 2004; Arai et al., 2006). The identification of TDP-43 as the major protein as the neuropathological hallmark lesions of patients with frontotemporal lobar degeneration with ubiquitinated inclusions (FTLD-U, which has been renamed as FTLD-TDP) and in amyotrophic lateral sclerosis (ALS) emphasizes the importance of TDP-43 in these overlapping neurodegenerative diseases (Neumann et al., 2006; Mackenzie et al., 2009). Furthermore, mutations in the TARDBP gene in familial and sporadic ALS have been reported, which suggests that abnormal TDP-43 alone is sufficient to cause neurodegeneration and underscores the role of TDP-43 in the pathogenesis of these related diseases (Kuhnlein et al., 2008; Rutherford et al., 2008; Daoud et al., 2009). The frequent co-existence of ALS and FTD in the same patient with a common abnormal protein inclusion suggests that these two are a continuum of the same neurodegenerative disorder, and some authors have proposed to re-classify FTLD-U and ALS under a common umbrella term TDP-43 proteinopathies (Forman et al., 2007). Clinically, it is important to ascertain the presence of co-existing FTD in ALS because its presence predicts a shorter survival time and more difficult management (Lomen-Hoerth, 2004; Olney *et al.*, 2005). The presence of cognitive impairments in ALS may also critically impair the individual's ability to make advanced medical directives and financial decisions, and recognizing these problems early may simplify the potential problems encountered in later stages of the disease.

Furthermore, the presence of co-existing tau-postive neurofibrillary tangle pathology in this case, although not extensive, likely have contributed to, and may have also hastened, the patient's cognitive decline and eventual demise. The subtle memory decline would have been overshadowed by the patient's executive dysfunction and behavioral changes, and would have been difficult to identify clinically. This highlights the importance of most mortem examination in these studies as we learn more about the different types of dementias. There is also an urgent need to develop better clinical biomarkers to accurately identify the different forms of proteinopathies in dementias as new disease modifying therapies emerge.

Take home messages

Our case clearly illustrates that cognitive symptoms are frequent but can be very subtle in early ALS. A high index of suspicion is needed to recognize dementia especially when the patient is already disabled by her motor deficits. The diagnosis of cognitive impairment and behavioral symptoms in an ALS patient is not only relevant in the academic research setting, but it also plays an important role when the patient wants to make advanced medical directives about various issues or in palliative planning in diseases like ALS and FTD. The importance of neuropathological examination is clearly demonstrated in our case where the presence of TDP-43 inclusions is the backbone of diagnosing FTD-ALS with TDP43. In addition, the presence of contributing secondary pathology is common in the elderly, especially Alzheimer's disease and cerebrovascular disease in which the underlying prevalence in the population is already high. As in our case there is co-existing Alzheimer's disease evidenced by bilateral hippocampal atrophy in MRI brain and presence of neurofibrllary tangles in hippocampus in neuropathology.

REFERENCES AND FURTHER READING

Ayala YM, Pantano S, D'Ambrogio A, *et al.* (2005). Human, Drosophila, and C.elegans TDP43: nucleic acid binding properties and splicing regulatory function. *J Mol Biol*, **348**, 575–88.

Brooks BR, Miller RG, Swash M, Munsat TL (2000). El Escorial revisited: revised criteria for the diagnosis of amyotrophic lateral sclerosis. *Amyotroph Lateral Scler Other Motor Neuron Disord,* **1,** 293–9.

Chaudhuri KR, Crump S, al-Sarraj S, Anderson V, Cavanagh J, Leigh PN (1995). The validation of El Escorial criteria for the diagnosis of amyotrophic lateral sclerosis: a clinicopathological study. *J Neurol Sci,* **129,** Suppl:11–12.

Forman MS, Trojanowski JQ, Lee VM (2007). TDP-43: a novel neurodegenerative proteinopathy. *Curr Opin Neurobiol,* **17,** 548–55.

Lomen-Hoerth C (2004). Characterization of amyotrophic lateral sclerosis and frontotemporal dementia. *Dement Geriatr Cogn Disord,* **17,** 337–41.

Lund & Manchester groups (1994). Clinical and neuropathological criteria for frontotemporal dementia. The Lund and Manchester Groups. *J Neurol Neurosurg Psychiatry,* **57,** 416–18.

Mackenzie IR (2007). The neuropathology of FTD associated With ALS. *Alzheimer Dis Assoc Disord,* **21,** S44–9.

Mackenzie IR, Neumann M, Bigio EH, *et al.* (2009). Nomenclature for neuropathologic subtypes of frontotemporal lobar degeneration: consensus recommendations. *Acta Neuropathol* **117,** 15–18.

McKhann GM, Albert MS, Grossman M, Miller B, Dickson D, Trojanowski JQ (2001). Clinical and pathological diagnosis of frontotemporal dementia: report of the Work Group on Frontotemporal Dementia and Pick's Disease. *Arch Neurol,* **58,** 1803–9.

Neary D, Snowden J, Mann D (2005). Frontotemporal dementia. *Lancet Neurol,* **4,** 771–80.

Neary D, Snowden JS, Gustafson L, *et al.* (1998). Frontotemporal lobar degeneration: a consensus on clinical diagnostic criteria. *Neurology,* **51,** 1546–54.

Neumann M, Sampathu DM, Kwong LK (2006). Ubiquitinated TDP-43 in frontotemporal lobar degeneration and amyotrophic lateral sclerosis. *Science,* **314,** 130–3.

Olney RK, Murphy J, Forshew D, *et al.* (2005). The effects of executive and behavioral dysfunction on the course of ALS. *Neurology,* **65,** 1774–7.

Ringholz GM, Appel SH, Bradshaw M, Cooke NA, Mosnik DM, Schulz PE (2005). Prevalence and patterns of cognitive impairment in sporadic ALS. *Neurology,* **65,** 586–90.

Strong MJ (2008). The syndromes of frontotemporal dysfunction in amyotrophic lateral sclerosis. *Amyotroph Lateral Scler,* **9,** 323–38.

Wang HY, Wang IF, Bose J, Shen CK (2004). Structural diversity and functional implications of the eukaryotic TDP gene family. *Genomics,* **83,** 130–9.

Progressive difficulty producing speech

Mariana Blanco and Morris Freedman

Clinical history – main complaint

E.B. presented as an 83-year-old man with a 3–4-year history of progressive speech difficulty. His main problem was finding words. For example, he said "I can't speak properly, my SPEAK is hard and I can't get out sentences." Speech was slurred at times and did not always make sense. He also stuttered. In addition, he had difficulty understanding what others were saying. Memory was reportedly good and he was independent in all activities of daily living except for finances. He was still driving without any difficulty.

General history

Past medical history was remarkable for hypertension and ischemic heart disease. Psychiatric history was unremarkable.

Family history

Family history revealed that his father suffered from late onset dementia.

Examination

General neurological exam was remarkable for bilateral cogwheeling in the upper extremities, rigid posture, and bilateral decreased arm swing. There was no asymmetry on motor examination. Snout, bilateral palmomental, and glabellar tap reflexes were positive. Graphesthesia was impaired.

Language examination showed that spontaneous speech was delayed and effortful with reduced fluency characterized by substitutions or misarticulation of words and long pauses. Syntax for verbal expression was impaired and speech was not always clear. Word finding difficulty and phonemic paraphasic

Case Studies in Dementia: Common and Uncommon Presentations, ed. S. Gauthier and P. Rosa-Neto. Published by Cambridge University Press. © Cambridge University Press 2011.

errors (e.g., "twenty tay" for 22 and "phisicate" for certificate) were present. Oral description of the Cookie Theft Picture from the Boston Diagnostic Aphasia Examination paralleled spontaneous speech in its decreased fluency and difficulty with phonology, e.g. "Well, a little child and he's. . . ah. . . I think. . . he might be a boy standing on. . . standing on. . . a STOOB to pick cookies and falling over for taking ah. . . these. . . from the KABNET. And there is a lady looking away from it and she has the dish and while she left the water running to the ground, the floor. . . and another dish. . . and. . . and. . . window with ka, kat, KUTTENS."

Repetition was intact for single one- and two-syllable words but impaired for sentences. Naming to confrontation was severely impaired. Errors included phonemic paraphasias (e.g. "harm" for harp), circumlocutions (e.g. "plant in a hot place, prickly" for cactus), semantic substitutions (e.g. "its what you eat" for pretzel) and phonologically related neologisms (e.g. "eleflator" for escalator).

Auditory comprehension for single words was intact. However, he struggled on sentences with higher grammatical complexity. He answered questions about paragraphs read to him at chance level.

Reading paragraph length material showed stuttering, as well as several sound and syllable additions and substitutions. He had difficulty reading irregular words, which he read with letter-to-sound correspondence. Errors for the most part consisted of regularizations indicating a pattern of surface dyslexia (e.g. "koir" for choir). Reading comprehension was spared for short and simple paragraphs only and overall testing of semantic knowledge showed good performance. On writing to dictation, spelling was mildly impaired for regular words and severely impaired for irregular sound-to-letter correspondence. Errors were consistent with surface dysgraphia. On frontal lobe testing, he had difficulty with planning, concentration, and abstract reasoning. There was perseveration on drawing alternating triangular and square figures. For the free-drawn clock, he was asked to draw a clock, put in the numbers and set the hands at ten after eleven. He showed frontal findings, i.e., he put the number "ten" in the "two" position and then set the hands on the "eleven" and the "ten." On the examiner clock, he was given a clock with a contour and numbers. He was asked to set the hands at "ten past eleven." He put the hands on the "ten" and the "eleven." Copy of a clock was relatively good, suggesting that posterior visuospatial function was preserved (see Fig. 14.1).

Memory was impaired but language problems likely contributed to his poor performance on testing. Attention was also impaired. He showed bilateral ideo-motor limb apraxia. There was no ideomotor apraxia for buccofacial or whole body commands.

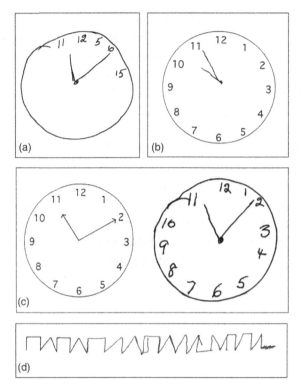

Fig. 14.1. Drawings at initial assessment; (a) Frontal findings on free-drawn clock, i.e., number "ten" in the "two" position and hands set at "eleven" and "ten." (b) Examiner's clock showing a frontal "stimulus pull" toward the number ten. (c) Clock copy was relatively good suggesting preservation of posterior visuospatial function. (d) Perseveration on drawing alternating triangular and square figures (frontal finding).

Special studies

Magnetic Resonance Imaging (MRI) of the brain showed diffuse atrophy. Single-Photon Emission Computed Tomography (SPECT) showed decreased perfusion in the left temporo-parietal region.

Diagnosis

The findings suggested a diagnosis of progressive non-fluent aphasia (PNFA). The possibility of corticobasal syndrome (CBS) was also raised. This was based on the features of parkinsonism and ideomotor apraxia found on the general neurological exam. However, the motor findings did not show the asymmetrical features typical of CBS.

Discussion

In 1982, Mesulam (2007) reported a series of patients presenting with atypical aphasia. Some had fluent speech, whereas others were non-fluent. There were comprehension deficits in some but not all. Mesulam reported these patients under the rubric of "Slowly Progressive Aphasia Without Generalized Dementia," but later proposed a change in terminology to "Primary Progressive Aphasia" (PPA). There are three variants of PPA: PNFA, semantic dementia, and logopenic progressive aphasia. PNFA is the most common of these variants (Knibb *et al.*, 2006).

PNFA is a progressive disorder with expressive language as the dominant feature. Other aspects of cognition are intact or relatively preserved. There is insidious onset and gradual progression. Spontaneous speech is non-fluent and effortful, with at least one of the following: agrammatism, phonemic paraphasias, and anomia (Neary *et al.*, 1998) (see Table 14.1).

E.B.'s speech was non-fluent, hesitant, and effortful. Agrammatism was observed with incorrect word order and misuse of small grammatical words. There were phonemic paraphasias, i.e. sound-based errors that include incorrect phoneme use and transposition of letters. Patients with PNFA tend to repeat parts of words, particularly the first consonant. Difficulty repeating words is also characteristic of this syndrome. Reading is non-fluent and effortful, with frequent paralexias or sound-based errors. Writing is also effortful, with spelling errors and features of agrammatism. Variable degrees of anomia may occur but there is relative sparing of single word comprehension. Sentence comprehension is impaired for the most difficult syntactic constructions such as negative passives (e.g. the girl was not hit by the boy) (Amici *et al.*, 2006).

It is important to note in E.B.'s case the presence of surface dyslexic and dysgraphic errors in reading and writing. Although surface dyslexia and dysgraphia are listed as supportive diagnostic features of SD, this is not the case for PNFA (Neary *et al.*, 1998). Nevertheless, their presence does not rule out PNFA.

Behavioral changes reflecting a decline in social conduct, as in frontotemporal dementia (FTD), may occur late in the disease. This contrasts with the profile in semantic dementia in which behavioral changes, similar in quality to FTD, may occur earlier in the illness (Rosen *et al.*, 2006).

Patients with PNFA may perform poorly on verbal memory tasks due to their language impairment. There should be no evidence of a severe perceptual or visuospatial disorder. With progression, frontal executive dysfunction may appear on testing, as was observed in E.B. General neurological exam may reveal diffuse motor slowing, reduced motor dexterity, mild rigidity, and limb apraxia (Neary *et al.*, 1998; Amici *et al.*, 2006).

Table 14.1. The clinical diagnostic features of progressive non-fluent aphasia

Clinical profile: disorder of expressive language is the dominant feature initially and throughout the disease course. Other aspects of cognition are intact or relatively well preserved.

I. Core diagnostic features (all must be present)
A. Insidious onset and gradual progression
B. Non-fluent spontaneous speech with at least one of the following:
  • Agrammatism
  • Phonemic paraphasias
  • Anomia

II. Supportive diagnostic features
A. Speech and Language
  1. Stuttering or oral apraxia
  2. Impaired repetition
  3. Alexia, agraphia
  4. Early preservation of word meaning
  5. Late mutism

B. Behavior
  1. Early preservation of social skills
  2. Late behavioral changes

C. Physical signs
  1. Late contralateral primitive reflexes
  2. Akinesia
  3. Rigidity
  4. Tremor

D. Investigations:
  1. Neuropsychology: non-fluent aphasia in the absence of severe amnesia of perceptuospatial disorder
  2. Electroencephalography (EEG): normal or minor asymmetric slowing
  3. Brain imaging (structural and/or functional): asymmetric abnormality predominantly affecting dominant (usually left) hemisphere

Source: Copyright © 1998 by AAN Enterprise, Inc. Modified with permission from Lippincott, Williams and Wilkins (Neary *et al.*, 1998).

Regarding demographics, age of onset is between 62 and 65 years of age. The male : female ratio is 1:2 and the duration of isolated speech problems is approximately 4 years. Average time from onset of symptoms to death has been reported as 6.8 years (Ogar and Gorno-Tempini, 2009).

CBS was considered within the differential diagnosis in E.B.'s case. This disorder is associated with progressive cortical (e.g., alien limb phenomena, cortical sensory loss, visual or sensory hemineglect), and asymmetrical extrapyramidal dysfunction (Boeve *et al.*, 2003). Studies have described a spectrum involving PNFA and CBS in the same patient at different stages of the disease (Knibb *et al.*, 2006). PNFA is often the presenting clinical picture of CBS and may thus precede the emergence of extrapyramidal features. In the case example presented above, the clinical suspicion of CBS was based on the neurological exam findings, i.e., rigidity, limb apraxia, and cortical sensory loss (agraphesthesia). However, the motor findings did not show the asymmetrical features that are typical of this disorder. Progressive supranuclear palsy (PSP) is another disorder with parkinsonism that may show initial symptoms consistent with PNFA. As the disease progresses, a vertical supranuclear gaze palsy and prominent postural instability with falls may develop.

Investigations that may help in the assessment of PNFA include MRI, SPECT, and positron emission tomography (PET). Although the results of these studies may be normal, left fronto-temporal atrophy may be seen on MRI. Left frontal hypometabolism on PET has also been documented (Nestor *et al.*, 2003). Although damage occurs more on the left side than the right, bilateral involvement may be seen with progression of disease. The electroencephalogram should be normal or show minor asymmetric slowing (Neary *et al.*, 1998).

A variety of neuropathological changes have been associated with PNFA. The most common are non-Alzheimer tauopathies (e.g. corticobasal degeneration, PSP, Pick-body positive findings) (Knibb *et al.*, 2006). Alzheimer pathology has also being identified in PNFA, with some reports showing these in up to 30% of cases. In these patients, the distribution of AD pathology may be unusual, showing a frontotemporal pattern (Knibb *et al.*, 2006; Ogar and Gorno-Tempini, 2009). Other neuropathological changes that have been associated with PNFA are non-specific cellular changes (DLDH), Creutzfeldt–Jakob disease, Lewy body disease, and FTD with motor neuron disease (Ogar and Gorno-Tempini, 2009).

Few studies have examined efficacy of treatment in PNFA. Speech therapy is aimed at preserving communication skills and improving the level of communication as much as possible, and may offer modest benefit, particularly early in the course of disease. Several reports, usually case studies, have documented several techniques used for treatment in PNFA (Ogar and Gorno-Tempini, 2009).

Antidepressants such as serotonin-reuptake inhibitors, bupropion, and trazodone have been used to treat the behavioral and mood changes that occur in PPA in general (Ogar and Gorno-Tempini, 2009; Vossel and Miller, 2008; Amici *et al.*, 2006), but the evidence for their use is limited. Studies using bromocritpine and galantamine were carried out in a mixed group of patients, without reporting data on the different variants of PPA. For bromocriptine, the results over the course of 7 weeks in PPA patients showed mild slowing of progression in language symptoms (Reed *et al.*, 2004). Galantamine has also been studied in PPA and showed a trend of efficacy (Vossel and Miller, 2008). One limitation outlined in the galantamine trial was that there could have been a possible admixture of patients with AD in the PPA group. This might explain the trend that was observed with this medication. The evidence to support drug treatment in PNFA is limited. Further studies are clearly needed.

Take home messages

PNFA is the most common of the three variants of PPA and is a subtype of FTLD.

The core clinical features of PNFA are insidious onset, gradual progression, and non-fluent spontaneous speech with at least one of the following: agrammatism, phonemic paraphasias, anomia.

PNFA may be associated with CBS.

REFERENCES AND FURTHER READING

Amici S, Gorno-Tempini ML, Ogar JM, Dronkers NF, Miller BL (2006). An overview on Primary Progressive Aphasia and its variants. *Behav Neurol*, **17**, 77–87.

Boeve BF, Lang AE, Litvan I (2003). Corticobasal degeneration and its relationship to progressive supranuclear palsy and frontotemporal dementia. *Ann Neurol*, **54**, Suppl 5, S15–19.

Knibb JA, Xuereb JH, Patterson K, Hodges JR (2006). Clinical and pathological characterization of progressive aphasia. *Ann Neurol*, **59**, 156–65.

Mesulam MM (2007). Primary progressive aphasia: a 25-year retrospective. *Alzheimer Dis Assoc Disord*, **21**, S8–S11.

Neary D, Snowden JS, Gustafson L, *et al.* (1998). Frontotemporal lobar degeneration: a consensus on clinical diagnostic criteria. *Neurology*, **51**, 1546–54.

Nestor PJ, Graham NL, Fryer TD, Williams GB, Patterson K, Hodges JR (2003). Progressive non-fluent aphasia is associated with hypometabolism centred on the left anterior insula. *Brain*, **126**, 2406–18.

Ogar JM, Gorno-Tempini ML (2009). *The Behavioral Neurology of Dementia*, Cambridge, UK, New York: Cambridge University Press.

Reed DA, Johnson NA, Thompson C, Weintraub S, Mesulam MM (2004). A clinical trial of bromocriptine for treatment of primary progressive aphasia. *Ann Neurol*, **56**, 750.

Rosen HJ, Allison SC, Ogar JM, *et al.* (2006). Behavioral features in semantic dementia vs other forms of progressive aphasias. *Neurology*, **67**, 1752–6.

Vossel KA, Miller BL (2008). New approaches to the treatment of frontotemporal lobar degeneration. *Curr Opin Neurol*, **21**, 708–16.

Young man with progressive speech impairment and weakness

Aiman Sanosi, Ian R. A. Mackenzie, and Ging-Yuek Robin Hsiung

Clinical history – main complaint

Mr. J is a 54-year-old right-handed man brought to medical attention by his daughter because of progressive speech difficulty over the last 2 years.

General history

Mr. J actually denied having any problems himself. However, the collateral history obtained from his daughter suggested that his speech fluency has declined and he was much slower to respond to conversations. For example, when he was asked a question, it would take him about 10–20 seconds to actually think of the answer, and when he did respond, his speech revealed a paucity of words with frequent word finding difficulty. The daughter also noticed that there was a change in his speech pattern as he was making more syntax errors with increased hesitancy. There was no obvious problem with reading and writing, although he was never a good writer. There was no history of word or phrase repetition either spontaneously or in response to questions. His comprehension of speech and knowledge of meaning of the words were relatively intact.

One year prior to presentation, his daughter has noticed some changes in his behavior. For example, he seem to be more impulsive with his shopping habits, as he was spending money on items that he did not really need, or on things that were way over his budget. She felt that there was a definite decline in judgment over his financial matters. In addition, the daughter said that he was more disorganized and easily distractible. For example, he was involved in three minor motor vehicle accidents in the past year. The patient explained that, in one instance, he was backing up out of a parking space; but he bumped into another car because he could not see that the car had moved into an adjacent parking space. In another situation, he said that he rear-ended another car because he was

Case Studies in Dementia: Common and Uncommon Presentations, ed. S. Gauthier and P. Rosa-Neto. Published by Cambridge University Press. © Cambridge University Press 2011.

not paying full attention when the other car in front of him stopped suddenly. No significant injury to any parties occurred with these minor vehicle accidents.

The daughter also mentioned increased impulsivity, aggression, and frequent frustration when things were not working out right. He seemed to have limited insight as he was not aware of his symptoms, and was apparently unconcerned about the social and financial consequences of his poor choices. These symptoms were insidious in onset, gradually progressing over time with no fluctuation.

His memory was mostly intact, as he was able to remember conversations as well as day-to-day activities. He has never been lost, and he has no problems recognizing faces. There was no history of hallucination, delusion, emotional liability, or mood changes. His sleep was good without any interruption, snoring, nightmare, or any abnormal movements at bedtime. His appetite was stable, and there was no food fads or unusual cravings. He remained intact with personal hygiene and grooming.

His general health was reasonably good except for some bilateral knee pain, presumably from osteoarthritis. He was on some medications for pain control. Otherwise, there was no history of head injury, and no evidence of any vascular risk factors.

He finished a grade XII education. Afterwards, he had a year of collage and then went to apprentice school as a carpenter. Since he finished his apprenticeship, he was working as a carpenter most of his life.

He had been married, but was separated from his wife about 8 years prior to presentation. Circumstances related to the breakdown of this marriage were not elaborated, although his daughter felt that his indifference to her mother's emotional need was a contributing factor. He had two daughters from his marriage. He had been a heavy drinker when he was younger, but not in the last 10 years. He had never smoked.

Family history

Mr. J's mother had dementia and passed away by the age of 57. A maternal uncle (mother's brother) also had a history of dementia and passed away at the age of 76. Her two remaining sibling are alive and well in their 70s and 80s.

Mr. J was the second born of three siblings. His older sister, 57, was alive and well and had no children. His younger sister, 53, had long-standing history of a mild but stable learning disability, which was felt to be secondary to childhood onset epilepsy.

Examination

He was co-operative during examination and not under stress, but appeared emotionally blunt. He was well dressed and in good hygiene. He did not exhibit any abnormal behavior, stereotypic, or utilization behavior. There was no evidence of echolalia or perseveration. His general physical examination was normal (BP = 130/80, with a regular pulse of 80. On cognitive assessment: He scored 29/30 on MMSE and 93/100 on 3MS. He lost one point with copying pentagon in the MMSE. He lost another point in the 3MS from verbal fluency, coming up with nine animals in 30 seconds, but lost most points with abstraction/similarities as he scored only 1/6. He did quite well with clock drawing test scoring 15/15.

On the Montreal Cognitive Assessment (MoCA), he scored 24/30. He lost points with naming (missing the rhinoceros, and he incorrectly called the camel a giraffe). He scored 3/5 with delayed recall, but was able to recall the other two words with categorical cueing and multiple-choice cueing. He had clear difficulties with phonemic verbal fluency, coming up with only two words beginning with "f" after a minute. He also lost points with sentence repetition. On the Frontal Assessment Battery, he scored 16/18 as he lost a point with verbal fluency again, only coming up with six words beginning with "s" after a minute, and made an error in the Go/No Go finger tapping test.

Cranial nerve examination: showed intact visual acuity and field. Pupils were symmetrical and reactive to light. Fundoscopy exam was normal with no evidence of papilledema. EOM movements were intact. No diplopia, nystagmus. However, there was a slight slowing of saccades. He had intact vertical and horizontal gaze. No facial muscle weakness or asymmetry. Hearing was intact bilaterally. Uvula was central and moving. Tongue showed no atrophy, weakness, or fasciculation. Motor examination: he had no abnormal posture, skin pigmentation, foot drop, or fasciculation. He had full proximal and distal strength 5/5 throughout all four extremities. His tone was normal. The reflexes were +2 symmetrically with no evidence of clonus. Planter responses were flexor. Primitive reflexes were absent. Sensory exam showed intact position, vibration, and pinprick sensation. Co-ordination examination was intact with no evidence of dysdiadokinesia, pass pointing, intention tremor, or positive rebound. His walking gaits as well as tandem walk were intact, and Romberg test was unremarkable.

Special studies

Blood work including blood count, liver function, electrolytes, renal function, Ca, thyroid function, folate, and B12 were in the normal range. MRI showed atrophy of both frontal lobes greater than expected for his age (Fig. 15.1). Temporal lobes were said to be normal in size.

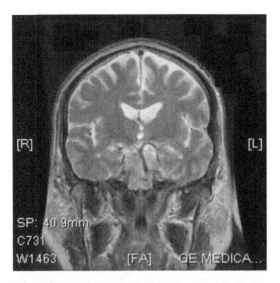

Fig. 15.1. A coronal T2 MRI image of the patient's brain demonstrating left greater than right cortical atrophy and widening of the sulci in the frontal lobes.

Diagnosis

The patient was clinically diagnosed with frontotemporal dementia with non-fluent progressive aphasia as well as behavioral symptoms.

Follow-up

One year later, the patient developed progressive weakness, especially on the left side of the body. He had fallen a few times when he stumbled and tripped on his toes. He also noticed that his left hand was getting weaker and he started to develop difficulty buttoning his clothes with his left hand. He was also unable to carry heavy objects with his left hand and things were slipping out of his fingers. He had also developed increasing difficulty with his speech and slurring of words. He noticed progressive difficulty swallowing solid food as well as occasional choking with water. His movements were also getting slower, and it took him two to three times as long to get dressed and groomed.

Apparently, he also developed symptoms of depression with decreased appetite, weight loss, difficulty falling asleep, decreased initiative to do things, and generally feeling down. He had been started on Bupropion 150 mg (SSRI) as well as Trazodone 100 mg by his family physician, which resulted in some improvement in sleep.

On cognitive assessment, he scored 27/30 on the MMSE and 93/100 on the 3MS. He was able to perform a mental reversal task. With short-term memory, he missed one word but recalled with categorical cueing. He was fully oriented to time and place. He had no problem with naming body parts. His animal verbal fluency was still 10/10. However, he had a lot of difficulties with abstractions, and his descriptions of the similarities were concrete. He lost one point with sentence repetition and another point with reading and obeying. With the second delayed recall, he scored 9/9. With the clock-drawing test, he scored 13/15 as he did not put all numbers on the clock properly. With the Frontal Assessment Battery, he scored 15/18. He had difficulty with phonemic lexical fluency, getting four words starting with the letter "s" after 1 minute, and lost another point with inhibitory control finger tapping. It took him a long time to learn the Luria hand sequence, but after six cycles, he was able to repeat the sequence independently.

On the general neurological examination, there were some clear changes from the first visit. He developed a masked face with decreased facial expression. He was very slow to respond. His words and speech were quite hypophonic and slurred. There was bilateral facial weakness, and weakness with whistling, blowing, as well as tongue protrusion. His jaw jerk was brisk. There was new tongue atrophy and fasciculation. He had nasal speech.

On strength testing, neck flexors and extensors were weak, 4/5. He was still reasonably good on confrontation at 5/5 on the right side, but on the left side, he was clearly weaker 4+/5 and there was also evidence of muscle fasciculation in his arm as well as thigh muscles. There was increased tone with spasticity in four limbs. Reflexes were pathologically increased +3 with no clonus. Plantar responses were extensors bilaterally. Sensory as well as co-ordination examinations were relatively intact.

NCS and EMG

Sensory and motor nerve conduction studies were normal. EMG needle electromyography showed mixed denervation pattern in the right FDI and left biceps with 2+ fasciculation potentials, positive sharp waves, and fibrillations. Motor units were polyphasic with increase sharp waves.

Further information from family history

After records from the patient's mother and maternal uncle were reviewed, his mother apparently had a behavioral variant of FTD, but suddenly declined rapidly when she developed muscle weakness 2 years later. She did not have formal electrodiagnostic testing for her muscle weakness. His uncle had a more protracted course with mixed behavioral and language problems, but no neuromuscular weakness was reported.

Final impression

His clinical diagnosis was changed to FTD-ALS syndrome based on his clinical presentation, EMG as well as the positive family history. The patient was started on Riluzole.

Over the next 3 months, speech pathology assessment suggested that it was unsafe for him to swallow, and a PEG-tube was inserted. Six months later, he died from PEG-tube infection and complications with sepsis.

External examination of the formalin-fixed brain showed no obvious cerebral atrophy or no focal lesions. The base of the brain was unremarkable apart from mild patchy atherosclerosis. Serial coronal sections through the cerebral hemispheres showed a normal ventricular system and deep gray structures. Sections of the brainstem and cerebellum were also unremarkable apart from mild loss of pigmentation of substantia nigra.

On microscopic examination, sections of cerebral neocortex showed mild degree of neuronal loss and reactive gliosis. Bielschowsky silver stain demonstrated moderate numbers of diffuse senile plaques but no neuritic plaques or neurofibrillary tangles. No tau or alpha-synuclein immunoreactivity was found. Moderate numbers of Ubiquitin and TDP-43 immunoreactive neuronal cytoplasmic inclusions and short dystrophic neurites were present in all cortical layers (Fig. 15.2(a)). Some of the inclusions are dense and compact while others have more granular appearance (Fig. 15.2(b)). No intranuclear inclusions were identified. A section of the hippocampus also showed Ubiquitin/TDP-43 positive inclusions in the dentate granule cell (Fig. 15.2(c)). Ubiquitin immunoreactive pathology was also present in the striatum (Fig. 15.2(d)). Sections of upper brainstem were unremarkable. The hypoglossal nucleus showed mild neuronal loss with some reactive gliosis and microglial activation. Section of the spinal cord showed decrease myelination of the cortical spinal tracts and a significant dropout of anterior horn cells. Many of the remaining neurons contain Ubiquitin/TDP-43 positive cytoplasmic inclusions, which had either filamentous or granular morphology. TDP-43 positive glial inclusions were also present. The cerebellum was unremarkable.

Pathological diagnosis

Frontotemporal lobar degeneration with motor neuron disease associated with TDP-43 inclusions (FTLD-TDP).

Discussion

Frontotemporal dementia (FTD) is a neuropathologically and clinically heterogeneous disorder characterized by focal degeneration of the frontal and/or temporal lobes. It is considered to be the third most common cause of cortical dementia, following Alzheimer's disease and Lewy body dementia (Neary *et al.*, 2005). It can be classified into three prototypic neurobehavioral syndromes: the behavioral variant of FTD, progressive non-fluent aphasia, and semantic dementia. Although most of the cases of FTD are sporadic, a positive family

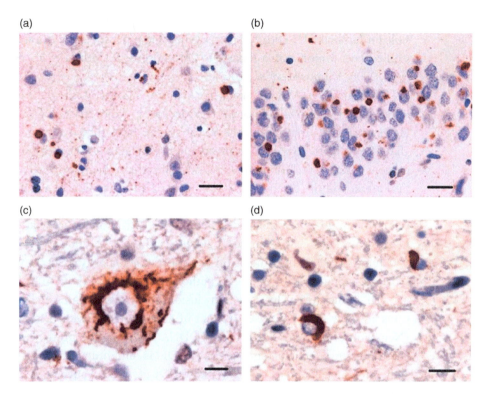

Fig. 15.2. Low magnitude (scale bar = 15 microns) micrographs showing multiple neuronal cytoplasmic inclusions and neurites (stained reddish brown) were observed in the frontal cortex (a), hippocampal dentate granule layer (b). High power magnification (scale bar = 5 microns) micrographs showing a spinal cord motor neuron (c) and glial cytoplasmic inclusions in cerebral white matter (d) containing TDP-43-immunoreactive filamentous cytoplasmic inclusions, stained reddish brown).

history is common in FTD, with up to 43% reporting a first-degree relative affected by a similar disorder (Gass *et al.*, 2006). Since the discovery of genetic forms of FTD, the clinical spectrum of FTD has been broadening (Boeve *et al.*, 2006). In families with FTD associated with tau mutations, in addition to the FTD spectrum of cognitive changes, Parkinsonism is often found in affected members (Behrens *et al.*, 2007; Josephs *et al.*, 2007). In families with progranulin mutations, some affect family members exhibited corticobasal syndrome (to distinguish them from corticobasal degeneration associated with tau-positive pathology), while some family members were clinically diagnosed with Alzheimer's disease prior to autopsy (Bruni *et al.*, 2007; Wider *et al.*, 2008; Kelley *et al.*, 2009). FTD associated with progranulin mutations have characteristic ubiquitin-positive, TDP-43 positive neuronal intranuclear inclusions (Mackenzie *et al.*, 2006). However, patients with progranulin mutations do not usually develop motor neuron diseases (Schymick *et al.*, 2007). The search for the gene responsible for familial FTD with ALS is actively being pursued, and a number of recent studies have demonstrated linkage to chromosome 9 (Morita *et al.*, 2006; Vance *et al.*, 2006; Valdmanis *et al.*, 2007).

Pathologically in ALS, the skein-like inclusion immunopositive for ubiquitin in lower motor neurons has been regarded as a major pathological hallmark. However, recent immunohistochemical studies have shown that neuronal and glial TDP-43 pathology is widespread and present in multiple areas of the central nervous systems, including the nigro-striatal system, the neocortical and allocortical areas, and the cerebellum (Geser *et al.*, 2009; Nishihira *et al.*, 2009). These findings suggest that ALS does not selectively affect only the motor system, but rather is a multi-system neurodegenerative TDP-43 proteinopathy affecting both neurons and glial cells (Arai *et al.*, 2010; Nishihira *et al.*, 2009).

While TDP-43 protein inclusions comprises the majority of all frontotemporal lobar degeneration with ubiquitin pathology (FTLD-U), about 10% of FTLD-U are TDP-43 negative. The protein inclusions in these remaining 10% of FTLD-U cases are now found to be a product of a gene called fused in sarcoma (FUS) (Neumann *et al.*, 2009). FUS is also a DNA/RNA-binding protein with striking structural and functional similarities to TDP-43, and mutations in FUS has been shown to cause familial ALS (Kwiatkowski *et al.*, 2009; Vance *et al.*, 2009). Like TDP-43, FUS is also implicating alterations in RNA processing as a key event in ALS pathogenesis, and further underscores the molecular link between FTLD and ALS (Lagier-Tourenne and Cleveland, 2009).

[*Note:* For comparison, refer to the case of a lady with weakness, fasciculations, and failing memory: the neuropathology in both of these cases is basically identical, but presentation is quite different. This case has an autosomal dominant family history, and presented with behavioral and language problems years before the onset of motor symptoms. By contrast, the other is apparently sporadic, and presented with mostly motor symptoms at first, while the cognitive symptoms came later].

Take home messages

A substantial proportion of FTD subjects may develop ALS, which adversely affect the survival of patients. Therefore, it is important to monitor motor symptoms in patients with FTD. Recent studies emphasized the overlapping role of TDP-43 in the pathogenesis of FTD and ALS, and there are also autosomal dominant forms of FTD-ALS suggesting the presence of another gene responsible for this disease

REFERENCES AND FURTHER READING

Arai T, Hasegawa M, Nonoka T, *et al.* (2010). Phosphorylated and cleaved TDP-43 in ALS, FTLD and other neurodegenerative disorders and in cellular models of TDP-43 proteinopathy. *Neuropathology*, **30**(2), 170–81.

Behrens MI, Mukherjee O, Tu PH, *et al.* (2007). Neuropathologic heterogeneity in HDDD1: a Familial frontotemporal lobar degeneration with ubiquitin-positive inclusions and progranulin mutation. *Alzheimer Dis Assoc Disord*, **21**, 1–7.

Boeve BF, Baker M, Dickson DW, *et al.* (2006). Frontotemporal dementia and parkinsonism associated with the IVS1+1G->A mutation in progranulin: a clinicopathologic study. *Brain*, **129**, 3103–14.

Bruni AC, Momeni P, Bernardi L, *et al.* (2007). Heterogeneity within a large kindred with frontotemporal dementia: a novel progranulin mutation. *Neurology*, **69**, 140–7.

Gass J, Cannon A, Mackenzie IR, *et al.* (2006). Mutations in progranulin are a major cause of ubiquitin-positive frontotemporal lobar degeneration. *Hum Mol Genet*, **15**, 2988–3001.

Geser F, Martinez-Lage M, Kwong LK, Lee VM, Trojanowski JQ (2009). Amyotrophic lateral sclerosis, frontotemporal dementia and beyond: the TDP-43 diseases. *J Neurol*, **256**, 1205–14.

Josephs KA, Ahmed Z, Katsuse O, *et al.* (2007). Neuropathologic features of frontotemporal lobar degeneration with ubiquitin-positive inclusions with progranulin gene (PGRN) mutations. *J Neuropathol Exp Neurol*, **66**, 142–51.

Kelley BJ, Haidar W, Boeve BF, *et al.* (2009). Prominent phenotypic variability associated with mutations in Progranulin. *Neurobiol Aging*, **30**, 739–51.

Kwiatkowski TJ, Jr, Bosco DA, Leclerc AL, *et al.* (2009). Mutations in the FUS/TLS gene on chromosome 16 cause familial amyotrophic lateral sclerosis. *Science*, **323**, 1205–8.

Lagier-Tourenne C, Cleveland DW (2009). Rethinking ALS: the FUS about TDP-43. *Cell*, **136**, 1001–4.

Mackenzie IR, Baker M, Pickering-Brown S, *et al.* (2006). The neuropathology of frontotemporal lobar degeneration caused by mutations in the progranulin gene. *Brain*, **129**, 3081–90.

Morita M, Al-Chalabi A, Andersen PM, *et al.* (2006). A locus on chromosome 9p confers susceptibility to ALS and frontotemporal dementia. *Neurology*, **66**, 839–44.

Neary D, Snowden J, Mann D (2005). Frontotemporal dementia. *Lancet Neurol*, **4**, 771–80.

Neumann M, Rademakers R, Roeber S, Baker M, Kretzschmar HA, Mackenzie IR (2009). A new subtype of frontotemporal lobar degeneration with FUS pathology. *Brain*, **132**, 2922–31.

Nishihira Y, Tan CF, Toyoshima Y, *et al.* (2009). Sporadic amyotrophic lateral sclerosis: widespread multisystem degeneration with TDP-43 pathology in a patient after long-term survival on a respirator. *Neuropathology*, **29**, 689–96.

Schymick JC, Yang Y, Andersen PM, *et al.* (2007). Progranulin mutations and amyotrophic lateral sclerosis or amyotrophic lateral sclerosis-frontotemporal dementia phenotypes. *J Neurol Neurosurg Psychiatry*, **78**, 754–6.

Valdmanis PN, Dupre N, Bouchard JP, *et al.* (2007). Three families with amyotrophic lateral sclerosis and frontotemporal dementia with evidence of linkage to chromosome 9p. *Arch Neurol*, **64**, 240–5.

Vance C, Al-Chalabi A, Ruddy D, *et al.* (2006). Familial amyotrophic lateral sclerosis with frontotemporal dementia is linked to a locus on chromosome 9p13.2–21.3. *Brain*, **129**, 868–76.

Vance C, Rogelj B, Hortobagyi T, *et al.* (2009). Mutations in FUS, an RNA processing protein, cause familial amyotrophic lateral sclerosis type 6. *Science*, **323**, 1208–11.

Wider C, Uitti RJ, Wszolek ZK, *et al.* (2008). Progranulin gene mutation with an unusual clinical and neuropathologic presentation. *Mov Disord*, **23**, 1168–73.

Case 16

Personality disintegration – it runs in the family

Jette Stokholm, Peter Johannsen, Jørgen E. Nielsen, and Anders Gade

Clinical history – main complaint

A 50-year-old man was referred for dementia evaluation a few months after losing his job as head of a department in a large company. According to colleagues his behavior and personality had gradually changed over a couple of years. Formerly responsible, correct, and always on time, he now neglected appointments and deadlines and spent most of a workday playing games on his computer. He had stopped caring about his personal appearance and hygiene; he let his hair and nails grow, stopped shaving, and wore the same jeans and T-shirt for days. During the summer he attended several music festivals, which he had never shown any interest in earlier, and was wearing caps and badges from these events. He had been given several warnings and moved to less demanding tasks, but the problems persisted, and he showed no sign of understanding when these were pointed out to him. When asked to resign from his job, he was offended but unconcerned about the causes and consequences. Although convinced that he was healthy and well functioning, he willingly accepted to participate in dementia evaluation.

His family described marked changes in his social behavior and empathy over perhaps 2 to 3 years. He no longer showed any interest in their well-being and in general was inconsiderate towards other people. He would address strangers and ask inappropriate personal questions and he would comment on people in public, often being quite rude and very loud. Playing golf, he broke the rules and acted as if he was the only player on the course. At dinner, he would pile up loads of food on his plate and eat it in haste. After finishing his meal, he would just leave the table and sit down to watch TV. He spent most of the day in front of the TV following different shows at different channels and had no trouble keeping track of the time and place of these. If anybody asked him to take part in the daily chores or pointed out the inappropriateness of his behavior to him, he became irritated and might stick out his tongue at them, but otherwise just ignored them.

Case Studies in Dementia: Common and Uncommon Presentations, ed. S. Gauthier and P. Rosa-Neto. Published by Cambridge University Press. © Cambridge University Press 2011.

When left alone, he generally seemed to enjoy himself and would often burst into laughter without any obvious reason.

The family also described that the patient withdrew from all social activity and that conversation with him was increasingly difficult. He almost never initiated a conversation and got lost in details and associations when trying to explain things. He would often search for words, but had no trouble understanding what was said, as long as it didn't require verbal abstraction. He no longer understood irony or sarcasm and had lost his sense of humor. Even though he was forgetful in his everyday life, his memory for what had happened recently was perfect and detailed.

He was physically well, but as he ate more, had developed a preference for sweets, and had stopped exercising, he had gained more than 10 kilos in weight over a year.

General history

The patient had 12 years of education and a successful career in business administration. He was divorced at the age of 47 and had three grown-up children from this marriage.

At the age of 44, the patient had suffered a minor concussion due to a fall on his bike. Otherwise there was no history of head trauma or neurological diseases. He took no medication and had no history of former alcohol abuse. He had smoked 8–10 cigarettes a day for several years.

Family history

There were several cases of early onset dementia on the maternal side in the patient's family. His mother, an aunt, his grandfather, and possibly also a great grandfather had all died around the age of 60 after 7–10 years of progressive changes in behavior, personality, and cognitive functions.

Examination

Physical examination was unremarkable with BP 120/70 and heart rate 60. Also the neurological examination was normal apart from marked behavioral abnormality. The patient was constantly grinning, apparently finding the neurological tests very funny. On the MMSE he scored 29/30 points, while on the EXIT25, a screening test for frontal lobe dysfunction, he scored 31/50 points. The average for healthy elderly subjects is 10/50 points (Royall et al., 1992) and for patients with mild dementia (primarily Alzheimer's disease and vascular dementia) 17/50 points (Stokholm et al., 2005).

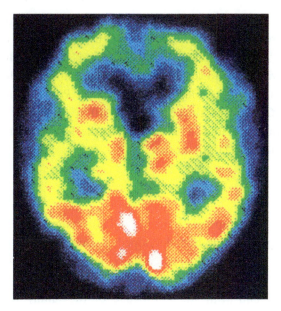

Fig. 16.1. A transaxial slice of the Tc99-HMPAO-SPECT scan showing marked reduction of cerebral blood flow anteriorly in both frontal lobes (at the top of the image).

Special studies

An MRI scan was initially described with white matter lesions in the temporal and parietal lobes, but no focal atrophy. A revised report also described cortical atrophy of the frontal lobes.

An HMPAO-SPECT scan of cerebral blood flow showed marked hypoperfusion of both frontal lobes (Fig. 16.1).

Neuropsychological testing showed intact abilities in most cognitive domains, but impairment on all tests of frontal lobe function. Verbal abstract thinking was the most severely impaired: responses to proverbs and "similarities" were extremely concrete. Also non-verbal problem solving was clearly impaired. In the modified version of Wisconsin Card Sorting Test, the patient showed a marked tendency to perseverate in former categories. In fluency tests (both verbal and non-verbal) production was clearly reduced and there were examples of rule breaking and perseveration. On language tests, his use of words and concepts was vague and careless, but without real aphasic symptoms (Boston naming: 54/60). His scores on memory tests were excellent (Rey´s complex figure: 25/36, Picture recall: 22/30) and his visuoperceptual and spatial abilities were fully preserved.

To evaluate an aspect of social cognition, the patient was tested with a paper version of the emotional hexagon (Sprengelmeyer *et al.*, 1996), a test of recognition of the six basic emotions in facial expressions made more difficult by morphs

(90/10%; 70/30%) of two emotions each. Also on this test he achieved a perfect score. During the neuropsychological examination the patient was constantly humming, tapping his foot, and making repetitive sounds such as "dum, dum, dum." He cooperated willingly and seemed very satisfied with his performances.

Sequencing of the tau-encoding *Microtubule Associated Protein Tau* (*MAPT*) gene revealed a *c.*1907C > T substitution in exon 10, a previously described pathogenic missense mutation in *MAPT* confirming the FTLD diagnosis (Ref: http://www.molgen.ua.ac.be/FTDMutations).

Diagnosis

The diagnosis of the Frontotemporal Dementia (FTD) was given based on the dominant clinical symptoms that had developed gradually over a couple of years: apathy, disinhibition, loss of social conduct, impaired empathy, stereotypic behavior, neglect of self-care, altered eating pattern, and impaired insight. At the time of referral and with the knowledge of the family history, the diagnosis was quickly established, but at this time the patient had already had symptoms for about 2 years and fulfilled the clinical criteria for FTD (McKhann *et al.*, 2001).

The neuropsychological profile with significant impairment on frontal lobe tests in the absence of amnesia, aphasia, and spatial disorders supported this diagnosis, as did the frontal atrophy on the MR scan, the frontal hypoperfusion on the SPECT-CBF scan, and the molecular–genetic analysis.

Follow-up

At the 1-year follow-up, the patient's language had markedly deteriorated, and he was now clinically aphasic, constantly searching for words, getting stuck in sentences, and using the same words and phrases again and again. His attention was poor and he was very easily distracted by environmental stimuli such as people walking by outside. When he noticed a paper on the desk, he started reading aloud from it. He clearly remembered the staff and the different examinations a year earlier, including many of the short neuropsychological tests. He still seemed joyful and completely unaffected by his symptoms. In the emotional hexagon, he now showed a severe deficit in emotional face recognition.

The family described a heavy increase in alcohol consumption. The patient would empty whatever was in the house. At one point when he was out of wine, he had found the spare key to the neighbors' house and let himself in to find a bottle, which he drank while watching their TV. He had accepted to hand in his driver's license, but on a few occasions he "borrowed" other people's cars to go for a short ride.

Two years after the diagnosis the patient moved into a nursing home. At this point he was almost mute. Occasionally, he would repeat what other people were saying (echolalia), but more often he was just grunting and humming. He exhibited a number of stereotypic behaviors such as knocking at tables and the walls, and tapping his feet in certain rhythms. He was extremely apathetic and spent most of the day in front of TV in his room, where he preferred to watch children's programs. Some days he would suddenly leave the nursing home to visit friends or family members. He was still able to find his way around town, and on several occasions he managed to take the train or a bus to visit his children in other towns.

The patient died at the nursing home 5 years after the diagnosis was established, which suggests a survival of 7 to 8 years after the initial symptoms.

Discussion

Frontotemporal Lobar Degeneration (FTLD) is used here as the general label for neurodegenerative diseases involving primarily the anterior regions of the brain. In other literature terms such as Pick´s disease (Kertesz and Munoz, 1998) and frontotemporal dementia (FTD) (Hodges, 2007) are preferred.

The patient presented here is a prototypical example of the behavioral variant of FTLD, exhibiting most of the characteristic features of this clinical subtype. With the characteristic symptoms and a family history of dementia with similar features, the diagnosis in this case was very easy to establish. Unfortunately, only few patients present with so many characteristic and isolated symptoms of frontal lobe dysfunction and even fewer with a well documented family history. Often, patients are referred with fewer and less specific symptoms, and many bvFTLD-patients have been through psychological or psychiatric treatment before the correct diagnosis is established.

Social withdrawal, inactivity, and loss of interest and motivation are often misinterpreted as depression, and self-centered behavior may be regarded as a sign of midlife crises or marital problems. Also, sudden development of alcohol abuse is typically thought to reflect a personal crisis when seen in middle-aged people. The symptoms, which primarily separate patients with bvFTLD in an early phase from patients with psychological or psychiatric problems, are socially inappropriate behavior, loss of empathy, and lack of insight. Relatives report that the patient frequently will say or do things that make them feel embarrassed, while the patient himself seems totally unaware that he is breaking social rules and causing other people distress. Psychiatric patients seldom act directly tactless and are more often oversensitive to other people's reaction. Another major concern often raised by the relatives is that the patient has become "cold hearted."

He/she may seem indifferent to what happens to other people, and even dramatic events may not cause emotional reactions. Such patients may react with irritability or aggression when disrupted in their doings, but they never exhibit anxiety, grief, or deeper concerns. This is very different from most psychiatric patients, who are often tormented by negative emotions.

One of the core symptoms of bvFTLD is the lack of insight into the disease. Lack of insight is also typical for psychotic patients, but not for patients with milder psychiatric disorders. Some patients may feel that their concentration or memory is poor or may report unspecific physical symptoms, most are totally unaware of the behavioral changes and about a third of the patients deny being ill (Pijnenburg et al., 2004). The pervasive lack of insight may be illustrated by the following explanation given by our patient during a clinical conference: "*My mother became ill at about the age of 52, and she died some years later from her dementia disease. My mother's sister also became ill with this same disease at about the age of 50. And my maternal grandfather developed this dementia disease slightly after the age of 50, so I know my risk. Fortunately I have this contact with the Memory Clinic, so if I were to develop the same symptoms, I know whom to contact. Fortunately that has not been the case so far.*"

As in all dementia evaluations, information from an informant can be crucial. For bvFTLD, this is even more the case as subtle behavioral changes and changes in social conduct cannot be revealed by testing and is therefore dependent on reliable information. As seen in the present case, the patient's insight in the situation is most often poor to non-existent stressing this further. In these cases it might be necessary to talk to the relative without the presence of the patient in order to get the full and detailed story, as the spouse may feel embarrassed or fear the patient's reaction.

Another diagnostic challenge concerns the classification of patients in different FTLD-subtypes. Many patients present with a combination of behavioral and language-related symptoms that don't fit any of the three clinical subgroups described by Neary et al. in 1998. This reflects that the underlying pathological distribution in most cases is less selective than the descriptions of the clinical syndromes might suggest. In clinical practice it is therefore often necessary to base the sub-classification on the dominant symptoms. In some of the first descriptions of the behavioral form of FTLD it was suggested that patients should be subclassified into those with disinhibited and those with apathetic behavior (Snowden et al., 1996), but both features often co-exist and are environmentally dependent (Kipps et al., 2007).

Neuropsychological testing can be a great help in the diagnostic process, identifying a profile of frontal lobe dysfunction. In other cases, however, the neuropsychological examination may be normal in spite of profound behavioral disturbances (in patients with predominantly orbital or ventromedial prefrontal pathology), or test results may be generally poor as a result of the patient's difficulties in cooperating. BvFTD-patients often have difficulty concentrating; they constantly get distracted from the tasks and start talking about other things. They work superficially and carelessly, answer questions without deeper reflection, and omit to check their response. It might therefore be more useful to look at the qualitative performance than at the actual test scores when evaluating the neuropsychological profile of patients with possible bvFTD.

Newer research suggests that, instead of measuring cognitive functions when evaluating bvFTD-patients, focus should be on measuring changes in social conduct and emotion processing. Deficits in various aspects of social cognition have been demonstrated in patients with bvFTD (Lough *et al.*, 2006; Gregory *et al.*, 2002; Snowden *et al.*, 2003), but so far only few clinically useful tests exist. In this case we only used one test of social cognition; the emotional hexagon. Deficits in the ability to recognize facial expressions have been described in patients with bvFTD (Lavenu *et al.*, 1999; Keane *et al.*, 2002) with the speculation that this might contribute to the impairments in social behavior. Our patient, however, obtained a perfect score on this test at the first visit, although his behavior was already socially very inappropriate. This, of course, does not rule out the possibility that inefficient use of emotion recognition in guiding behavior, or impaired recognition of social and complex emotions (which we did not test), may contribute to early behavioral changes in bvFTD.

A preserved memory, as demonstrated in the patient presented here, was earlier considered a hallmark for FTD, but several recent reports indicate that episodic memory may be severely disturbed even in the early stages (e.g., Graham *et al.*, 2005). Even so, preserved episodic memory certainly is a strong argument against Alzheimer's disease.

Structural (CT and MRI) and functional (SPECT or PET) neuroimaging can assist in establishing the diagnosis, but in the early phases of the disease normal scans cannot rule out a neurodegenerative disorder. However, atrophy (or hypoperfusion) localized anteriorly in the frontal and temporal lobes supports the diagnosis. For some FTD subtypes, the atrophy can be localized to one side – most often the left anterior temporal region. This is not always mentioned in routine clinical descriptions.

A family history of a similar disease exists in 25%–40% of FTD cases, indicating a strong genetic component, and genetic counseling should be offered and mutation screening considered in families with a clear family history of FTD. Mutations in two genes on chromosome 17, *MAPT* and *GRN*, are associated with autosomal dominant inherited FTD, accounting for approximately 10% of FTD cases each, while mutations in *CHMP2B*, *FUS*, and *TARDBP*, *VCP*, are much rarer causes of FTD.

Take home messages

Cognitive decline is not always the first or dominant sign of a neurodegenerative disease.

The possibility of familial dementia should be considered in all FTD-cases.

REFERENCES AND FURTHER READING

Cairns NJ, Bigio EH, Mackenzie IR, et al. (2007). Neuropathologic diagnostic and nosologic criteria for frontotemporal lobar degeneration: consensus of the Consortium for Frontotemporal Lobar Degeneration. *Acta Neuropathol (Berl)*, **114**(1), 5–22.

Graham A, Davies R, Xuereb R, et al. (2005). Pathologically proven frontotemporal dementia presenting with severe amnesia. *Brain*, **128**, 597–605.

Gregory C, Lough S, Stone V, et al. (2002). Theory of mind in patients with frontal variant frontotemporal dementia and Alzheimer's disease: theoretical and practical implications. *Brain*, **125**, 752–64.

Hodges JR, ed. (2007). *Frontotemporal Dementia Syndromes*. Cambridge, UK: Cambridge University Press.

Keane J, Calder AJ, Hodges JR, Young AW (2002). Face and emotion processing in frontal variant frontotemporal dementia. *Neuropsychologia*, **40**, 655–65.

Kipps CM, Knibb, JA, Hodges JR (2007). Clinical presentations of frontotemporal dementia. In Hodges JR., ed. *Frontotemporal Dementia Syndromes*. Cambridge, UK: Cambridge University Press.

Lavenu I, Pasquier F, Lebert F, Petit H, van der Linden M (1999). Perception of emotion in frontotemporal dementia and Alzheimer disease. *Alzheimer Disease and Associated Disorders*, **13**, 96–101.

Lough S, Kipps CM, Treise C, Watson P, Blair JR, Hodges JR (2006). Social reasoning, emotion and empathy in frontotemporal dementia. *Neuropsychologia*, **44**, 950–8.

McKhann GM, Albert MS, Grossman M, Miller B, Dickson D, Trojanowski JQ (2001). Clinical and pathological diagnosis of frontotemporal dementia: report of the Work Group on Frontotemporal Dementia and Pick's Disease. *Arch Neurol*, **58**, 1803–9.

Pijnenburg YAL, Gillissen F, Jonker C, Scheltens P (2004). Initial complaints in frontotemporal lobar degeneration. *Dementia and Geriatric Cognitive Disorders*, **17**(4), 302–6.

Rosen HJ, Allison SC, Schauer GF, Gorno-Tempini ML, Weiner MW, Miller BL (2005). Neuroanatomical correlates of behavioural disorders in dementia. *Brain*, **128**, 2612–25.

Royall DR, Mahurin RK, Gray KF (1992). Bedside assessment of executive cognitive impairment: the executive interview. *J Am Geriatr Soc*, **40**, 1221–6.

Snowden JS, Neary D, Mann D (1996). *Fronto-Temporal Lobar Degeneration: Fronto-Temporal Dementia, Progressive Aphasia, Semantic Dementia.* New York: Churchill Livingstone.

Snowden JS, Gibbons ZC, Blackshaw A, *et al.* (2003). Social cognition in frontotemporal dementia and Huntington's disease. *Neuropsychologia*, **41**(6), 688–701.

Sprengelmeyer R, Young, AW, Calder AJ, *et al.* (1996). Loss of disgust. Perception of faces and emotions in Huntington's disease. *Brain*, **119**, 1647–65.

Stokholm J, Vogel A, Gade A, Waldemar G (2005). The Executive Interview (EXIT25) as a screening test for executive dysfunction in patients with mild dementia. *J Am Geriatr Soc*, **53**(9), 1577–81.

Woman with complaints about her left arm

Yannick Nadeau, Mario Masellis, and Sandra E. Black

Clinical history main complaint

A 62-year-old right-handed lady consulted her family doctor when she noticed she was unable to use her knitting needle properly with her left hand. This "clumsiness" became progressively worse over several months. Her left arm would "no longer do what she wanted it to do."

In the following year, the lack of control of her left hand had become so profound that she was describing her hand as essentially useless for most tasks. She had to rely exclusively on her right hand to use utensils, to button her jacket, and to fold clothes. She denied any weakness or sensory deficits. There was no history of cognitive decline.

General history

Born in Hungary, she completed high school and 1 year of technical school before working as a medical secretary. She was previously healthy and was not taking any medication. Her past medical history was significant for appendectomy, cholecystectomy, and hysterectomy. She had stopped smoking more than 25 years before. She was drinking one to two glasses of wine daily.

Family history

Her mother died at age 71 of a hemorrhage secondary to an intracranial aneurysm; she previously had several strokes. Her father died at age 70 of emphysema. There was no family history of dementia or movement disorder.

Examination

Vital signs and general examination were normal.

Case Studies in Dementia: Common and Uncommon Presentations, ed. S. Gauthier and P. Rosa-Neto. Published by Cambridge University Press. © Cambridge University Press 2011.

She performed normally on cognitive testing. Cranial nerves were normal, including all extraocular movements. Power and bulk were normal in all muscle groups. Deep tendon reflexes were normal. Plantar responses were flexor. No sensory loss could be demonstrated. There was no abnormality on double simultaneous tactile stimuli, on testing stereognosis, or graphesthesia. There was no rigidity or bradykinesia. There was a mild action tremor of the left hand, without rest tremor. With her eyes closed, the fingers of her left hand showed very subtle pseudoathetotic movements. When she concentrated on a mental task, the fingers of her left hand would extend and abduct. She had moderate to marked apraxia of the left upper extremity. She had marked difficulty with coordinated, rapid, or alternating movements with her left hand. In the left lower extremity, these abnormalities were present but milder. Her only primitive reflex was grasping with the left hand. Gait stride and length was normal. However, there was an overflow dystonic posture of the left upper arm, which was held slightly abducted at the shoulder, and extended at the elbow and wrist with flexion of the fingers. Arm swing was absent on the left side.

Special studies

Her brain MRI showed mild atrophy in keeping with her age and an ECD Single Photon Emission Computerized Tomography (SPECT) scan was normal. Median somatosensory evoked potentials were normal. An EEG revealed bitemporal sharp wave discharges. These were non-specific, but compatible with increased cortical irritability. There was no slowing.

Diagnosis

The provisional diagnosis was Corticobasal Syndrome (CBS) based on the combination of subtle asymmetric extrapyramidal findings and prominent apraxia.

Follow-up

Three years after onset, she was no longer able to dress herself. She felt that her left arm had "a mind of its own," moving against her will. She would often have to hold it with her right hand. Stereognosis remained intact, but she had bilateral decreased graphesthesia. She showed signs of left-sided neglect. Deep tendon reflexes became mildly brisk on the left side. Signs of rigidity and apraxia were becoming evident in her right limbs. She was no longer able to write with her right hand. She had marked bilateral ideomotor apraxia, worse on the left side. She had no problem identifying tools and their use. She could

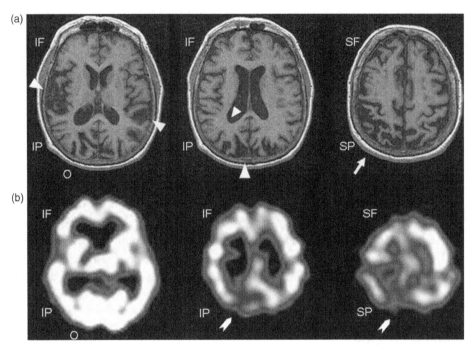

Fig. 17.1.   Repeat investigation done three years after onset. Axial T1-weighted MRI
(a) showed diffuse cortical and subcortical atrophy (triangles), slightly worse in the
posterior part of the right hemisphere (arrow). This region showed decreased
perfusion (arrow heads) on the brain SPECT (b) (IF inferior frontal, IP inferior
parietal, O occipital, SF superior frontal, SP superior parietal).

pantomime and imitate intransitive gestures, but not transitive gestures. She
could not imitate non-representational gestures. Praxis improved with actual
tool use, but it still remained abnormal. She had developed depressive symptoms that responded well to sertraline 100 mg/day. She scored 24/30 on the
Mini-Mental Status Exam (MMSE), losing 3 points for attention, 1 point for
recall and 2 points because she could not write or draw. She had trouble with
calculation and visuospatial skills. Her memory and her language remained
relatively unaffected. A repeat brain MRI done 3 years after onset showed
diffuse, severe parenchymal atrophy, worse in the posterior right hemisphere
(Fig. 17.1(a)). An ECD brain SPECT study showed moderately severe decreased
perfusion within the right parietal lobe, which extended into the right lateral
occipital lobe (Fig. 17.1(b)).

One year later, despite relatively stable cognition, she was dependent for all
activities of daily living. She had no useful function in her upper extremities.
Rigidity had progressed in all four limbs. She developed dysarthria, orofacial
apraxia, and oculomotor apraxia. The right arm demonstrated signs of alien limb,

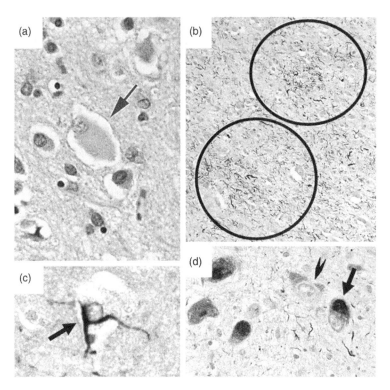

Fig. 17.2.   Autopsy of the patient showing finding consistent with corticobasal degeneration. (a) Balloon neurons (arrow) in the cortex (hematoxylin and eosin). (b) Astrocytic plaques (circles) in the cortex (Gallyas stain). (c) Glial coils (arrow) in the white matter (Gallyas stain). (d) Neurofibrillary tangles (arrow) next to a pigmented neuron (arrow head) in substantia nigra (Gallyas stain).

grabbing her left arm or touching her face against her will. Eventually, she developed severely increased tone in all limbs with generalized hyperreflexia. The last MMSE was done approximately 5 years after onset. She scored 17/25, losing 5 points for attention/calculation, 1 point for orientation, 1 point for recall, 1 point for reading and obeying; she was unable to hold the piece of paper to fold it, write a sentence or draw because of the motor symptoms.

She died at age 69, 7 years after onset. Autopsy confirmed the diagnosis of Corticobasal Degeneration (CBD). Macroscopically, there was diffuse atrophy, which was slightly more pronounced in the right parietal lobe. Besides severe dropout of neurons and gliosis in the neocortex, there were astrocytic plaques (Fig. 17.2(b)), tau positive inclusions reminiscent of Pick bodies, and balloon neurons (Fig. 17.2(a)). In the white matter, glial coils were observed (Fig. 17.2(c)). The changes in the basal ganglia were similar with loss of neurons, astrocytic plaques, and tau positive threads. In the midbrain, there was a moderate to marked dropout of pigmented neurons, without Lewy bodies. There were neurofibrillary tangles in the substantia nigra and a significant number of tau positive threads (Fig. 17.2(d)).

Discussion

CBS is an akinetic-rigid clinical syndrome characterized by lateralized motor and cognitive signs, such as rigidity, dystonia, spontaneous or stimulus-sensitive myoclonus, apraxia, alien limb phenomenon, cortical sensory loss, and aphasia.

This clinical syndrome has been associated with many pathological entities other than CBD, including Progressive Supranuclear Palsy (PSP), Alzheimer's disease, Creutzfeldt–Jakob disease, and many diseases in the spectrum of Fronto-temporal Lobar Degeneration (FTLD): Pick's disease, Frontotemporal Dementia (FTD) with ubiquitin-positive inclusions, FTD due to mutations of MAPT and PGRN (Wadia *et al.*, 2007).

Ante-mortem diagnosis can be difficult because proposed criteria lack sensitivity and specificity. Limb apraxia is considered a hallmark sign of CBS and the symptom most frequently associated with this disorder (Graham *et al.*, 2003). It has been estimated that 70% of CBS cases present with apraxia (Leiguarda *et al.*, 1994). However, this figure may be due to selection bias because apraxia is considered a distinguishing criterion for the diagnosis of CBS.

The useless arm is a very common presentation of CBS. It may be secondary to a combination of rigidity, bradykinesia, dystonia, alien limb phenomenon, and apraxia. In the case presented above, the initial neurological examination revealed only minor abnormalitie besides apraxia.

Ideomotor apraxia is the most frequent type of apraxia (Leiguarda *et al.*, 1994). It is the impairment in the execution of learned skilled movements, characterized by spatial and temporal errors (Petreska *et al.*, 2007). According to the traditional definition, apraxia affects equally both sides of the body despite unilateral pathology (usually in the language dominant hemisphere). However, apraxia in CBS is virtually always asymmetric, predominantly affecting one side, though the other side does eventually manifest the syndrome.

There is no single widely accepted neuropsychological model of ideomotor apraxia that can account for empirical evidence of all the observed modality-specific dissociations. Many models have in common two separate systems interacting in a complex, large-scale network: a conceptual system, which stores knowledge about gestures and tools, and an executive system, which is responsible for execution of movements (Stamenova *et al.*, 2009). Patients with CBS usually can recognize gestures and distinguish correctly performed from incorrectly performed movements. This suggests that CBS impairs production and execution, but not the conceptual knowledge of actions (Jacobs *et al.*, 1999). There is convincing evidence showing that patients with CBS have more difficulties imitating gestures than pantomiming to verbal command. There seems to be no clear difference between performance of meaningful and meaningless actions. However, for transitive meaningful gestures, use of the actual tool improves performance (Stamenova *et al.*, 2009).

Ideational apraxia is less frequent than ideomotor apraxia in CBS, but it has been documented (Kertesz *et al.*, 2000). Discussion of ideational apraxia is complicated by the heterogeneous definition of the phenomenon in the literature. The term is sometimes used for the disturbance in the conceptual organization of actions, and sometimes it is blended with conceptual apraxia, the loss of knowledge of how to use tools. Nevertheless, the typical errors in ideational apraxia are content errors secondary to loss of action concepts, as opposed to accuracy errors seen with ideomotor apraxia.

Limb-kinetic apraxia is impaired execution of simple distal movements. Movements appear coarse and unco-ordinated. It may be difficult to distinguish from Parkinsonism or dystonia. Its nature is debated in the literature. Some consider it an executive apraxia, while others argue it is a pure motor deficit because of its unilateral nature and lack of voluntary–automatic dissociation. Nevertheless, it is frequent in CBS and can lead to significant functional limitation.

As with apraxia, the definition of alien limb phenomenon is debated. It is considered a motor or a sensory-based phenomenon. It is generally described as an involuntary movement that appears to be directed or to conduct a task against the will of the patient. It can be a simple automatic movement like grasping any visible object, or more complex goal-directed actions like counteracting voluntary actions performed by the contralateral hand.

The progression of apraxia and other motor symptoms in CBS is variable. The symptoms usually remain strongly asymmetrical for at least 2 years before spreading to contralateral limbs (Boeve *et al.*, 2003). Buccofacial apraxia usually develops later in the progression of the disease. Eventually, there is generalization and disability becomes severe.

Traditionally, apraxia has been considered as a deficit that is only revealed during unnatural testing situations (like pantomime and imitation) without direct consequence in everyday life. Indeed, apraxic patients can frequently demonstrate preserved use of actual tools despite being unable to pantomime their use (Graham *et al.*, 1999). This apparent dissociation is explained by the fact that environmental cues provided by real context improve the execution of skilled movements. However, there is evidence that impaired pantomime is associated with clumsiness when handling actual objects. Also, a study of patients with left hemisphere stroke has shown a significant relationship between apraxia severity and dependency in physical functioning (Hanna-Pladdy *et al.*, 2003). The limitation of this methodology is that apraxia is rarely an isolated deficit in stroke patients. It is now recognized that apraxia in CBS can have important consequences on everyday life and independence, even before any significant cognitive decline or movement disorder is evident (Stamenova *et al.*, 2009).

Take home messages

A "useless upper limb" is a frequent initial complaint in CBS.

Apraxia can lead to significant functional impairment despite preserved cognition and few other motor signs.

Acknowledgments

This patient was enrolled in the Sunnybrook Dementia study, which is funded by the Canadian Institutes of Health Research. YN receives personal support from the LC Campbell foundation. MM receives salary support from the CIHR and Department of Medicine. SEB is supported by the Department of Medicine, Sunnybrook Research Institute and the Brill Chair in Neurology. We thank Dr. AE Lang for referring this patient and Dr. J Bilbao for the pathological diagnosis and for providing illustrative slides from this case.

REFERENCES AND FURTHER READING

Boeve BF, Lang AE, Litvan I (2003). Corticobasal degeneration and its relationship to progressive supranuclear palsy and frontotemporal dementia. *Ann Neurol*, **54**, S15–19.

Graham NL, Zeman A, Young AW, *et al.* (1999). Dyspraxia in a patient with corticobasal degeneration: the role of visual and tactile inputs to action. *J Neurol Neurosurg Psychiatry*, **67**, 334–44.

Graham NL, Bak TH, Hodges JR (2003). Corticobasal degeneration as a cognitive disorder. *Mov Disord*, **18**, 1224–32.

Hanna-Pladdy B, Heilman KM, Foundas AL (2003). Ecological implications of ideomotor apraxia: evidence from physical activities of daily living. *Neurology* **60**, 487–90.

Jacobs DH, Adair JC, Macauley B, *et al.* (1999). Apraxia in corticobasal degeneration. *Brain Cogn*, **40**, 336–54.

Kertesz A, Martinez-Lage P, Davidson W, *et al.* (2000). The corticobasal degeneration syndrome overlaps progressive aphasia and frontotemporal dementia. *Neurology*, **55**, 1368–75.

Leiguarda R, Lees AJ, Merello M, *et al.* (1994). The nature of apraxia in corticobasal degeneration. *J Neurol Neurosurg Psychiatry*, **57**, 455–9.

Petreska B, Adriani M, Blanke O, *et al.* (2007). Apraxia: a review. *Prog Brain Res*, **164**, 61–83.

Stamenova V, Roy EA, Black SE (2009). A model-based approach to understanding apraxia in corticobasal syndrome. *Neuropsychol Rev*, **19**, 47–63.

Wadia PM, Lang AE (2007). The many faces of corticobasal degeneration. *Parkinsonism Relat Disord*, **13 Suppl 3**:S336–40.

The aged brain: when the pieces don't fit

Bruno Franchi

Clinical history

Mary presented from her home to our Tertiary Hospital in early June of 2003 (age 96) having "stumbled to the ground" being unable to get up. It is unclear how she obtained help; however the Ambulance crew noted she was failing to complete her Activities of Daily Living (ADLs) at home. The house condition was very poor, being dirty with evidence she was not cooking or eating well. She was walking with a frame and receiving assistance from domiciliary care on a monthly basis. She was noted to have significant visual and hearing impairment.

She was admitted to the General Medical Unit and requested residential care placement. A social work review was obtained to get her approved for placement. On signing the paperwork, she was noted to be "lucid and adamant she does not want to live at home." Despite waiting for placement, she tired of waiting and discharged herself in early July. She was discharged with community supports ("GP Homelink"). No cognitive testing was undertaken during this admission.

She presented 8 weeks after discharge after a piece of paper she left on her heater caught fire. She let herself out of the house. Her neighbor called the Fire Department and the Ambulance service brought her to our tertiary hospital for assessment of smoke inhalation. Carboxyhemoglobin was 2% (<0.8%). No injury was sustained. She felt well and wanted to return home with her brother the next day. Her brother refused to take her home as he did not feel she was safe. She was admitted to the Geriatric Unit from Emergency for further assessment.

After admission to the Unit she continued to want to go home, despite the fact her home had too much smoke damage to habit. The community service did not accept her back into its program at her home as even with supports she was deemed "unable to cope."

Case Studies in Dementia: Common and Uncommon Presentations, ed. S. Gauthier and P. Rosa-Neto. Published by Cambridge University Press. © Cambridge University Press 2011.

General history

The Royal Adelaide Hospital's initial contact with Mary was in 1999, where at the age of 92 she was living independently at home with no services. She was mobilizing with a stick. She presented having tripped over a small table in her hallway whilst going to bed. She was able to drag herself to her phone and call her family for help. At that time, she had a documented past history of hypertension and anemia (for which she previously refused investigation). Investigation in the Emergency Department revealed an intertrochanteric fracture of her left hip. This was fixed with a left Austofix hip nail the next day. This admission was complicated by hematemesis and iron-deficient anemia was documented. She refused endoscopic investigation. Folate and B12 deficiency were diagnosed and treated.

She was described on discharge in 1999 as "a lovely 92-year-old woman." Nurses noted she was "co-operative and keen," mixing well with staff and clients.

She was transferred to a rehabilitation hospital and MMSE was 27/30, having lost 2 points in recall and one in construction. At that time her supportive brother initially voiced concern at her inability to look after herself in the home environment.

Self-reporting of her ability to perform ADLs was discrepant from descriptions by nursing staff. She could not provide a clear history of why she presented to hospital and felt she had returned home before moving to the rehabilitation facility. Occupational Therapy review in 1999 of ADLs revealed she was able to shower herself independently, and independent with dressing. Meal preparation was limited by physical, rather than cognitive, process deficits.

Further history from her brother revealed that, over the last 6 years he had been encouraging her to seek placement in residential care, which she initially accepted but each time refused at the last minute. He admitted to supporting her with shopping and banking issues. After discussion, she decided that moving into a residential facility would work, thus she was discharged into a low care facility 1 month later.

She represented to the Emergency Department 4 months later with chest pain, still living in the low care residential facility, stating that she was only there for respite and would return home soon. She had a 5-day admission having had a subendocardial myocardial infarct diagnosed.

Family history

There was no significant family history.

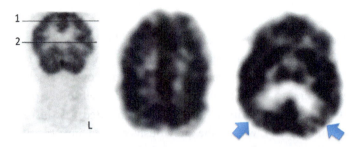

Fig. 18.1.   Reduction in FDG uptake in the posterior-inferior parietal lobes bilaterally (arrows) as well as mildly reduced relative FDG uptake in both medial temporal lobes (left worse than right). No abnormal FDG uptake is noted elsewhere, including in the rest of the cerebral cortex, including the frontal lobes, subcortical nuclear structures, and the cerebellum.

Examination

There were no remarkable findings in 2003 beyond significant frailty, blindness, and deafness on physical examination. MMSE was 17/23 – she recalled 3/3 objects, lost 4 points in calculation (subtraction task), and 2 points in orientation. Her blindness and deafness made assessments of the language functions difficult. Frontal Assessment Battery score was 14/18 with 1 point lost in similarities, 1 in lexical fluency, 1 in conflicting instructions and 1 in Go-No Go instructions.

Blood tests, including those routinely performed in a dementia screen, were unremarkable.

Functionally, on the ward she was able to shower with minimal assistance, only requiring encouragement to use soap. She was mobilizing with her frame and one stand-by assistant. She agreed to low level care placement.

Special studies

CT of her head confirmed general parenchymal volume loss with patchy decreased attenuation periventricularly. No significant areas of ischemia or space-occupying lesions were noted. PET scan was highly suggestive of a neurodegenerative process of Alzheimer's type. No scan evidence of frontal lobe dementia (Fig. 18.1).

Diagnosis

The clinical diagnosis prior to the PET scan being performed was frontotemporal dementia. The final clinical diagnosis after the PET scan and on discharge was that of Alzheimer's type dementia. She was not started on acetylcholine esterase therapy. She was discharged to a low level residential facility.

Follow-up

The next contact was in 2004 (Age 98) where her General Practitioner referred her to the Geriatric Unit (from home) for ongoing management. She had discharged herself from the hostel 9 weeks after her discharge from hospital in 2003. The G.P. documented she was not coping at home and was unhappy at being sent in. The District nurses were dressing a traumatic leg wound, having recently fallen. This was now complicated by cellulitis. She had lost weight and had poor hygiene. She was accepting Meals on Wheels (5 days a week), help from Domiciliary Care (7 days a week) and the District Nurses (7 days a week for medications and wound dressings). She was noted to perhaps have the occasional hallucination.

All of the support services had voiced concerns and were keen to move to the Guardianship Board to see her moved to residential care against her will. She commonly refused placement.

Her Domiciliary Care case worker described several issues; malnutrition with significant weight loss over 12 months and poor food safety, for example, cooking a chicken, placing it in the cupboard and eating it the next day. She was often forgetting to eat. There were times where there was no food in the house. She would frequently leave her doors unlocked. There were times her taps were found to be left on, flooding the floors on occasion. She had left food on the stove cooking and had left her oven on. She was not washing her clothes and refused to let others take her clothes for washing. She denied the clothes she was wearing were dirty, despite being fecally stained.

She was found on two occasions by staff half naked sitting on her heater. There were times the care workers could not get into the house, as sometimes the doors were all locked and she could not hear them knocking. They usually got in through the back door that was often left open. She had no cutlery or plates in the home as she threw them out when she finished using them. Her floors often had discarded food remnants on them.

She was re-admitted to the Geriatric Unit. "No meaningful history" was obtained from the patient. She refused to answer most questions, but was oriented to place.

Functionally, she tolerated food and fluids well, was continent, and most nursing assistance was related to setting up. Physiotherapists noted she was a high falls risk and suggested supervision with all ambulation. She continued to want to return home.

Abbreviated Mental Testing score was 9/10, failing the recall task. Mini-mental testing was 16/21 with 2 points lost in orientation, 3 points in calculation (spelling task) and none in recall. Frontal Assessment Battery score was 10/18 having difficulties with similarities (1 lost), Lexical fluency (1 lost), Motor series (2 points), Conflicting instructions (2 lost) and Go-No Go (2 lost). An MRI was obtained, revealing mild volume loss in the parietal and posterior temporal lobes.

A PET scan was repeated, and no significant difference was noted when compared to the previous films. She was discharged to a nursing home with the instruction that the Guardianship Board should be approached should she try to leave. Her medication list on discharge was aspirin, ramipril, frusemide, atenolol, FGF, and thyroxine. The final clinical diagnosis was frontotemporal dementia.

She presented to the Emergency Department from the Nursing Home in July of 2007 after slipping out of a chair. No cognitive assessment was undertaken and she was returned to the Nursing Home from the ED. The Ambulance service stated she was "difficult to assess due to patient's dementia." Interestingly, the medication list at this time revealed the addition of risperidone and pericyazine, the indication for which was unclear.

She died in the nursing home on the 15/5/2008. There was no post-mortem.

Discussion

This case is particularly interesting in that it does not on face value fit into one category of neurodegenerative disorders. In these cases, it is always worthwhile considering a diagnosis of vascular dementia, as one can rationalize each of the focal difficulties clinically as a "microinfarct." When considering her past history, it is evident she had hypertension and a myocardial infarction that would highlight the high likelihood that on pathological testing at post-mortem, there would have been a significant vascular burden. In all patients, especially those who present with cognitive dysfunction, vascular risk factors need to be addressed as a matter of priority.

One does try to place patients that present in an atypical manner into a particular pattern, especially since the potential benefits of acetylcholine esterase therapy are considered if a diagnosis of Alzheimer's dementia (and potentially the Dementia of Lewy Bodies) is made. Consideration should have been undertaken, given the findings on the PET scan, but when all was weighed up it was felt it was unlikely she would benefit.

It seems the clinical diagnosis of Alzheimer's dementia was not correct, given the preservation of her memory and orientation throughout her admissions. The failure to recall two of the three objects on MMSE in 1999 would be best rationalized as a short-term organic brain syndrome, delirium, as there was no other time where her formal memory tasks demonstrated significant compromise.

When her final admission to the Emergency Department is considered, she was seen to be "too demented" to give a rational history. This may have reflected a delirium at that time, or a deterioration in her cognition. The use of two antipsychotic agents suggests there was a degree of psychosis to her illness; however, there is a chance they were inappropriately prescribed to manage her wanting to leave.

One can be clear, however, that there was evidence of frontal lobe dysfunction throughout her admissions. She failed to recognize her risk in her lack of ability to safely care for herself demonstrating a lack of insight and judgment. The progressive prompting evident to a greater extent through all of her admissions with her preservation of memory suggests sequencing or initiation issues. There was no suggestion of behavioral disinhibition. Given there was progressive dysfunction, one would suggest an underlying neurodegenerative syndrome, although an increasing vascular burden could be postulated.

One can not over-emphasize the importance of her visual and hearing impairment. False beliefs related to misinterpretation of the environment due to significant visual impairment is known as Charles–Bonnet syndrome. Addressing the causes and ensuring staff manage poor vision and deafness with care and respect makes a significant difference to the affected individuals quality of life.

This case highlights the difficulties that can be faced in older patients that present with domains of dysfunction that do not fit traditional patterns. Her brother recognized the changes in Mary as far back as 1993, but during the admission in 1999 no significant deficits were noted. Her persistent wish to return home was respected, despite the fact she had set fire to her home and was failing with short-term high intensity community support afterward. Balancing impaired patients' wishes and risk for self-harm can be very difficult and often relies on the treating team's intrinsic beliefs.

Take home messages

Not all cases of dementia fit into classical diagnostic paradigms.

Balancing patient wishes and their safety is difficult, and the manner in which it is addressed is often dependent on the treating team's beliefs.

The potential benefit of cholinesterase inhibitors in late onset and advanced stages of AD must be carefully weighed against risks related to overall frailty.

FURTHER READING

Cramer C, Haan MN, Galea S, Langa KM, Kalbfleisch JD (2008). Use of statins and incidence of dementia and cognitive impairment without dementia in a cohort study. *Neurology*, **71**, 344–50.

Cukierman-Yaffe T, Gerstein HC, Williamson JD, *et al.* for the Action to Control Cardiovascular Risk in Diabetes-Memory in Diabetes (ACCORD-MIND) investigators (2009). Relationship between baseline glycemic control and cognitive function in individuals with type 2 diabetes and other cardiovascular risk factors. *Diabetes Care*, **32**, 221–6.

Debette S, Beiser A, Decarli C, *et al.* (2010). Association of MRI Markers of Vascular Brain Injury With Incident Stroke, Mild Cognitive Impairment, Dementia, and Mortality. The Framingham Offspring Study. Stroke, Feb 18. [Epub ahead of print]

Gorelick PB, Bowler JV (2010). Advances in vascular cognitive impairment. *Stroke*, **41**(2), e93–e98.

Kazui H, Ishii R, Yoshida T, *et al.* (2009). Neuroimaging studies in patients with Charles Bonnet Syndrome. *Psychogeriatrics*, **9**(2), 77–84.

Mendez MF, Shapira JS, McMurtray A, Licht E (2007). Preliminary findings: behavioral worsening on donepezil in patients with frontotemporal dementia. *Am J Geriatr Psychiatry*, **15**(1), 84–7.

Peters R, Beckett N, Forette F, *et al.* (2008). Incident dementia and blood pressure lowering in the HYpertension in the Very Elderly Trial COGnitive function assessment (HYVET-COG): a double-blind, placebo controlled trial. *Lancet Neurol*, **7**, 683–9.

Case 19

Hypersexuality in a 69-year-old man

Oscar L. Lopez and James T. Becker

Clinical history – main complaint

A 69-year-old man who developed a Kluver–Bucy syndrome (KBS) (i.e., hypersexuality, bulimia, hyperorality, placidity), pseudobulbar affect, depression, and psychosis after multiple cerebral ischemic lesions. At age 68, he experienced a left side hemiparesis of acute onset secondary to a pontine ischemic lesion. He was left with a mild left side weakness, instability with tendency to fall, and mild pseudobulbar affect; he had a tendency to cry in the absence of depression or external factors.

One year later, he developed headaches, dizziness (described as disequilibrium), and increased left side weakness. He became apathetic, socially withdrawn, docile, and had episodes of rage and verbal and physical violence. He tended to eat voraciously, stuffing food in his mouth. He compulsively put his fingers in his mouth and bit his cane, and he spent hours masturbating, regardless of the presence of family members. He also developed urinary incontinence. Nevertheless, he was able to read the newspaper and followed programs on TV. He gradually developed symptoms of major depression.

General history

High school graduate with history of hypertension and coronary artery disease. He lives with his wife.

Family history

Father died at age 70 and mother at age 78 of heart disease. No history of dementia was reported in his family.

Case Studies in Dementia: Common and Uncommon Presentations, ed. S. Gauthier and P. Rosa-Neto. Published by Cambridge University Press. © Cambridge University Press 2011.

Examination

Detailed neurological and cognitive evaluations were conducted beginning at age 71 (Lopez *et al.*, 1995). In his initial evaluation, he was oriented to person and place, and partially oriented to time. He had flat affect and a lack of emotional response to any type of stimuli. He had frequent outbursts of laughter, and overreacted and expressed fear to propioceptive stimuli (e.g., he cried and groaned when his blood was drawn, or when the sensory examination was performed). He was unable to interpret proverbs; his responses were inappropriate and concrete. He developed depressed mood, and met criteria for major depression.

There was minimal right facial weakness. He had lead-pipe rigidity in the right arm, and action-intention tremors in upper limbs. His strength was normal on the right, but there was moderate weakness (3/5) on the left. The deep tendon reflexes were normal on the right and hyperactive on the left. The plantar response was down going on the right, and neutral on the left. The cerebellar testing was significant for a mild dysmetria in the finger-to-nose maneuver. Stereognosis was abnormal and graphesthesia was preserved. He had difficulty naming the objects he touched. He had an unstable gait, and used a cane to ambulate.

The Mini-Mental State examination (MMSE) (Folstein *et al.*, 1975) score was 23, the Mattis Dementia Rating Scale (MDRS) (Mattis, 1976) score was 119, the Hachinski Ischemic Scale (Hachinski *et al.*, 1975) score was 13, the Hamilton Depression Scale (HDRS) (Hamilton, 1960) score was 16, and the Blessed Dementia Rating Scale (BDRS) for activities of daily living (Blessed *et al.*, 1968) was 10.

Special studies

Blood tests (cell blood count, metabolic panels, thyroid profile, and vitamin B12 levels) were essentially normal. His apolipoprotein genotype was 2/4. The MRI of the brain obtained at age 68 showed a pontine infarct. The MRI done at age 70 showed ischemic lesions in the right internal capsule, putamen, globus pallidus, and body of the caudate nucleus. In addition, he had smaller infarcts in the left putamen and globus pallidus (Lopez *et al.*, 1995). He had mild confluent deep white matter lesions, especially in parietal–occipital regions.

He had extensive neuropychological evaluations involving test of memory, language, visuospatial and visuoconstructional, and attention and executive functions (Lopez *et al.*, 1995). He had moderate to severe executive-attentional deficits. He performed abnormally on tests that required sustained attention, response to inhibition, or set shifting (e.g., Stroop test, Trail-making). Tests that examined the ability to organize and interpret visual information were also impaired. He failed in the Similarities test of the Weschler Adult Intelligence Test. His verbal and non-verbal memory were mildly impaired, as well as his autobiographical memory.

His speech was fluent with normal prosody, but he had errors in productive language, especially on tasks that required lexical–semantic processing. He performed abnormally on mental calculation tasks, and the Smell Identification Test was abnormal (Lopez *et al.*, 1995).

His copy of a complex geometric figure as well as his copy of two-dimensional figures showed a tendency to oversimplification. He was mildly impaired on the Visual Benton's Form Discrimination test. The Clock Drawing test was abnormal.

Diagnosis

The initial diagnostic impression was that this patient developed a complex and severe neuropsychiatric symptomatology associated with a dementia syndrome secondary to vascular disease, although the presence of a neurodegenerative disease could not be ruled out.

Follow-up

He was treated with carbamazepine for his KBS symptoms, which gradually subsided. He had no focal motor symptoms and did not experience new strokes. Although his symptoms of major depression improved at follow-up, there was an increase in the severity of the pseudobulbar affect, with significant episodes of inappropriate laughter. In addition, he developed persecutory delusions associated with irritability and agitation. He was treated with fluoxetine for the pseudobulbar and depressive symptoms, and risperidone and clonazepam for his delusions and episodes of agitation. He died 5 years after the onset of his behavioral symptoms, and 1 year after his last clinical evaluation. No autopsy was performed.

His cognitive symptoms remained stable or had minimal improvement over time. Figure 19.1 shows the MMSE and MDRS from baseline to his 36-month evaluation. His symptoms of depression improved, and his activities of daily living remained stable. Figure 19.2 shows the HDRS and BDRS for activities of daily living during the follow-up period.

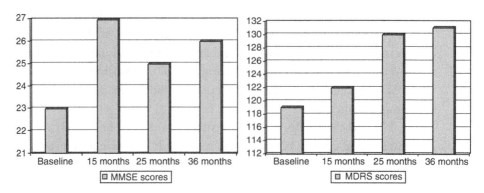

Fig. 19.1. Changes from baseline to 36 month follow-up in MMSE and MDSS scores.

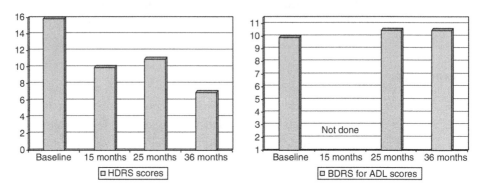

Fig. 19.2. Changes from baseline to 36 mo followup in the HDRS and BBRS for ADL.

Discussion

This patient presented with a significant neuropsychiatric symptomatology after several episodes of strokes. However, the severity of the vascular disease detected by MRI did not explain these symptoms, which initially led to the assumption that a cortical neurodegenerative disorder was also present. However, the course of his dementia was consistent with a vascular process, since his cognitive deficits improved or remained stable even after 3 years' follow-up. This is not what we expect from a progressive neurodegenerative disorder (e.g., Alzheimer's disease [AD] or frontotemporal dementia). The most interesting aspect of this patient was that he had persistent behavioral symptomatology in the context of a stable or improving cognitive syndrome.

The classification of vascular dementia can be divided into multiple etiological subtypes: (1) large vessel lesions, usually involving large infarcts affecting cortical, subcortical, or both regions, (2) strategically localized infracts, (3) small vessel disease, where patients have multiple small subcortical lesions, (4) hemorrhagic lesions, and (5) hyporefusion type, usually associated with ischemia in the watershed areas (Lopez *et al.*, 2004). The etiology of this patient's vascular dementia is clearly related to small vessel disease, and the vascular syndromes associated to this vascular mechanism are: lacunar state, Binswanger's disease, and thalamic dementia (Jellinger, 2002; Mahler and Cummings, 1991; Roman, 1985). Lacunar states and Binswanger's disease are sometimes difficult to distinguish, since both may be secondary to hypertensive or arteriosclerotic microangiopathy of lenticulostratiate and penetrating arterioles, and can cause similar neurological and psychiatric symptoms (Mahler and Cummings, 1991). Our patient had the typical symptoms associated with Binswanger's disease including, an initial stepwise deterioration, pseudobulbar affect, urinary incontinency, and gait disturbance. However, he did not exhibit extensive white matter lesions usually seen in this condition. Thus, we concluded that he suffered from a lacunar state, and not from Binswanger's disease.

Studies that attempted to establish a behavioral pattern among the different types of vascular dementia found that patients with small vessel vascular dementia had more apathy, aberrant motor behavior, and hallucinations than those with large vessel vascular dementia. By contrast, those with large vessel vascular dementia had more agitation and euphoria (Staekenborg *et al.*, 2009).

Although the ischemic lesions detected in this patient were localized in subcortical regions, he expressed multiple behavioral syndromes of cortical and cortical–subcortical etiology during the course of the disease (Cummings, 1993). It is important to note that cortical gray matter function is not always spared in patients with subcortical ischemic lesions. SPECT studies of patients with subcortical ischemic vascular dementia (SIVD) revealed decreased perfusion in cortical gray matter areas (Mielke *et al.*, 1992), and microinfarct-like lesions can be present in the gray matter of demented subjects (White *et al.*, 2002). Similarly, studies conducted with continuous arterial spin-labeled MRI showed that subjects with SIVD and AD had decreased blood flow in frontal and parietal regions, and there was an association between white matter lesions and frontal lobe blood flow only in the SIVD group (Schuff *et al.*, 2009). In addition, changes can be present in subcortical gray matter in patients with SIVD, both with and without ischemic lesions. It has been shown that the volume of the caudate nuclei are smaller in SIVD than in cognitively normal subjects with or without history of strokes (Looi *et al.*, 2009), which suggests a more widespread vascular damage than that revealed by diagnostic neuroimaging studies.

Multiple studies have shown increased prevalence of psychiatric symptoms after strokes (Angelelli *et al.*, 2004), and psychiatric symptoms are common in dementia (Lyketsos *et al.*, 2002; Steffens *et al.*, 2005), especially in AD (Lopez *et al.*, 2003) and vascular dementia (Ballard *et al.*, 2000). Studies from referral clinics have shown that mood-related symptoms are more frequent in vascular dementia than in AD (Lopez *et al.*, 2003; Staekenborg *et al.*, 2009) although some studies have not detected such difference (Thompson *et al.*, 2009). Binetti and colleagues (Binetti *et al.*, 1993) found that 45% of the patients with AD and 38% of the patients with vascular dementia had delusions, and the content (paranoid vs. misidentification) was similar in both syndromes. Importantly, in vascular dementia patients, delusions occurred mainly during the first year, and in those with higher MMSE scores.

Because psychotic symptoms are common in cortical neurodegenerative disorders (e.g. AD) (Lopez *et al.*, 2001, 2003), it might be expected that lesions to the cortical temporal-parietal lobes would be associated with psychosis in patients with vascular dementia (Levine and Finkelstein, 1982). Similarly, pathological laughing and crying is less frequent in AD than in vascular dementia (Lopez *et al.*, 2003; Robinson *et al.*, 1993; Starkstein *et al.*, 1995), and consequently, one expects more of these symptoms in vascular dementia. However, there are studies that have shown psychotic symptoms emerging from damage to subcortical structures (e.g., putamen (Kitabayashi *et al.*, 2006), brainstem dopaminergic nuclei (Nishio *et al.*, 2007)), and pathological laughing and crying can develop from lesions in either cortical or subcortical regions (Robinson *et al.*, 1993). Thus, psychotic symptoms and pseudobulbar affect can occur in both degenerative and vascular states, although the former appears to be more common in AD, and the latter in vascular dementia.

Fully developed or partial KBS have been described in multiple pathologies that affect the CNS, including head trauma (Lilly *et al.*, 1983), herpes encephalitis (Shoji *et al.*, 1979), Huntington's disease (Janati, 1985), adreno-leukodystrophy (Powers *et al.*, 1980), porphyria (Guidotti *et al.*, 1979), post-irradiation encephalopathy (Benito-Leon and Dominguez, 1998), and Whipple's disease (Leesch *et al.*, 2009). However, in this report, we discuss KBS in the context of the neurodegenerative disorders and vascular disease that occur in the elderly. The KBS was the most disturbing behavior manifested by this patient; hypersexuality, hyperorality, and placidity. He showed signs of hypermetamorphosis (an impulse to explore and touch), although he never exhibited visual agnosia, which is considered a component of the KBS in animal models and humans (Kluver and Bucy, 1937; Terzian and Ore, 1955). Although KBS has been reported in neurodegenerative disorders (e.g., frontotemporal dementia (Lilly *et al.*, 1983), AD (Kile *et al.*, 2009)), we believe that, in this patient, the KBS is due to repeated ischemic lesions to the amygdaloid nuclei and their connections (Carroll *et al.*, 2001; Chou *et al.*, 2008; Hayman *et al.*, 1998), which can disrupt frontal–temporal and temporal–hypothalamic connections; another recent case report showed that KBS was associated with bilateral thalamic infarcts (Muller *et al.*, 1999). The implication of disconnection and the role of visual agnosia in KBS have been extensively discussed in a previous publication (Lopez *et al.*, 1995). It is important to note that the use of anticonvulsants and antipsychotics successfully controlled this syndrome.

Take home messages

The evolution of the behavioral syndrome can be independent of the cognitive syndrome in patients with vascular dementia.

"Cortical" cognitive and behavioral syndromes can be present in patients with subcortical ischemic vascular dementia.

REFERENCES AND FURTHER READING

Angelelli P, Paolucci S, Bivona U, *et al.* (2004). Development of neuropsychiatric symptoms in poststroke patients: a cross-sectional study. *Acta Psychiatr Scand*, **110**(1), 55–63.

Ballard C, Neill D, O'Brien J, McKeith IG, Ince P, Perry R (2000). Anxiety, depression and psychosis in vascular dementia: prevalence and associations. *J Affect Disord*, **59**(2), 97–106.

Benito-Leon J, Dominguez J (1998). Kluver–Bucy syndrome in late delayed postirradiation encephalopathy. *J Neurol*, **245**(6–7), 325–6.

Binetti G, Bianchetti A, Padovani A, Lenzi G, De Leo D, Trabucchi M (1993). Delusions in Alzheimer's disease and multi-infarct dementia. *Acta Neurol Scand*, **88**(1), 5–9.

Blessed G, Tomlinson BE, Roth M (1968). The association between quantitative measures of dementia and senile changes in the cerebral white matter of elderly subjects. *Br J Psychiat*, **114**, 797–811.

Carroll BT, Goforth HW, Raimonde LA (2001). Partial Kluver–Bucy syndrome: two cases. *CNS Spectr*, **6**(4), 329–32.

Chou CL, Lin YJ, Sheu YL, Lin CJ, Hseuh IH (2008). Persistent Kluver–Bucy syndrome after bilateral temporal lobe infarction. *Acta Neurol Taiwan*, **17**(3), 199–202.

Cummings JL (1993). Frontal-subcortical circuits and human behavior. *Arch Neurol*, **50**, 873–80.

Folstein MF, Folstein SE, McHugh PR (1975). Mini-mental state: a practical method grading the cognitive state of patients for the clinician. *Psychiat Research*, **12**, 189–98.

Guidotti TL, Charness ME, Lamon JM (1979). Acute intermittent porphyria and the Kluver–Bucy syndrome. *Johns Hopkins Med J*, **145**(6), 233–5.

Hachinski VC, Iliff LD, Zihka E, *et al.* (1975). Cerebral blood flow in dementia. *Arch Neurol*, **32**, 632–7.

Hamilton M (1960). A rating scale for depression. *J Neurol, Neurosurg, Psychiatry*, **23**, 56–62.

Hayman LA, Rexer JL, Pavol MA, Strite D, Meyers CA (1998). Kluver–Bucy syndrome after bilateral selective damage of amygdala and its cortical connections. *J Neuropsychiatry Clin Neurosci*, **10**(3), 354–8.

Janati A (1985). Kluver–Bucy syndrome in Huntington's chorea. *J Nerv Ment Dis*, **173**(10), 632–5.

Jellinger KA (2002). The pathology of ischemic–vascular dementia: an update. *J Neurol Sci*, **203–204**, 153–7.

Kile SJ, Ellis WG, Olichney JM, Farias S, DeCarli C (2009). Alzheimer abnormalities of the amygdala with Kluver–Bucy syndrome symptoms: an amygdaloid variant of Alzheimer disease. *Arch Neurol*, **66**(1), 125–9.

Kitabayashi Y, Narumoto J, Otakara C, Hyungin C, Fukui K, Yamada K (2006). Schizophrenia-like psychosis following right putaminal infarction. *J Neuropsychiatry Clin Neurosci*, **18**(4), 561–2.

Kluver H, Bucy PC (1937). "Psychic blindness" and other symptoms following bilateral temporal lobectomy in rhesus monkeys. *Am J Physiol*, **119**, 352–3.

Leesch W, Fischer I, Staudinger R, Miller DC, Sathe S (2009). Primary cerebral Whipple disease presenting as Kluver–Bucy syndrome. *Arch Neurol*, **66**(1), 130–1.

Levine DN, Finklestein S (1982). Delayed psychosis after right temporoparietal stroke or trauma: relation to epilepsy. *Neurology*, **32**(3), 267–73.

Lilly R, Cummings JL, Benson DF, Frankel M (1983). The human Kluver–Bucy syndrome. *Neurology*, **33**(9), 1141–5.

Looi JC, Tatham V, Kumar R, *et al.* (2009). Caudate nucleus volumes in stroke and vascular dementia. *Psychiatry Res*, **174**(1), 67–75.

Lopez OL, Becker JT, Klunk W, Dekosky S (1995). The nature of behavioral disorders in human Kluver–Bucy syndrome. *Neuropsychiat Neuropsychol Behav Neurol*, **8**(3), 215–21.

Lopez OL, Smith G, Becker JT, Meltzer CC, DeKosky ST (2001). The psychotic phenomenon in probable Alzheimer's disease: a positron emission tomographic study. *J Neuropsychiatry Clin Neurosci*, **13**, 50–5.

Lopez OL, Becker JT, Sweet RA, *et al.* (2003). Psychiatric symptoms vary with the severity of dementia in probable Alzheimer's disease. *J Neuropsychiatry Clin Neurosci*, **15**(3), 346–53.

Lopez OL, Kuller LH, Becker JT (2004). Diagnosis, risk factors, and treatment of vascular dementia. *Curr Neurol Neurosci Rep*, **4**(5), 358–67.

Lyketsos CG, Lopez O, Jones B, Fitzpatrick AL, Breitner J, DeKosky S (2002). Prevalence of neuropsychiatric symptoms in dementia and mild cognitive impairment: results from the cardiovascular health study. *J Am Med Assoc*, **288**(12), 1475–83.

Mahler ME, Cummings JL (1991). Behavioral neurology of multi-infarct dementia, *Alzheimer Dis Assoc Disord*, **5**(2), 122–30.

Mattis S (1976). Mental status examination for organic mental syndrome in the elderly patient. In Bellak L, Karuso TB, eds. *Geriatric Psychiatry*. New York: Grune & Stratton.

Mielke R, Herholz K, Grond M, Kessler J, Heiss W-D (1992). Severity of vascular dementia is related to volume of metabolically impaired tissue. *Arch Neurol*, **49**, 909–13.

Muller A, Baumgartner RW, Rohrenbach C, Regard M (1999). Persistent Kluver-Bucy syndrome after bilateral thalamic infarction. *Neuropsychiatry Neuropsychol Behav Neurol*, **12**(2), 136–9.

Nishio Y, Ishii K, Kazui H, Hosokai Y, Mori E (2007). Frontal-lobe syndrome and psychosis after damage to the brainstem dopaminergic nuclei. *J Neurol Sci*, **260**(1–2), 271–4.

Powers JM, Schaumburg HH, Gaffney CL (1980). Kluver–Bucy syndrome caused by adreno-leukodystrophy. *Neurology*, **30**(11), 1231–2.

Robinson RG, Parikh RM, Lipsey JR, Starkstein SE, Price TR (1993). Pathological laughing and crying following stroke: validation of a measurement scale and a double-blind treatment study. *Am J Psychiatry*, **150**(2), 286–93.

Roman GC (1985). The identity of lacunar dementia and Binswanger disease. *Med Hypotheses*, **16**(4), 389–91.

Schuff N, Matsumoto S, Kmiecik J, *et al.* (2009). Cerebral blood flow in ischemic vascular dementia and Alzheimer's disease, measured by arterial spin-labeling magnetic resonance imaging. *Alzheimer's Dement*, **5**(6), 454–62.

Shoji H, Teramoto H, Satowa S, Satowa H, Narita Y (1979). Partial Kluver–Bucy Syndrome following probably herpes simplex encephalitis. *J Neurol*, **221**(3), 163–7.

Staekenborg SS, Su T, van Straaten EC, *et al.* (2009). Behavioural and psychological symptoms in vascular dementia; differences between small and large vessel disease. *J Neurol Neurosurg Psychiatry*, **81**(5), 547–51.

Starkstein SE, Robinson RG, Berthier ML, Price TR (1988). Depressive disorders following posterior circulation as compared with middle cerebral artery infarcts. *Brain*, **111**, 375–87.

Starkstein SE, Migliorelli R, Teson A, *et al.* (1995). Prevalence and clinical correlates of pathological affective display in Alzheimer's disease. *J Neurol, Neurosurg, Psychiatry*, **59**(1), 55–60.

Steffens DC, Maytan M, Helms MJ, Plassman BL (2005). Prevalence and clinical correlates of neuropsychiatric symptoms in dementia. *Am J Alzheimer's Dis Other Demen*, **20**(6), 367–73.

Terzian H, Ore GD (1955). Syndrome of Kluver and Bucy; reproduced in man by bilateral removal of the temporal lobes. *Neurology*, **5**(6), 373–80.

Thompson C, Brodaty H, Trollor J, Sachdev P (2009). Behavioral and psychological symptoms associated with dementia subtype and severity. *Int Psychogeriatr*, 1–6.

White L, Petrovich H, Hardman J, *et al.* (2002). Cerebrovascular pathology and dementia in autopsied Honolulu-Asia Aging Study participants. *Ann NY Acad Sci*, **977**, 9–23.

Case 20

Man with fluctuating confusion

Uwe Ehrt, Robert Perry, and Dag Aarsland

Clinical history – main complaint

Mr. K was a 75-year-old retired sailor in very good overall physical condition. At the first assessment, Mr. K reported a gradual cognitive decline, subjectively described as memory impairment, during the last 2 years. His spouse confirmed cognitive impairment, and noted some functional impairment, with considerable fluctuations in his cognitive performance. The spouse also reported that Mr. K had developed apathy; he was no longer interested in news or taking part in chores at home, and some irritability.

General history

He had a pacemaker due to atrial fibrillation, and was treated with warfarin and also with atorvastatin because of hyperlipidemia. He had recently been referred to cardiologic examination because of hypotension. There was no history of psychiatric or other neurological disorders, and psychotropic drugs had not been used.

Family history

One brother and one sister had suffered from dementia, and another sister suffered from tremor, but none of these family members had been formally diagnosed.

Examination

Cognitive testing confirmed memory impairment and also revealed visuospatial impairment. Mini-Mental State Examination (MMSE) score was 22 (orientation 8/10, subtracting sevens 1/5, short-term memory 2/3; he was unable to draw pentagons). He failed completely on the ten-point clock drawing test (score = 0),

Case Studies in Dementia: Common and Uncommon Presentations, ed. S. Gauthier and P. Rosa-Neto. Published by Cambridge University Press. © Cambridge University Press 2011.

the Dementia Rating Scale (DRS) was 104 out of 142 (memory 33/37; Initiation and perseveration 12/37; Construction 6/6; Conceptualization 38/39; Memory 15/25). Additionally, he suffered from mild expressive aphasia, with a Boston Naming Test score of 36/60. The total Neuropsychiatric Inventory (NPI) score was 8, and the NPI-Q score was 3 (anxiety, apathy, aberrant motor behavior). NPI-Q is a questionnaire based on the 12 NPI items (each scored 0–3) completed by an informant, was 31. He was referred to the movement disorders clinic because of tremor and dizziness.

Special studies

Blood tests did not show any abnormalities. Standard computer tomography of the brain revealed normal features. MRI was contraindicated due to pacemaker.

Initial diagnosis

The neurologist diagnosed intermittent mild right-sided parkinsonism in upper body, with tremor and bradykinesia, but no rigor. Walking was near normal, but he was unsteady on turning and had a pathological pull-test. In addition, cognitive impairment was noted. No specific treatment was started and the patient was referred for psychiatric examination.

Follow-up

Six months later, the patient's improvement continued. He was able to walk outside his home by himself (with some overall slowness), but was more active, socially engaged, and interested in his surroundings. He was remaining in good physical condition, and exercised every day. His testing performance was stable or even improved: MMSE 24/30, Boston Naming Test 43. Clock-Drawing-Test 7/10.

After 12 months, the patient's condition remained relatively stable, although with some increase in the tremor. His MMSE score was 25 of 28 (unable to draw or write due to tremor), and verbal memory testing had declined. However, he remained physically active, with a near normal walking ability.

18 months after treatment commenced, mild worsening of memory and tremor was noted, MMSE score was reduced to 19, and NPI-Q had increased to 6 (anxiety, irritability, aberrant motor activity). Anxiety was noted to be related to distress when he was left alone. He was seen again by his movement disorders specialist, who noted that both tremor and bradykinesia was markedly improved.

At 2 years' evaluation, a marked cognitive and motor worsening was noted. Motor symptoms such as worsening gait, stooped posture, and falls had developed. Cognitive fluctuations had developed. MMSE score was 18, clock drawing 0, and NPI-Q had increased to 13 (delusion, agitation, depression, anxiety, apathy, irritability, aberrant motor activity, daytime sleepiness). There had been one episode of visual hallucinations, and one episode with facial agnosia where he did not recognize his spouse. Verbal agitation and depression were noted, as well as increased daytime sleepiness. A trial with L-DOPA was prematurely withdrawn due to gastrointestinal side effects. Apraxia had developed, and he was now in need of daytime care.

The situation remained relatively stable during the next year, with no major changes in the treatment regime. At assessment 3 years after the first evaluation, activities of daily living had deteriorated further, episodes of confusion were common. There were occasional visual hallucinations, where he would see people, but these episodes were not very distressing for the patient. Episodes with loss of consciousness emerged. His MMSE score had declined to 16.

After 4 years he was admitted to a nursing home. He had frequent and vivid hallucinations (seeing see people and animals), and also occasionally had auditory hallucinations – not voices but sounds including doors being shut. His hallucinations were sometimes distressing and frightening. There were episodes with fainting, which occurred weekly. His affective and cognitive states fluctuated for no obvious reason. At assessment, the Unified Parkinson's Disease Rating Scale (UPDRS) motor subscale total score was 36, with marked tremor and bradykinesia. L-DOPA treatment was initiated by the neurologist, but had to be stopped again because of side effects (confusion), but later restarted and continued at a small dose of 100 mg/d. Antipsychotic treatment with quetiapine 12.5 mg was recommended. However, he died less than 5 years after initial examination.

At autopsy, he was diagnosed as having Lewy body disease with cortical and subcortical Lewy bodies, and with moderate levels of neurofibrillary tangles in the medial temporal lobe and hippocampus (Braak stage III) and mild amyloid plaques (CERAD score 1/5; not amounting to Alzheimer's disease). It is also of interest that there was moderate demyelination in the white matter (assessed semiquantitatively as grade 2 out of 4).

Discussion

This case presented with asymmetric parkinsonism, and cognitive impairment was noted at the time of diagnosis. Thus, the most important differential diagnoses were possible: dementia associated with Lewy Bodies (DLB) or Dementia associated with Parkinson's disease (PDD). DLB is characterized clinically by dementia accompanied by idiopathic parkinsonism, cognitive fluctuation, and persistent visual hallucinations (McKeith *et al.*, 2005). PDD and DLB have similar clinical presentation as well as underlying brain changes, and differentiation between the two syndromes is entirely based on the relative timing of parkinsonism and cognitive impairment. Currently, an arbitrary cut-off is set at 1 year, i.e., if dementia occurs before or within 1 year after onset of parkinsonism, a diagnosis of DLB is made, whereas PDD is diagnosed if dementia occurs after more than 1 year of motor parkinsonism. This situation is, however, complicated by emerging evidence that mild cognitive impairment may be found in a substantial proportion of PD patients at time of diagnosis.

Cognitive profile

The cognitive profile in DLB is characterized by attentional, executive, and visuoperceptual impairments, whereas memory is usually relatively spared early in disease course (Metzler–Baddeley, 2007). The cognitive profile of our patient was characteristic. One striking feature was that, although initially the MMSE score was in the mildly impaired range, with a score of 22, he failed completely on the clock drawing test. This combination of a marked impairment of executive and visuo-constructive impairment with relatively spared memory, language, and orientation, which has been described in several studies, is likely related to the early involvement of fronto-subcortical circuits and the dorsal and ventral visual pathways. As is usually the case, as the disease progressed, his performance on the MMSE became more impaired, suggesting that the subcortical changes were superimposed by more pronounced cortical lesions. Another typical feature was the relatively early occurrence of cognition and consciousness fluctuations. Fluctuating cognition is very characteristic for DLB and is listed as a core feature in the clinical criteria for DLB.

Apathy

Neuropsychiatric features are more common in DLB than in Alzheimer's disease patients. The most characteristic feature is visual hallucinations, which however occurred relatively late in this patient. The most striking neuropsychiatric feature in our patient was the early occurrence of apathy, characterized by reduced interest and motivation in goal-directed activities, indifference, and flattened affect. The patient had lost interest in activities that had previously been pleasurable, and he became much more passive, which was distressing for his spouse. Together with depression, anxiety, and hallucinations, apathy is among the most common neuropsychiatric symptoms in DLB, and several studies have shown that while apathy per definition is not associated with much suffering by the patient, it is among the most distressing symptoms for caregivers. In addition, he had increased daytime sleepiness, which is the most common sleep problem in DLB after REM-sleep behavioral disorder.

Imaging

Due to the implanted pacemaker, CT scans, but not MRI scans, were available and the findings were normal. The typical MRI imaging pattern in DLB includes global brain volume loss, a predominantly subcortical pattern of cerebral atrophy, and relative preservation of the medial temporal lobe compared to Alzheimer's disease. This has convincingly been shown in several studies comparing groups of patients with DLB and Alzheimer's disease (Beyer *et al.*, 2007). However, in single case investigations, due to low specificity, CT or MRI imaging do not usually aid in the diagnosis, and structural imaging therefore still mainly serves to identify vascular or other structural secondary morbidity. The most important imaging technique for the diagnosis of DLB is dopamine transporter SPECT to detect typical pre-synaptic nigro-striatal pathology. Dopamine transporter SPECT can distinguish between Alzheimer's disease and probable and, importantly, even possible DLB at high sensitivity and specificity (O'Brien *et al.*, 2009 (Fig. 20.1). In a case with clear-cut spontaneous parkinsonism early in the disease however, this test is unlikely to be beneficial.

Treatment

Currently, there are no licensed treatments for DLB. There is however convincing evidence of marked cholinergic deficits in DLB, associated with both cognitive impairment and hallucinations (Aarsland *et al.*, 2004), and there is some evidence that cholinesterase inhibitors are useful for cognition and neuropsychiatric symptoms in DLB (Aarsland *et al.*, 2004). The only placebo-controlled trial provided support for the hypothesis that these drugs can improve symptoms in DLB (McKeith *et al.*, 2000). Our patient was treated with donepezil, which was associated with improvement in several symptom domains, including cognition and apathy. There was even some evidence that parkinsonism improved, although no change in motor symptoms were found in the randomized trial. Several attempts were made to improve motor symptoms in our patient with L-DOPA, although there was no clear evidence of benefit. There are no systematic studies of the effect of L-DOPA in DLB, but there is some preliminary evidence supporting a trial of L-DOPA in patients with DLB and prominent parkinsonism.

Neuropathology

The key neuropathologic features of DLB are neuronal inclusions consisting mainly of alpha-synuclein and ubiquitin. In our case, the neuropathological diagnosis confirmed the clinical diagnosis of DLB, and thus the final diagnosis

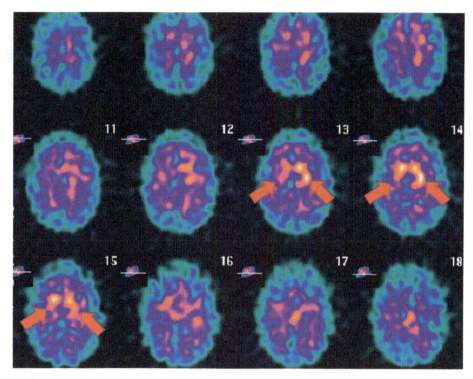

Fig. 20.1. Dopamine transporter TRODAT SPECT in LDB reveals marked bilateral loss of striatal uptake (red arrows) due to nigrostriatal degeneration.

was definite DLB. Using alpha-synuclein staining, Lewy bodies were detected in subcortical regions including brainstem, as well as neocortical frontal, temporal, and parietal regions. In addition, there was some Alzheimer-type pathology, including neurofibrillary tangles, with a Braak and Braak stage of III, and a low density of amyloid plaques in the neocortex (both of these changes may be found in "normal" elderly people) and occasional neurofibrillary tangles in the frontal lobe. The combination of Lewy body and mild Alzheimer-type pathology is common in DLB, and is associated with a less characteristic clinical DLB syndrome compared to the relatively few cases with pure Lewy body pathology. Moderate white-matter demyelination may relate to episodes of hypotension detected clinically, or be associated with disrupted cholinergic mechanisms.

Take home messages

This patient initially presented with hypotension, demontrating that cardiac autonomic failure can be an early phenomenon in DLB.

The typical cognitive profile with predominant executive and visuospatial impairment was demonstrated by the failed clock drawing combined with a relatively high MMSE score.

The case demonstrates the wide variety of psychiatric symptoms which commonly occur in DLB, including apathy and visual hallucinations.

REFERENCES AND FURTHER READING

Aarsland D, Mosimann UP, McKeith IG (2004). Role of cholinesterase inhibitors in Parkinson's disease and dementia with Lewy bodies. *J Geriatr Psychiatry Neurol*, **17**, 164–71.

Ballard CG, Jacoby R, Del Ser T, *et al.* (2004). Neuropathological substrates of psychiatric symptoms in prospectively studied patients with autopsy-confirmed dementia with lewy bodies. *Am J Psychiatry*, **161**, 843–9.

Beyer MK, Larsen JP, Aarsland D (2007). Gray matter atrophy in Parkinson disease with dementia and dementia with Lewy bodies. *Neurology*, **69**, 747–54.

Kaufer DI, Cummings JL, Ketchel P, *et al.* (2000). Validation of the NPI-Q, a brief clinical form of the Neuropsychiatric Inventory. *J Neuropsychiatry Clin Neurosci*, **12**, 233–9.

McKeith I, Del Ser T, Spano P, *et al.* (2000). Efficacy of rivastigmine in dementia with Lewy bodies: a randomised, double-blind, placebo-controlled international study. *Lancet*, **356**, 2031–6.

McKeith IG, Dickson DW, Lowe J, *et al.* (2005). Diagnosis and management of dementia with Lewy bodies: third report of the DLB Consortium. *Neurology*, **65**, 1863–72.

Metzler-Baddeley C (2007). A review of cognitive impairments in dementia with Lewy bodies relative to Alzheimer's disease and Parkinson's disease with dementia. *Cortex*, **43**, 583–600.

Molloy SA, Rowan EN, O'Brien JT, McKeith IG, Wesnes K, Burn DJ (2006). Effect of levodopa on cognitive function in Parkinson's disease with and without dementia and dementia with Lewy bodies. *J Neurol Neurosurg Psychiatry*, **77**, 1323–8.

O'Brien JT, McKeith IG, Walker Z, *et al.* (2009). Diagnostic accuracy of 123I-FP-CIT SPECT in possible dementia with Lewy bodies. *Br J Psychiatry*, **194**, 34–9.

Case 21

Man with post-operative cognitive impairment

Gustavo C. Román and Carlos Bazán III

Reson for consultations

A 47-year-old Caucasian man was referred due to memory problems and depression following surgical treatment of aortic dissection 1 year earlier. After surgery, he was unable to return to work and began receiving disability benefits.

History

One year ago this man arrived at the ER complaining of chest pain radiating to the back and abdomen, head and neck, and blurred vision with visual "spots." He provided a reasonable history; speech and cursory neurological examination were normal. Despite no previous history of hypertension his Blood Pressure (BP) was 160/90 mm Hg. He became confused and hypotensive (systolic BP: 70 mm Hg). He was not tachycardic and extremities were warm with good femoral pulses. Myocardial infarction was ruled out. Computerized Tomography (CT) of the chest showed aortic dissection starting in the aortic root and extending to the arch and descending aorta with exit around T12. The aortic valve was not involved. Hemopericardium was confirmed by 2D echocardiogram.

He immediately underwent successful surgical treatment complicated by bradycardia and hypotension requiring admission to the Coronary Care Unit (CCU). In the immediate post-operative period he became agitated and self-extubated himself; later, in the CCU, he was found to have episodic twitching of the right side of the face and the right hand. On initial neurological examination, there was limited movement of his right upper limb but frequent convulsive movements on the right leg were present. He was treated with a loading dose of 20 mg/kg of fosphenytoin intravenously. An Electroencephalogram (EEG) revealed numerous partial seizures originating from the left frontal region, consistent with non-convulsive status epilepticus.

Case Studies in Dementia: Common and Uncommon Presentations, ed. S. Gauthier and P. Rosa-Neto.
Published by Cambridge University Press. © Cambridge University Press 2011.

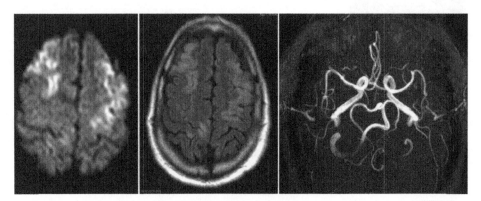

Fig. 21.1. Diffusion-weighted image demonstrates bilateral frontal lobe gyriform hyperintensity in a watershed infarct distribution (left). FLAIR MRI shows gyriform T2 hyperintensity in a watershed infarct distribution in both frontal lobes with effacement of the involved sulci (center). 3D time of flight MRA (right) demonstrates symmetric flow through the branches of the middle and anterior cerebral arteries. A posterior communicating artery is present on the right side measuring approximately 1.7 mm in diameter. The left posterior communicating artery is not seen.

Magnetic Resonance Imaging (MRI) of the brain (Fig. 21.1) showed bilateral acute frontoparietal cortical infarcts in the watershed anterior and middle cerebral artery parasagittal distribution, consistent with hypoxic brain injury. A 3-D time of flight MR angiogram (MRA) (Fig. 21.1) showed intracranial internal carotid arteries of normal caliber and appearance. The visualized middle, anterior, and posterior cerebral arteries were normal.

The right vertebral artery was tortuous and crossed the midline before becoming the basilar artery. The right vertebral artery was dominant. The left vertebral artery ended in a posterior inferior cerebellar branch. The basilar artery was normal. MRA of the circle of Willis was normal but the left posterior communicating artery was not visualized.

The week following the surgery

His neurological examination revealed an alert and cooperative patient responding very slowly to questions and simple orders. There was perseveration and slow speed of psychomotor processing; short-term memory deficits, and executive dysfunction with abnormal Luria's kinetic melody tests. His speech was fluent with frequent episodes of anomia consistent with mild expressive aphasia. Cranial nerves were normal including normal visual fields and no facial weakness. He had a residual mild left hemiparesis that affected more the leg than the arm or the hand. Ankle and knee reflexes were brisk bilaterally and symmetrically, with bilateral Hoffman and Babinski signs and a few beats of ankle clonus on the left. Light touch sensation was decreased in the left lower limb. He was able to walk with support and exhibited scissoring of the left leg.

One month following the surgery

In rehabilitation, his speech and motor deficits had improved, but he continued to present rare, short episodes of seizure activity, and multiple staring episodes and absences, despite anticonvulsant treatment (Dilantin,® Keppra®). EEG continued to be abnormal with frequent sharp delta transients in the left temporal region, with intermittent, irregular theta and delta slowing in the left temporal area. He was discharged home on anticonvulsant medications to continue the rehabilitation treatment as an outpatient.

His previous level of cognitive function had declined despite minimal motor and speech deficits and better seizure control; at home, he was no longer independent and required help with basic and instrumental activities of daily living; he became depressed, tearful, and apathetic. Six months after surgery, it was clear that he could not return to his previous work and was declared permanently incapacitated due to sequelae of ischemic stroke from the peri- and post-operative hypotensive brain insult.

Previous medical history

Previous history of knee arthritis and chronic low back pain; he smoked 1.5 packs per day for 20 years. He drank socially and denied history of drug use.

He gained weight and became obese due to inactivity and excessive eating; 3 months earlier was diagnosed with obstructive sleep apnea. The nocturnal polysomnographic (PSG) study showed obstructive apneas and hypopneas; these were more frequent and severe during REM sleep and diminished severely REM sleep percentage. The Respiratory Distress Index (RDI) was 75 apneas per hour with oxygen desaturations (SaO_2) as low as 72%. During the PSG, the severe obstructive sleep apnea syndrome improved with nasal Continuous Positive Airway Pressure (CPAP) treatment.

General history

Patient had 12 years of formal education and was living with his wife and children. His birth history and early developmental milestones were normal. He was the youngest of five sisters and one brother. Patient was right-handed and English was the only language he spoke. He completed high school and technical courses. He worked as a supervisor in a service company.

Family history

Family history was non-contributory.

Examination

Approximately 1 year after the surgery, the patient was overweight (BI index 31.5). He looked older than his chronological age, tired, and sleepy, casually dressed with good grooming and hygiene. General physical examination was within normal limits, afebrile, pulse: 83/min, BP: 122/69 mm Hg. He was a good historian and had accurate recollection of his surgery 1 year earlier. His speech was slow, clear, and without abnormalities; he had no difficulty understanding conversational speech and task instructions. Insight and judgment were good. His mood was depressed with a congruent affect. His train of thought was linear and logical without delusions or hallucinations. He made good eye contact and exhibited appropriate interpersonal skills. He denied recent seizures and was compliant with his antiepileptic medications. He complained of frequent arousals at night and had been unable to use his nasal CPAP. He continued to snore, was usually tired upon awakening in the morning, and complained of excessive daytime sleepiness.

On cognitive examination he complained of forgetfulness and problems with even simple tasks at home. He was able to provide general information regarding his home address and telephone number, social security number, names of children and close and distant relatives, education and past history. MMSE = 28/30 (he failed to remember 2/3 objects spontaneously, but did it with clues); verbal fluency for animals = 10/min (reduced for educational level); he was unable to do Luria's kinetic melody hand tasks after repeated trials. Otherwise, his general neurological examination revealed normal cranial nerves, including visual fields by confrontation. He had residual spasticity of the left leg and walked with a cane. The remainder of the examination was non-focal and non-contributory. Frontal release signs were not present.

Special studies

Recent laboratory tests included normal complete blood count and chemistry laboratory examinations. Repeat brain MRI 6 months after the acute events showed reduction of edema and ischemia in the areas previously affected (Fig. 21.2).

Neuropsychological evaluation included a neurobehavioral status examination, face-to-face neurocognitive testing, and computer-administered measures.

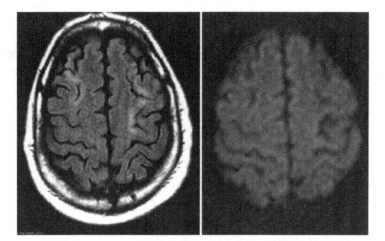

Fig. 21.2. MRI FLAIR (left) obtained 6 months later demonstrates residual T2 hyperintensity in the bilateral frontal lobes in a watershed infarct distribution. There is less swelling of the affected frontal lobe gyri with increased sulcal prominence. Diffusion-weighted image (right) obtained 6 months later show resolution of the watershed infarct hyperintensity within the bilateral frontal lobes.

He was calm, co-operative and engaged in the interview. There was no agitation or retardation. He was co-operative with good effort on all tasks.

Tests results demonstrated average intellectual abilities, consistent with pre-morbid functioning based on reading skills; significant discrepancy between verbal comprehension (average to high-average) and processing speed (low to borderline). Results indicated prominent executive dysfunction, slowed processing speed and visual memory problems with substantial decline from pre-morbid levels. On verbal memory, he demonstrated a flat learning curve, but his ability to recall information after a delay was within normal limits. Regarding visual memory, his ability to copy a figure was within normal limits, with impaired ability to remember and copy the figure after a short and long delay. On the Minnesota Multiphasic Personality Inventory (MMPI), he endorsed a high level of distress, symptoms of depression, and feelings of isolation from others.

Diagnosis

This patient illustrates the clinical manifestations of *hypoperfusive dementia* and he fulfilled NINDS-AIREN diagnostic criteria for *vascular dementia* (Román *et al.*, 1993) including: (1) presence of dementia; (2) evidence of stroke; and (3) a temporal relation between the first two conditions. First, he fulfilled criteria for *dementia* as evidenced by decline in cognitive function from a previous normal level, with involvement of memory and two other cognitive domains (executive function and processing speed); loss of independence and functional impairment. Second, he presented *brain imaging (MRI) evidence of bilateral frontal ischemic stroke* in a typical watershed distribution resulting from hypotension due to acute aortic dissection, surgical repair, and immediate post-operative course. MRA absence of stenosis or Cerebrovascular Disease (CVD) of intracranial blood vessels supports this diagnosis. Third, cognitive problems, dementia, and disability occurred as a result of the ischemic stroke.

He presented also *post-stroke vascular depression* manifested by apathy, sadness, tearfulness, changes in mood, recurrent and fleeting suicidal ideation, and problems coping with his incapacity to work, as well as adjusting to the loss of income and lack of responsibility.

Finally, untreated *sleep apnea syndrome* probably worsened his cognitive deficits and depression. Seizures were under control with medication and played no major role on cognitive deficits.

Discussion

Despite effective auto-regulation of cerebral blood flow (CBF), acute and severe systemic arterial hypotension may result in ischemic brain infarction (Román, 2004), as in the patient illustrated here. Despite his relatively young age, and the absence of extracranial and intracranial CVD, he had watershed infarction as a result of relentless hypotension following aortic dissection. Heavy smoking could have impaired the effective maintenance of CBF (Hossain *et al.*, 2009).

Watershed infarctions

Watershed or boundary zone infarcts occur with less severe hypotension in patients with impaired collateral circulation due to severe, extensive, or multiple atheromatous stenoses of the cerebral arteries. In general, elderly patients are more susceptible to watershed infarcts than younger subjects are. Lesions typically affect cortical areas at the junction of large-vessel arterial territories as demonstrated here (Fig. 21.1) and resulted in *status epilepticus.*

A competent Circle of Willis is the main mechanism of brain protection against hypotension and blockage of cerebral arteries. The Anterior Communicating Artery (ACoA), via the proximal segment of the Anterior Cerebral Artery (ACA), provides hemispheric cerebral blood flow from the contralateral Internal Carotid Artery (ICA). Bisschops *et al.* (2003) showed that, in cases of unilateral ICA occlusion, collateral flow via the ACoA protected from internal border zone infarcts ipsilateral to the occluded ICA. In some cases of watershed infarction ipsilateral to ICA atherosclerosis, recurrent microembolism may be an aggravating factor (Momjian-Mayor and Baron, 2005).

The Basilar Artery (BA) supplies collateral flow to the anterior circulation through the Posterior Communicating artery (PCoA), via the proximal segment of the Posterior Cerebral Artery (PCA), with reversal of flow. According to Schomer and colleagues (1994), absence of a PCoA measuring at least 1 mm in diameter is associated with increased risk of watershed infarction. Our patient had no visible left PCoA.

The ophthalmic artery provides potential collateral flow to the ICA from the ipsilateral external carotid artery. In chronic situations, leptomeningeal vessels develop collaterals between distal branches of the Middle Cerebral Artery (MCA) and PCA.

There are five markers of brain hemodynamic failure: orthostatic limb shaking, blurry vision on exposure to heat, leptomeningeal and ophthalmic collateral circulation on angiography, watershed infarction, and impaired vasodilatation with acetazolamide. Only orthostatic limb shaking was predictive of increased stroke risk. Visual deficits in the patient reported here could be construed as early manifestations of decreased cerebral perfusion.

Typical areas of ischemia involve the cortex posterior to the intraparietal sulcus at the boundaries between ACA and MCA. The central white matter, between the deep territories of the ACA and MCA is often involved; as well as the periventricular white matter fed by long-penetrating end-arterioles. In the elderly, hypoperfusive brain lesions resulting from cardiac failure or hypotension produce *incomplete white matter infarction*, similar to that observed at the penumbra of large infarcts (Pantoni *et al.*, 1996).

Moody and colleagues (1990) studied the anatomical patterns of microcirculation that explain the susceptibility of certain cerebral areas to hypoperfusion. Brain areas irrigated by short penetrating arteries tolerate better hypotension and hypoperfusion. These resistant areas include cerebral cortex, subcortical arcuate fibers, corpus callosum, and claustrum, external and extreme capsules. The latter three receive dual circulation and are highly resistant to hypotensive and hypoperfusive injuries.

In addition to white matter lesions, *watershed cortical microinfarcts* due to cerebral hypoperfusion in the elderly worsen the clinical manifestations of Alzheimer's disease. Watershed cortical microinfarcts are ten times higher in Alzheimer's disease than in controls (Miklossy *et al.*, 2003). Congophilic angiopathy is an important risk factor (Suter *et al.*, 2002).

Hippocampal sclerosis

Hippocampal sclerosis is a localized form of ischemia and atrophy observed in very old demented subjects, particularly in those with cardiac disease (Dickson *et al.*,

1994; Corey-Bloom *et al.*, 1997). The hippocampal arteries arise mainly from the PCA and anterior choroidal artery. Straight arteries from the hippocampal arteries enter Ammon's horn through the dentate gyrus and then branch out at right angles in a rake-like pattern. As a result, the CA1 sector is poorly vascularized. *Mesial temporal lobe sclerosis* or *hippocampal sclerosis* was originally observed in patients with epilepsy, gliosis and atrophy of Ammon's horn, recurrent seizures or *status epilepticus* and anoxia. Another cause is perinatal ischemia in the distal PCA territory at the time of birth.

Hippocampal sclerosis in the elderly is characterized by selective neuronal loss in the CA1 sector of the hippocampus extending into the subiculum, without cavitation (Leverenz *et al.*, 2002). Crystal *et al.* (1993) postulated that the cause of hippocampal sclerosis in the elderly is probably systemic hypoperfusion with hypoxia–ischemia; Vinters *et al.* (2000) suggested that it may result from ischemia due to intrinsic CVD. These two hypotheses are complementary and not mutually exclusive.

Vascular depression

New-onset depression – particularly after 60 years of age – may have a neurological etiology. Depression frequently follows clinically eloquent strokes. Post-Stroke Depression (PSD) occurs in about 33% of all stroke survivors. Seventy patients with a single ischemic stroke. Patients with PSD had statistically significant larger brain infarcts that involved predominantly the basal ganglia and the posterior corona radiata. The highest risk for PSD was with left pallidum lesions. There is a high frequency of Executive Dysfunction (ED) in patients with vascular lesions. 158 stroke patients were further classified in four groups: (1) depression with executive dysfunction (DED); (2) depression without ED, (3) ED without depression; and (4) absent depression and normal executive function. Lesions of left frontal–subcortical circuits were associated with DED [OR = 1.6 95% CI 1.1–2.5]. These studies have confirmed that interruption of pre-frontal-subcortical circuits originating in dorsolateral pre-frontal cortex, orbitofrontal cortex, or anterior cingulate cortex, caused by ischemic strokes at the level of caudate, pallidum, thalamus, or their subcortical-cortical loops in the white matter, significantly increase risk of PSD and ED. These studies support the concept of "vascular depression" or "depression-executive dysfunction syndrome of late life."

Apathy

Apathy can be defined as a quantitative reduction of voluntary, goal directed behaviors and classify the possible pathogenesis of apathy in three groups:

emotional–affective, cognitive, and auto-activation, corresponding to disruptions at different levels of the pre-frontal subcortical circuits. Apathy can be a symptom of depression, but it also occurs in pure neurological conditions such as limbic lesions, Parkinson's disease, vascular depression, and vascular dementia

Take home messages

Neuropsychiatric cortical or subcortical symptoms are commonly associated with vascular cognitive dementia.

Vascular depression is an important neuropsychiatric aspect associated with vascular dementia.

REFERENCES AND FURTHER READING

Bisschops RH, Klijn CJ, Kappelle LJ, *et al.* (2003). Collateral flow and ischemic brain lesions in patients with unilateral carotid artery occlusion. *Neurology*, **60**, 1435–41.

Corey-Bloom J, Sabbagh MN, Bondi MW, *et al.* (1997). Hippocampal sclerosis contributes to dementia in the elderly. *Neurology*, **48**, 154–60.

Crystal HA, Dickson DW, Sliwinski MJ, *et al.* (1993). Pathological markers associated with normal aging and dementia in the elderly. *Ann Neurol*, **34**, 566–73.

Dickson DW, Davies P, Bevona C, *et al.* (1994). Hippocampal sclerosis: a common pathological feature of dementia in very old (greater than 80 years of age) humans. *Acta Neuropathol*, **88**, 212–21.

Hossain M, Sathe T, Fazio V, *et al.* (2009). Tobacco smoke: a critical etiological factor for vascular impairment at the blood–brain barrier. *Brain Res*, **1287**, 192–205.

Leverenz JB, Agustin CM, Tsuang D, *et al.* (2002). Clinical and neuropathological characteristics of hippocampal sclerosis. *Arch Neurol*, **59**, 1099–106.

Miklossy J (2003). Cerebral hypoperfusion induces cortical watershed microinfarcts which may further aggravate cognitive decline in Alzheimer's disease. *Neurol Res*, **25**, 605–10.

Momjian-Mayor I, Baron JC (2005). The pathophysiology of watershed infarction in internal carotid artery disease: review of cerebral perfusion studies. *Stroke*, **36**, 567–77.

Moody DM, Bell MA, Challa VR (1990). Features of cerebral vascular pattern that predict vulnerability to perfusion or oxygenation deficiency: an anatomical study. *Am J Neuroradiol*, **11**, 431–9.

Pantoni L, Garcia JH, Gutierrez JA (1996). Cerebral white matter is highly vulnerable to ischemia. *Stroke*, **27**, 1641–7.

Román GC (2004). Brain hypoperfusion: a critical factor in vascular dementia. *Neurological Research*, **26**, 454–8.

Román GC, Tatemichi TK, Erkinjuntti T, *et al.* (1993). Vascular dementia: diagnostic criteria for research studies. Report of the NINDS-AIREN International Workshop. *Neurology,* **43**, 250–60.

Schomer DF, Marks MP, Steinberg GK, *et al.* (1994). The anatomy of the posterior communicating artery as a risk factor for ischemic cerebral infarction. *N Engl J Med,* **330**, 1565–70.

Suter OC, Sunthorn T, Kraftsik R, *et al.* (2002). Cerebral hypoperfusion generates cortical watershed microinfarcts in Alzheimer disease. *Stroke,* **33**, 1986–92.

Vinters HV, Ellis WG, Zarow C, *et al.* (2000). Neuropathologic substrates of ischemic vascular dementia. *J Neuropathol Exp Neurol,* **59**, 931–45.

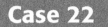

Case 22

Penicillin for dementia in a young man

Huali Wang and Xin Yu

Clinical history – main complaint

A 41-year-old man was referred to memory clinic because of memory loss, poor verbal expression, loss of interest, and blunted response to environment within the last 6 months. Irritability and slow behavioral response was first noted around 2 years before he was referred. At that time, the diagnosis of depression had been recorded in other hospitals and antidepressants were prescribed. But he reported poor response to antidepressants. Later on he developed prominent and persistent blunted emotion, and deteriorated memory and language ability. He also suffered occasional muscle alertness during sleep. In the past 6 months, he had difficulty in communication, and could not function well in the workplace.

General history

He received around 5 years of schooling education. He was a driver in a power plant. Lives with his wife and their only child.

Had been drinking for many years, around 1.5 liter beer per day. He stopped drinking around 1 month before he was referred to the memory clinic. No significant physical and mental changes were noted after he stopped drinking. No chronic medical problem. No medications.

Family history

No family history of dementia or memory loss. His aunt was diagnosed with psychosis.

Examination

BP 120/80 mmHg; pulse 84 bpm, regular. No sign of peripheral arterial disease. No skin lesions. The size of pupils was normal. No major neurological abnormalities

Case Studies in Dementia: Common and Uncommon Presentations, ed. S. Gauthier and P. Rosa-Neto. Published by Cambridge University Press. © Cambridge University Press 2011.

Table 22.1. Cognitive performance and neuropsychiatric evaluation before, 6 months, and 18 months after penicillin therapy

	Before therapy	6 months after therapy	18 months after therapy
General cognitive function			
MMSE	16/30	19/30	21/30
CASI	57/100	67/100	73/100
Memory			
CCNB Immediate memory	3/10	7/10	6/10
CCNB 5-min delayed recall	0	5/10	6/10
CCNB 30-min delayed recall	6/10	7/10	5/10
BVRT visual memory	5	12	4
BVRT delayed recall	0	2	1
Executive function			
Verbal fluency	8	12	15
Stroop test (color-word)	24	33	31
Color trail making test 2	310"	165"	150"
Attention and Speed of Information processing			
PASAT (# of correct response)	21/50	24/50	23/50
Trail-making A	82"	62"	63"
Color trail-making test 1	100"	66"	90"
Visuospatial function			
CERAD Construction praxis	3/4	3/4	3/4
Visual reproduction	23/41	29/41	25/41

Notes: MMSE: mini-mental status examination; CASI: cognitive abilities screening instrument; CCNB: cross-cultural neuropsychological battery; BVRT: Benton visual retention test; PASAT: paced auditory serial addition test; CERAD: consortium to establish a registry for Alzheimer's disease.

were noted except for minor difficulty in bilateral finger-to-nose test, and rapid alternating movement.

Special studies

Cognitive status was evaluated by the mini-mental state examination (MMSE) and a detailed neuropsychological battery for assessment of memory, language and executive function, attention, and concentration. The examination documented moderate dementia (MMSE = 16/30) with moderate amnesia and dysexecutive syndrome. Neuropsychological tests (Table 22.1) showed evidence of cognitive impairment of multiple domains, including memory, executive function, and attention and speed of information processing. Visuospatial

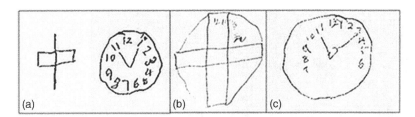

Fig. 22.1. Clock drawing tests performed (a) at initial visit, (b) 6-month and (c) 18-month after penicillin therapy. (a) The patient wrote a Chinese character before he drew the clock, since he had some difficulty in understanding the test instructions. (b) The subject drew two interacting rectangles (similar to the constructional praxis test in ADAS-Cog) within the circle, though he had not been administered the ADAS-Cog on this visit. His performance was very poor in clock drawing. (c) The patient drew a circle and wrote all numbers correctly. Though he put the numbers in wrong places, it was clear that he split the clock into two parts. Then he marked the time wrongly if based on the place of number, but seemed right on the "real" clock.

function was relatively preserved. Clock drawing test (CDT) suggested the patient had difficulty in understanding the instruction, and moderate executive dysfunction (Fig. 22.1(a)).

Significant apathy was presented based on interview with his wife, using Neuropsychiatric Inventory (NPI). Difficulty in sleep was also reported.

Laboratory workups including a complete blood count and differential, serum electrolytes and glucose, hepatic and renal function tests, thyroid function tests, serum B_{12} and folate levels, and an ECG were normal. The serum test for human immunodeficiency virus (HIV) was negative.

He was serologically positive for syphilis (Rapid Plasma Reagin (RPR) test positive, *Treponema Pallidum* Particle Agglutination (TPPA) titer = 1:128). Cerebrospinal Fluid (CSF) was clear with cell count 40/μL (normal 0–8/μL); leukocytes 6/μL, elevated level of protein 74.7 mg/dL (normal range 15.0–45.0 mg/dL), and normal level of glucose 3.13 mmol/L (2.50–4.50 mmol/L) and chloride 124 mmol/L (120–132 mmol/L). The glucose test and Pandy test in CSF were positive. The TPPA test and RPR test in CSF were positive, establishing the diagnosis of neurosyphilis.

A magnetic resonance imaging (MRI) scan was performed. 3D high-resolution anatomical images acquired with T1-weighted magnetization-prepared rapidly acquired gradient-echo sequence (3D-MPRAGE) showed significant generalized cerebral atrophy, particularly in bilateral medial temporal lobe and hippocampus (Fig. 22.2(a)). Fluid-Attenuated Inversion Recovery (FLAIR) images showed minor non-specific periventricular white matter hyperintensity.

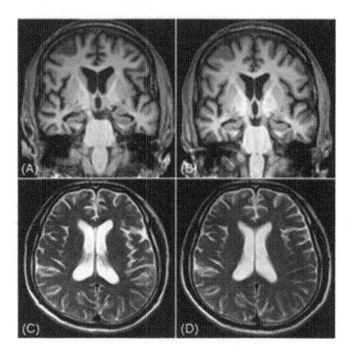

Fig. 22.2.   MRI performed (a),(c) before and (b),(d) 6-months after penicillin therapy. Note stable medial temporal lobe and hippocampus atrophy in high resolution T1 weighted MRI (a),(b). FLAIR MRI images (d),(c) shows only minor non-specific white matter hyperintensities.

Diagnosis

The initial diagnostic impression was dementia associated with neurosyphilis.

Follow-up

He received 3-week penicillin therapy at an Infectious Diseases Hospital. During the follow-up check-up 3 months after penicillin therapy, the serum RPR was negative.

His family reported modest improvement in his behavior. He started talking with his family, though sometimes losing his temper. His sleep was not recovered. When he was presented to memory clinic, he could say hello to the doctor, and sometimes join the discussion with doctors. However, inappropriate word finding was noted during the interview. He also exhibited slight europhia.

At 6 months after the penicillin therapy, his cognitive performance was slightly improved as shown in Table 22.1. Performance of verbal fluency and color trail-making test 2 was improved dramatically, suggesting executive function was restored after antisyphilitic therapy.

The follow-up MRI scan was unaltered compared with the initial visit. (Fig. 22.2)

Approximately 18 months after the penicillin therapy, he consulted the Infectious Diseases Hospital for a follow-up check-up of syphilis status.

He remained serologically positive for syphilis (RPR titer = 1:32, TPPA test was positive). The CSF was clear. The level of protein in CSF was decreased to normal (Pandy test negative, and level of protein 43.50 mg/dL (8.00–43.00)). The levels of glucose (2.92 mmol/L (2.50–4.50)) and chloride [125.10 mmol/L (120.0–132.0)] were normal. The cell in CSF was 220/uL and leukocyte 50. The syphilis tests in CSF were positive (RPR positive 1:2; TPPA positive).

General cognitive function was continuously improved. Executive function and memory were sustained after penicillin therapy. However, it was noted that his visual memory declined from visit 2 (6 months after penicillin therapy). It remains unclear whether the decline of visual memory was associated with the positive CSF syphilis test or attributed to progressive brain atrophy. It was worthwhile continuing follow-up of this patient.

Discussion

In this case, the patient exhibited three major syndromes: cognitive impairment, apathy, and minor neurological symptoms. Global cognitive impairment met the criteria for the diagnosis of dementia. As the patient was very young, the subtype diagnosis of dementia needed careful and extensive differential diagnosis. Apathy syndrome developed initially alerted the impairment of emotional circuit in the pre-frontal lobe. The most common causes for global cognitive impairment and apathy are neurodegenerative diseases such as Alzheimer's disease, frontal–temporal lobe atrophy, and recurrent episodes of cerebrovascular events such as post-stroke cognitive impairment and apathy. Neuroimaging examinations could help identify brain abnormalities, including medial temporal lobe and hippocampal atrophy in AD, lobular atrophy in frontal and temporal lobe in FTD, and clinically significant infarcts or hemorrhage for cerebrovascular events. On MRI images, there were significant medial temporal and hippocampal atrophy and enlargement of ventricles equivalent to the moderate to severe degree of atrophy on a visual rating scale (Wahlund et al., 2000). A combination of mini-mental state examination and medial temporal lobe atrophy ratings yields sensitivity and specificity greater than 85% in distinguishing AD from non-AD dementia. Thus, MTL atrophy is included in the recently NINCDS-ADRDA research criteria for AD (Dubois et al., 2007). But his age and minor neurological abnormalities were very atypical for AD. This prompted further syphilis testing, although his wife was concerned due to the social stigma of syphilis and the absence of inappropriate sexual relationship.

Neurosyphilis is known for causing dementia, but usually focal neurological abnormalities are present. Executive dysfunction (Gurses *et al.*, 2007; Mehrabian *et al.*, 2009), memory loss, and impairment in attention have been previously reported (Mehrabian *et al.*, 2009). This case presented multiple domain cognitive impairment particularly in memory, executive function and attention, while visuospatial function was relatively preserved. Theoretically, cognitive impairment can be improved as a clinical response to penicillin treatment. Verbal fluency was improved after penicillin treatment, suggesting executive function may be sensitive to anti-syphilitic therapy.

Neurosyphilis was easily overlooked in an affected patient with psychiatric symptoms who lacked overt neurologic signs (Kohler *et al.*, 2000; Lee *et al.*, 2009). Depression was reported when the limbic system was affected (Fujimoto *et al.*, 2001). Apathy has not yet been described in neurosyphilis and has been underrecognized not only by informants, but by the clinicians as well. Pre-frontal and temporal regions are differentially associated with apathy and disinhibition. Successful execution of complex social behaviors relies on the integration of social knowledge and executive functions, represented in the pre-frontal cortex, and reward attribution and emotional processing, represented in mesolimbic structures (Zamboni *et al.*, 2008). Apathy in this case may be attributed to generalized brain atrophy, and is related to executive dysfunction.

Neurosyphilis mimics different types of neuropsychiatric disorders, including pre-senile dementia. Mimicking AD radiologically was rarely described (van Eijsden *et al.*, 2008). With generalized cerebral atrophy involving medial temporal lobe and hippocampus, this case may easily be misdiagnosed. Medial temporal lobe atrophy involving hippocampus may be a poor prognostic sign in general paresis (Kodama *et al.*, 2000). Two years before antisyphilitic therapy, this patient experienced prominent progressive generalized cerebral atrophy, especially in medial temporal lobe and hippocampus. The brain atrophy was not improved after penicillin therapy. The radiological findings indicate a poor neurological and neurocognitive prognosis. Just as noticed, the CSF and serum syphilis tests remained positive at 18-month follow-up visit, suggesting an inadequate response to penicillin treatment and poor long-term outcome.

Even patients with classic cognitive impairment of Alzheimer's disease may actually have another, treatable disorder (Barrett, 2005). To minimize the misdiagnosis of a potentially reversible cognitive disorder, this case suggests that routine syphilis screening in young patients with cognitive impairment and psychiatric symptoms is indicated.

Take home messages

Although medial temporal atrophy is an excellent predictor for AD in elderly patients with cognitive impairment, in young-adulthood dementia due to neurodegenerative disorder is uncommon and other underlying causes should be sought.

Co-occurence of young-onset cognitive impairment and pronounced apathy raises the alertness for syphilis testing.

As medial temporal lobe and hippocampal atrophy may predict poorer prognosis in neurosyphilis, dementia associated with neurosyphilis may be persistent.

REFERENCES AND FURTHER READING

Barrett AM (2005). Is it Alzheimer's disease or something else? 10 disorders that may feature impaired memory and cognition. *Postgrad Med*, **117**(5), 47–53.

Dubois B, HH Feldman, Jacova C, *et al.* (2007). Research criteria for the diagnosis of Alzheimer's disease: revising the NINCDS-ADRDA criteria. *Lancet Neurol*, **6**(8), 734–46.

Fujimoto H, Imaizumi T, Yoshida H, *et al.* (2001). Neurosyphilis showing transient global amnesia-like attacks and magnetic resonance imaging abnormalities mainly in the limbic system. *Intern Med*, **40**(5), 439–42.

Gurses C, Kurtuncu M, Jirsch J, *et al.* (2007). Neurosyphilis presenting with status epilepticus. *Epileptic Disord*, **9**(1), 51–6.

Kodama K, Okada S, Komatsu N, *et al.* (2000). Relationship between MRI findings and prognosis for patients with general paresis. *J Neuropsychiatry Clin Neurosci*, **12**(2), 246–50.

Kohler CG, Ances BM, Coleman AR, *et al.* (2000). Marchiafava-Bignami disease: literature review and case report. *Neuropsychiatry Neuropsychol Behav Neurol*, **13**(1), 67–76.

Lee CH, Lin WC, *et al.* (2009). Initially unrecognized dementia in a young man with neurosyphilis. *Neurologist*, **15**(2), 95–7.

Mehrabian S, Raycheva MR, Petrova E, *et al.* (2009). Neurosyphilis presenting with dementia, chronic chorioretinitis and adverse reactions to treatment: a case report. *Cases J*, **2**, 8334.

van Eijsden P, Veldink JH, Linn FH, *et al.* (2008). Progressive dementia and mesiotemporal atrophy on brain MRI: neurosyphilis mimicking pre-senile Alzheimer's disease? *Eur J Neurol*, **15**(2), e14–5.

Wahlund LO, Julin P, Johansson S-E, *et al.* (2000). Visual rating and volumetry of the medial temporal lobe on magnetic resonance imaging in dementia: a comparative study. *J Neurol Neurosurg Psychiatry*, **69**(5), 630–5.

Zamboni G, Huey ED, Krueger F, *et al.* (2008). Apathy and disinhibition in frontotemporal dementia: Insights into their neural correlates. *Neurology*, **71**(10), 736–42.

Thiamine for dementia in a young woman

Christian Schmidt, Steffen Plickert, David Summers,
and Inga Zerr

Clinical history – main complaint

A 39-year-old woman was reported to the "German National Reference Center
for the Surveillance of Transmissible Spongiform Encephalopathies" (NRC). She
suffered from rapidly progressive dementia having developed in less than
3 months, visual disturbances including temporary total anopsia, hallucinations,
ataxia, and vegetative dysregulation.

Past clinical history

Twelve weeks before being admitted to a neurology department and being
reported to the NRC, she underwent elective tonsillectomy for recurrent infections. Thereafter, she suffered from persistent severe dysphagia. She didn't report
to a physician until she was re-admitted to a gastroenterology unit in week 9 after
surgery due to recurrent emesis, dehydration, and 25 kg weight loss. Routine
diagnostic work up (sonography, endoscopy, abdominal CT, blood tests) didn't
reveal the symptoms' etiology. From then on, rapidly progressive dementia,
hallucinations, temporary anopsia, ataxia, dysphonia, formal thought disorder,
nystagmus, and later somnolence developed within 4 weeks. The patient was
referred to a psychiatric unit and eventually to a neurology department in week
12 after surgery.

Cerebral MR imaging was performed (Fig. 23.1). Due to the findings, the
patient was reported to the NRC as suspected variant CJD.

General history

The patient's medical history comprised allergic asthma, hyperlipidemia, nasal
sinus surgery (4 and 6 years before), and pulmonary embolism (15 years before).
She neither abused alcohol, nicotine, or illicit drugs nor did she take any

Case Studies in Dementia: Common and Uncommon Presentations, ed. S. Gauthier and P. Rosa-Neto.
Published by Cambridge University Press. © Cambridge University Press 2011.

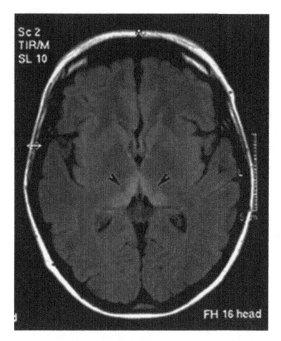

Fig. 23.1.   Axial brain section in FLAIR MR Imaging. The bilaterally hyperintense dorsomedial thalami appear as the so called "Hockey Stick Sign" (or "Pulvinar Sign") due to the characteristic hyperintensities' shape.

medication before. She had never received blood transfusions, heterologous grafts, or growth hormones. She lived in Germany, had never been abroad for a long time and had never visited the UK. She had no regular contact with cattle.

Family history

The family's medical history comprised allergies, asthma, psoriasis, cerebrovascular disease, colon cancer, but no early onset dementia or other significant neurological or psychiatric disorder. No early deaths within the family were reported.

Examination

By the time of admission to the reporting hospital (week 12 after tonsillectomy), the main signs and symptoms were: impaired memory (Mini-Mental Status Examination MMSE 22/30), formal thought disorder, avolition, visual hallucinations and visual disturbances, intermittent somnolence, dysphonia, high amplitude spontaneous nystagmus, flaccid paraparesis of the lower extremities (inability to stand or walk), dysmetria and ataxia as well as intention tremor especially affecting the upper extremities, tachycardia, and urinary incontinence.

Special studies

Imaging: MRI FLAIR imaging (Fig. 23.1) revealed the "Hockey Stick Sign", also known as the "Pulvinar Sign." The MRI of the spine was normal. Sonography of extra- and intracranial vessels excluded stenoses or dissection. Abdominal CT and endoscopy having been performed 4 weeks earlier had not shown signs of malignancy.

Electrophysiology: generalized theta-activity but neither epileptic potentials nor triphasic waves were recorded on EEG. Neurography detected signs of acute axonal damage.

Laboratory (blood): within normal range were celiac disease associated antibodies, paraneoplastic antineuronal antibodies, and thyreoperoxidase antibodies. Vitamin B1 level was 54 ng/mL (range: 20–100 ng/mL), erythrocyte transketolase activity 38 U/L (range: 60–85 U/L).

Genetics: PRNP gene, codon 129: methionine/valine heterozygosity.

Laboratory (CSF): no signs of hemorrhage, acute, or chronic inflammation. Proteins 14–3–3 negative. Tau 110 pg/mL (not elevated).

Diagnosis

The combination of rapidly progressive dementia, psychosyndrome, ataxia, visual disturbances, and the Pulvinar Sign revealed by MRI as well as the exclusion of encephalitis or many other possible causes of that symptom constellation made the involved physicians consider a prion disease – namely variant Creutzfeldt–Jakob disease – as a differential diagnosis. Therefore, the patient was reported to the NRC.

Just before a NRC counseling physician visited the patient, a probatory treatment with high dose Vitamin B1 and magnesium was started. After that, the patient gradually improved. Hence the final diagnosis of Wernicke's encephalopathy was established. Initially, this was not strongly considered a differential diagnosis because the patient did not misuse alcohol. Special laboratory testing (erythrocyte transketolase activity) supported the diagnosis later on.

Follow-up

The patient responded well to the therapy. The cognitive and psychiatric status improved, the motor symptoms were regressing. The patient started to eat again.

Five weeks after admission to the reporting hospital (week 17 after surgery), the patient could be transferred to a rehabilitation unit. In week 18 after surgery, the patient still had some minor cognitive impairment, but was again able to sit and control bowel and bladder function.

Discussion

Rapidly progressive dementia, the "Hockey Sticks" (MRI Pulvinar Sign) and the exclusion of encephalitis led to the differential diagnosis of variant Creutzfeldt–Jakob disease (vCJD) in the first place. Wernicke's disease was not as strongly considered initially since the patient was non-alcoholic.

vCJD is a transmissible prion disease associated with Bovine Spongiform Encephalopathy (BSE) (Will et al., 1996). Patients are often young – median 30yrs of age – and mainly present with progressive psychiatric symptoms, dementia, ataxia, and visual disturbances (Zeidler et al., 1997a, b). A core diagnostic finding is the so-called "Hockey Stick Sign" also known as the "Pulvinar Sign" on cerebral MR imaging (Collie et al., 2003; Zeidler et al., 2000). It is characterized by bilaterally hyperintense pulvinar nuclei of the thalamus on FLAIR or DWI MRI (Summers et al., 2004). In adequate clinical context its sensitivity is 78%–90% and specificity almost 100% for vCJD (Tschampa et al., 2007). Its radiological differential diagnoses comprise thalamic infarction, top-of-the-basilar ischemia, MV2 subtype of sporadic CJD, post-infectious encephalitis, cat scratch disease, Alper's syndrome and Wernicke's disease (Doss et al., 2003; Haik et al., 2002; Krasnianski et al., 2006; Nolli et al., 2005; Weidauer et al., 2003; Zeidler et al., 2000).

Wernicke's Encephalopathy (WE) is a neurologic condition characterized by cognitive impairment, nystagmus, defective oculomotor function, and ataxia (Donnino et al., 2007). Korsakov's psychosis can be present as a co-morbidity. Due to the symptomatology it is a differential diagnosis to prion diseases (Bertrand et al., 2009). The estimated prevalence in Germany, home country to the patient presented here, is approx. 0.3%–0.8% (Sechi and Serra, 2007). Thiamine (Vitamin B1) deficiency is considered the disease's cause often found in malnourished alcoholic patients.

The patient presented here had no history of alcohol or drug abuse. Her thiamine levels were always low but in a normal range. Therefore, WE had not been the first differential diagnosis. Nonetheless, the patient had suffered from malnutrition and weight loss due to dysphagia and recurrent emesis. The rapid development of a variety of neuropsychiatric disorders to the full extent of WE have been described in non-alcoholic patients, especially after weight loss due to gastric surgery and/or hyperemesis (Dallal et al., 2006; Fandino et al., 2005; Makarewicz et al., 2007; Sechi, 2008; Singh and Kumar, 2007).

Table 23.1. Differential diagnoses of rapidly progressive dementia

Degenerative	Inflammatory	Others
• Alzheimer's dementia • Lewy body dementia • Frontotemporal dementia • Parkinson's disease • Multisystem atrophy • Corticobasal degeneration • Progressive supranuclear palsy	• Hashimoto's Encephalopathy • Multiple sclerosis • vasculitis/collagenosis • Sarcoidosis • antibody mediated and/or paraneoplastic autoimmune encephalitis (antibodies, e.g., VGKC, Yo, Hu, Mac, CV2c, GAD, Neuropil, Adenylate kinase, glial, NR1, NR2, Amphiphysin, Ri) • Celiac disease associated Encephalopathy	• psychiatric disease • malignancy • non-antibody mediated paraneoplastic encephalopathies • toxic (e.g., alcohol induced encephalopathy, lithium intoxication, methotrexate toxicity and other drug or heavy metal induced encephalopathies) • metabolic and/or genetic and/or other degenerative encephalopathies (e.g., M. Wilson, Huntington's disease, orthochromatic leukodystrophia, M. Niemann-Pick C, osmotic myelinolysis, hyperparathyroidism, Fahr's disease, hereditary prion disease) • vascular disease • vitamin deficiency (e.g., Wernicke's disease) • infectious encephalitis (e.g., Herpes encephalitis, PML, SSPE and other esp. viral diseases, prion diseases) • CSF circulation disturbances (e.g., normal pressure hydrocephalus)

Notes: Compiled from Bertrand *et al.* (2009), Geschwind *et al.* (2008), Heinemann *et al.* (2007), Kelley *et al.* (2009), Walker (2007) and clinical experience at the NRC-TSE, Germany.

Although the thiamine levels were normal, erythrocyte transketolase activity was decreased indicating thiamine deficiency and suggesting WE. Erythrocyte transketolase is a thiamine-dependent enzyme involved in the pentose phosphate pathway (Pearce, 2008). This case shows once more that determination of that enzyme's activity can be a helpful tool for the clinician. Thiamine deficiency can also cause neuropathies and Beri Beri disease (Angstadt *et al.*, 2005; Koike *et al.*, 2008; Walker and Kepner, 2009). Hence tachycardia, dysphonia, parapareses with areflexia as well as the compatible neurography findings could have been signs of overlapping Beri Beri – and at the same time, because untypical in vCJD, of great differential diagnostic importance.

Hypothetically, the disease of the patient described had developed as follows. Initially the tonsillectomy caused dysphagia leading to malnutrition and depletion of the thiamine reserve, which normally lasts for approximately 18 days (Sechi and Serra, 2007). The possibly genetically predisposed (Sechi and Serra, 2007) patient then developed first signs of WE. Dysphagia is even described as one of its rare early symptoms (Karaiskos *et al.*, 2008). Therefore, it can be speculated that the patient entered a self-sustaining vicious cycle of dysphagia, hyperemesis, and malnutrition. Thence the patient's cognitive, neurologic, and autonomous status declined. After probatory treatment was initiated, the symptoms responded very well to thiamine and magnesium supplements.

The main lesson to learn from this clinical case is to consider WE as an easily treatable differential diagnosis of rapidly progressive dementias (Table 23.1). The obvious "Hockey Stick Sign" in MR imaging almost misled the involved physicians, since it was isolated while WE typical periaqueductal lesions as well as signal alterations of the corpora mammillaria were not present.

Take home messages

Wernicke's Encephalopathy should always be considered a treatable differential diagnosis of rapidly progessive dementia.

Isolated, so called "typical" findings such as the Pulvinar Sign on MRI should always only be interpreted in the clinical context. Otherwise one can easily be misled in the differential diagnostic process.

The Hockey Stick Sign (Pulvinar Sign) can occur on cerebral MR Imaging in Wernicke's Disease patients.

Wernicke's encephalopathy can occur in non-alcoholic patients especially in those with substantial weight loss.

Measurement of erythrocyte transketolase activity is of high diagnostic value regarding WE.

Exclusion of treatable causes of dementias should be performed thoroughly and pertinaceously in order to avoid misdiagnosis of fatal diseases with their far reaching consequences for patients and relatives.

Acknowledgments

The case study presented here is based on an article accepted for publication in *CNS Spectrums* (07/2009) (Schmidt C, Plickert S, Summers D, Zerr, I: "Pulvinar sign in Wernicke's encephalopathy"). We gratefully appreciate *CNS Spectrums'* permission allowing the authors to publish that case study in this book in a modified form.

REFERENCES AND FURTHER READING

Angstadt JD, Bodziner RA, (2005). Peripheral polyneuropathy from thiamine deficiency following laparoscopic Roux-en-Y gastric bypass. *Obes Surg*, **15**(6), 890–2.

Bertrand A, Brandel JP, Grignon Y, *et al.* (2009). Wernicke encephalopathy and Creutzfeldt–Jakob disease. *J Neurol*, **256**(6), 904–9.

Collie DA, Summers DM, Sellar RJ, *et al.* (2003). Diagnosing variant Creutzfeldt–Jakob disease with the Pulvinar sign: MR imaging findings in 86 neuropathologically confirmed cases. *Am J Neuroradiol*, **24**(8), 1560–9.

Dallal RM (2006). Wernicke encephalopathy after bariatric surgery: losing more than just weight. *Neurology*, **66**(11), 1786.

Donnino MW, Vega J, Miller J, Walsh M (2007). Myths and misconceptions of Wernicke's encephalopathy: what every emergency physician should know. *Ann Emerg Med*, **50**(6), 715–21.

Doss A, Mahad D, Romanowski CAJ (2003). Wernicke encephalopathy: unusual findings in nonalcoholic patients. *J Comput Assist Tomogr*, **27**(2), 235–40.

Fandiño JN, Benchimol AK, Fandiño LN, Barroso FL, Coutinho WF, Appolinário JC (2005). Eating avoidance disorder and Wernicke–Korsakoff syndrome following gastric bypass: an under-diagnosed association. *Obes Surg*, **15**(8), 1207–10.

Geschwind MD, Shu H, Haman A, Sejvar JJ, Miller BL (2008). Rapidly progressive dementia. *Ann Neurol*, **64**(1), 97–108.

Haïk S, Brandel JP, Oppenheim C, *et al.* (2002). Sporadic CJD clinically mimicking variant CJD with bilateral increased signal in the Pulvinar. *Neurology*, **58**(1), 148–9.

Heinemann U, Krasnianski A, Meissner B, *et al.* (2007). Creutzfeldt–Jakob disease in germany: a prospective 12-year surveillance. *Brain*, **130**(5), 1350–9.

Karaiskos I, Katsarolis I, Stefanis L (2008). Severe dysphagia as the presenting symptom of Wernicke–Korsakoff syndrome in a non-alcoholic man. *Neurol Sci*, **29**(1), 45–6.

Kelley BJ, Boeve BF, Josephs KA (2009). Rapidly progressive young-onset dementia. *Cogn Behav Neurol*, **22**(1), 22–7.

Koike H, Ito S, Morozumi S, *et al.* (2008). Rapidly developing weakness mimicking Guillain-Barré syndrome in Beriberi neuropathy: two case reports. *Nutrition*, **24**(7–8), 776–80.

Krasnianski A, Schulz-Schaeffer WJ, Kallenberg K, *et al.* (2006). Clinical findings and diagnostic tests in the MV2 subtype of sporadic CJD. *Brain*, **129**(9), 2288–96.

Makarewicz W, Kaska L, Kobiela J, *et al.* (2007). Wernicke's syndrome after sleeve gastrectomy. *Obes Surg*, **17**(5), 704–6.

Nolli M, Barbieri A, Pinna C, Pasetto A, Nicosia F (2005). Wernicke's encephalopathy in a malnourished surgical patient: clinical features and magnetic resonance imaging. *Acta Anaesthesiol Scand*, **49**(10), 1566–70.

Pearce JMS (2008). Wernicke–Korsakoff encephalopathy. *Eur Neurol*, **59**(1–2), 101–4.

Sechi G (2008). Prognosis and therapy of Wernicke's encephalopathy after obesity surgery. *Am J Gastroenterol*, **103**(12), 3219.

Sechi G, Serra A (2007). Wernicke's encephalopathy: new clinical settings and recent advances in diagnosis and management. *Lancet Neurol*, **6**(5), 442–55.

Singh S, Kumar A (2007). Wernicke encephalopathy after obesity surgery: a systematic review. *Neurology*, **68**(11), 807–11.

Summers DM, Collie DA, Zeidler M, Will RG (2004). The pulvinar sign in variant Creutzfeldt–Jakob disease. *Arch Neurol*, **61**(3), 446–7.

Tschampa HJ, Zerr I, Urbach H (2007). Radiological assessment of Creutzfeldt–Jakob disease. *Eur Radiol*, **17**(5), 1200–11.

Walker FO (2007). Huntington's disease. *Lancet*, **369**(9557), 218–28.

Walker J, Kepner A (2009). Wernicke's encephalopathy presenting as acute psychosis after gastric bypass. *J Emerg Med*,

Weidauer S, Nichtweiss M, Lanfermann H, Zanella FE (2003). Wernicke encephalopathy: MR findings and clinical presentation. *Eur Radiol*, **13**(5), 1001–9.

Will RG, Ironside JW, Zeidler M, *et al.* (1996). A new variant of Creutzfeldt–Jakob disease in the UK. *Lancet*, **347**(9006), 921–5.

Zeidler M, Johnstone EC, Bamber RW, *et al.* (1997a). New variant Creutzfeldt–Jakob disease: psychiatric features. *Lancet*, **350**(9082), 908–10.

Zeidler M, Stewart GE, Barraclough CR, *et al.* (1997b). New variant creutzfeldt-jakob disease: neurological features and diagnostic tests. *Lancet*, **350**(9082), 903–7.

Zeidler M, Sellar RJ, Collie DA, *et al.* (2000). The pulvinar sign on magnetic resonance imaging in variant Creutzfeldt–Jakob disease. *Lancet*, **355**(9213), 1412–18.

Case 24

Dizziness in someone with HIV

Nicholas W. S. Davies and Bruce J. Brew

Clinical history – main complaint

A 57-year-old right-handed man presents with a 1-year history of poor balance, increasing forgetfulness, and difficulties following conversations. His initial problem is that of intermittent episodes of dysequilibrium accompanied by nausea, particularly on standing or looking upwards. Between these short-lived attacks, he notices imbalance and a tendency to veer to one side when walking. After referral to a neurologist, the clinical diagnosis of a peripheral vestibular disorder is made. Subsequently, he reports slowing of his typing skills, deterioration in his handwriting and word finding difficulties, although none of his family or friends has noticed these problems. He describes feeling apathetic, but not depressed. Furthermore, he suffers increasingly frequent migrainous headaches with visual aura as well as urinary frequency and hesitancy.

General history

He is educated to higher degree level and works in a management position. He was diagnosed human immunodeficiency virus (HIV) positive 24 years before. He took anti-retroviral drugs for 6 years, only halting due to side effects 7 years before the onset of his neurological symptoms. His nadir CD4 count is 450 cells/μL. He is a non-smoker, drinks alcohol modestly, and does not use illicit drugs.

Family history

There is a family history of malignancy in two first-degree relatives. His mother suffers from Parkinson's disease.

Case Studies in Dementia: Common and Uncommon Presentations, ed. S. Gauthier and P. Rosa-Neto. Published by Cambridge University Press. © Cambridge University Press 2011.

Examination

The mini-mental test score is 30. Neurological examination reveals saccadic pursuit eye movements but no nystagmus, impaired fine finger movements, depressed ankle jerks, and impaired vibration and temperature sensation in both distal lower limbs. Tandem gait is markedly impaired. The vestibular ocular reflexes and vestibular ocular reflex suppression are normal and the Semont test, whilst provoking symptoms, leads to no nystagmus. General physical examination is unremarkable.

Special studies

MRI shows no focal atrophy or marked white matter change. However, MR spectroscopy of the deep frontal white matter and striatum reveals mildly reduced N-acetyl aspartate creatine ratios, mildly increased choline creatine ratios, but normal myoinositol creatine ratios.

Neuropsychological tests show evidence of impaired auditory attention span, auditory working memory, speed of information processing, psychomotor tracking, and cognitive flexibility.

His routine bloods tests including treponemal serology are unremarkable. His CD4 count is 640 cells/μL (above 500 cells/μL is normal) and plasma HIV-1 viral load is 57512 copies/mL. Cerebrospinal fluid (CSF) examination is abnormal. The CSF white blood cell count is elevated at 35 cells/μL of which polymorphonuclear cells predominated, CSF protein is 1.01 g/L, and CSF glucose 2.9 mmol/L compared with 5.5 mmol/L in blood. CSF neopterin is 122 nmol/L (normal range 0–13 nmol/L) and CSF beta-2-microglobulin 6.41 mg/L (normal range 0–2.2 mg/L). Gram's stain and India ink preparations reveal no organisms on microscopy and CSF Cryptococcal antigen is negative. CSF HIV viral load is 235832 copies/mL and resistance testing reveals fully sensitive HIV-1 subtype B (Fig. 24.1).

Diagnosis

AIDS dementia complex stage 1 or HIV associated neurocognitive disorder.

Follow-up

Combined anti-retroviral therapy (CART) consisting of high dose abacavir, lamivudine, and nevirapine is commenced. A repeat lumbar puncture performed 4 weeks after starting therapy showed the following improvements: CSF white cell count 6 cells/μL, CSF protein 0.80 g/L, CSF viral load 200 copies/mL, CSF

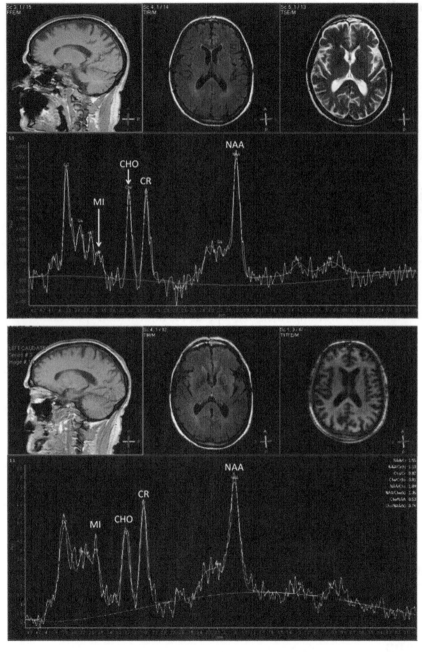

Fig. 24.1.   Magnetic resonance spectroscopy of the left caudate nucleus at presentation (above) and after 6 months antiretroviral therapy (below) showing initially mild reduction in the NAA creatine ratio and mild increase in choline creatine ratio, the latter that normalizes after 6 months. However, a rise in myoinositol creatine ratio is seen following 6 month's treatment. MI = myoinositol, CHO = choline, CR = creatine, NAA = *N*-acetyl aspartate.

neopterin 49 nmol/L and CSF beta-2-microglobulin 4.6 mg/L. After 6 months' treatment the patient notes substantial improvement in balance, headache frequency, energy levels, concentration, and memory. Neurological examination shows resolution of the gait and fine finger movement impairments. Repeat neuropsychological assessment demonstrates improvement in speed of information processing and psychomotor speed, cognitive flexibility, delayed visual recall, unstructured verbal learning, semantic fluency, and abstraction. However, many of these domains remain at levels beneath those expected pre-morbidly. Plasma HIV viral load by now is below the limit of assay detection (<50 copies/mL). Repeat MR spectroscopy shows improvement in the choline creatine ratios, but increase in the myoinositol creatine ratios, possibly reflecting gliosis.

Discussion

HIV is a human retrovirus that causes progressive immunosuppression accompanied by marked depletion of CD4 positive T-lymphocytes. Its neurological manifestations result either from direct infection of the nervous system by the virus or from CNS opportunistic infection, facilitated by immunosuppression, such as by JC virus or *Toxoplasma gondii*.

HIV associated neurocognitive disorder (HAND)

HAND is the currently approved term that encompasses the neurocognitive syndromes caused by HIV. HAND varies in severity from the asymptomatically neurocognitively impaired to those with dementia (Antinori *et al.*, 2007). Previously HIV neurocognitive impairment was classified into AIDS Dementia Complex stages 1 to 4 (Price and Brew, 1988), where stage 1 included those with milder deficits that did not preclude them from work. Prior to the advent of CART approximately 30% of patients with late-stage AIDS were demented. In the resource-rich world, since the arrival of CART, the incidence of dementia has fallen, but the prevalence has risen due to increased survival. Furthermore, the phenotype of HAND has altered with milder and fluctuating cognitive impairment increasingly recognized (Antinori *et al.*, 2007). Risk factors for the development of HIV dementia (HAD) include: persistently high viral load, low nadir CD4 cell count, increasing age and female sex, low body mass index, anaemia, and intravenous drug abuse (McArthur *et al.*, 2005).

Symptoms and signs

HAD is a subcortical dementia characterized by memory deficits, psychomotor slowing and behavioral changes (Brew, 2001). Cortical symptoms can occur later in the disease process. Typically, the symptoms evolve over months, but more acute presentations are reported. Patients usually have preserved insight into their condition and are able to describe their symptoms. The majority of patients report impaired concentration and often relate having to re-read passages or losing the thread of a conversation. Motor dysfunction is typically prominent with over half of patients noting increased clumsiness, particularly related to fine finger movements, for example, with the use of a keyboard or with handwriting. Increased apathy is common and accompanied by social withdrawal such as reduced interest in friends or hobbies. However, the dysphoria of depression is often absent. Rarely (~5%), the presenting feature of HAD is mania. On examination, impairment of smooth pursuit and saccadic eye movements, action tremor, brisk deep tendon reflexes, and frontal release signs can be found. Gait disturbance is frequent, often with marked impairment of heel-to-toe walking. Symptoms and signs of myelopathy and neuropathy become more frequent with increasing duration of HAD; however, urinary frequency and signs of a distal symmetrical sensory neuropathy are common at presentation. The mini-mental test score is usually unimpaired early in the disease process as the disorder is predominantly subcortical but often response times are slowed. Up to one-third of patients report increasing headache frequency with the onset of HAD.

Pathogenesis

The CNS damage underlying HAND occurs secondarily to the direct toxic action of virus-produced proteins and as a consequence of immune activation. It is thought that the bloodstream is the route of entry of HIV to the brain. Significantly, the majority of HIV found within the CNS is macrophage-tropic indicating that carriage within infected monocytes is likely to represent the "Trojan horse." HIV is able to infect a variety of cells within the CNS, including astrocytes, but productive infection occurs only within microglia and macrophages. The burden of histopathological change falls within the basal ganglia, and deep white matter. Affected brain tissue shows microscopically activated glia, occasional multinucleated giant cells, myelin pallor, loss of pyramidal cells, and evidence of synaptodendritic injury (Ellis *et al.*, 2009).

Investigations

Investigations are required to exclude CNS opportunistic infections and to establish definitively the diagnosis of HAD. Principle amongst these is neuroimaging with the modality of MRI; however, current imaging techniques underestimate HIV-related CNS damage when compared to post-mortem studies. The typical changes are of atrophy affecting both cortical and subcortical structures, which late in the disease can result in the appearance of *ex vacuo* hydrocephalus.

Deep white matter structures show frequently confluent, high-signal-intensity changes without mass effect on T2 FLAIR. These represent interstitial water rather than demyelination. Magnetic resonance spectroscopy can aid diagnosis by demonstrating reduced *N*-acetyl aspartate levels in keeping with neuronal injury, elevated choline secondary to astrocytosis, and elevated myoinositol (Thurnher and Donovan Post, 2008). Typically, areas of interest studied include the deep frontal white matter and caudate nuclei.

Patients presenting with suspected HAD should undergo CSF examination. CSF can show mild perturbations in CSF white cell count and protein levels, but hypoglychorrhachia is uncommon. Intrathecal immune activation is indicated by elevated levels of CSF neopterin and ß-2-microglobulin; the former being produced by activated monocytes, macrophages, and microglia, and the latter predominantly from cytotoxic T-lymphocytes (Brew and Letendre, 2008). Neither marker is specific for HAD. CSF HIV viral load correlates well with HAD severity in untreated patients. However, in CART-treated patients, HAD can occur despite the CSF HIV viral load being beneath assay detection limits. In some HAD patients, especially in those with previous exposure to antiretroviral drugs, HIV resistance patterns may differ between plasma and CSF; therefore in the presence of detectable viral load, testing should be performed on samples from both compartments.

Formal neuropsychological assessment aids but is not essential in the diagnosis of HAND.

Treatment and assessment of response

CART has transformed management of HIV. Currently, seven classes of antiretroviral drugs are licensed for treatment, each of which has a different mode of action and a range of side effects. Treatment of HIV requires combination use of drugs to which the virus is sensitive in order to prevent the development of resistance. However, treatment of HIV within the CNS requires specific attention, as the ability of different drugs to penetrate the CNS varies considerably. Drug regimens with a higher CNS penetration are associated with greater levels of suppression of CSF HIV viral load, which in turn is associated with more marked improvement in neuropsychological performance (Letendre *et al.*, 2004). Improvements in HAD associated with CART include not only suppression of CSF viral load but falls in CSF neopterin and ß-2-microglobulin, improvement and sometimes resolution of MRI white matter changes and MRS findings, although the latter may take in excess of 9 months. Furthermore, serial neuropsychological assessments are of particular use in monitoring response to therapy.

Learning points

This case illustrates several clinical learning points. First, the patient developed cognitive impairment despite a CD4 cell count at a level for which the probability of opportunistic infection is low and when CART would not routinely be initiated. Whilst the patient was not on CART at presentation, he had previously received antiretroviral treatment. It is recognized that, for patients on CART developing HAD, nadir CD4 cell count is of more predictive value for the development of cognitive impairment rather than the value at presentation (Robertson *et al.*, 2007). Second, at presentation the viral load was substantially greater when measured in the CSF than plasma demonstrating the importance of considering the CNS as an immunologically separate compartment. Third, in the early stages of HAD, symptoms other than memory impairment or motor dysfunction, such as dysequilibrium, can be domin-ant, yet the classical features of HAD can be found if sought. Fourth, the initial CSF revealed a polymorphonuclear pleocytosis, which though uncommon and alerts the clinician to other opportunistic infections, is not incompatible with the diagnosis of HAD. Fifth, the case illustrates that MR spectroscopy is a useful imaging adjunct to the diagnosis of HAD, particularly when routine MRI brain sequences show no typical abnormalities. Finally, the case illustrates that with appropriate CNS-penetrating CART substantial neurological improvement can occur.

Take home messages

HAD can occur at CD4 cell counts indicative of only moderate immunosuppression.

Appropriate CNS-penetrating CART can lead to substantial clinical improvement in HAD.

Magnetic resonance spectroscopy can aid clinical diagnosis of HAD.

REFERENCES AND FURTHER READING

Antinori A, Arendt G, Becker JT, *et al.* (2007). Updated research nosology for HIV-associated neurocognitive disorders. *Neurology*, **69**, 1789–99.

Brew BJ (2001). AIDS dementia complex. In *HIV Neurology*. New York: Oxford University Press, pp. 74–7.

Brew BJ, Letendre SL (2008). Biomarkers of HIV related central nervous system disease. *Int Rev Psychiatry*, **20**, 73–88.

Ellis RJ, Calero P, Stockin MD (2009). HIV infection and the central nervous system: a primer. *Neuropsychol Rev*, **19**, 144–51.

Letendre SL, McCutchan JA, Childers ME, *et al.* (2004). Enhancing antiretroviral therapy for human immunodeficiency virus cognitive disorders. *Ann Neurol*, **56**, 416–23.

McArthur JC, Brew BJ, Nath A (2005). Neurological complications of HIV infection. *Lancet Neurol*, **4**, 543–55.

Price RW, Brew BJ (1988). The AIDS dementia complex. *J Infect Dis*, **158**, 1079–83.

Robertson KR, Smurzynski M, Parsons TD, *et al.* (2007). The prevalence and incidence of neurocognitive impairment in the HAART era. *AIDS*, **21**, 1915–21.

Thurnher MM, Donovan Post MJ (2008). The uses of structural neuroimaging in the brain in HIV-1 infected patients. In *The Spectrum of Neuro-AIDS Disorders: Pathophysiology, Diagnosis and Treatment*. Washington: ASM Press, pp. 247–72.

Case of young man smoking pot but with a mother who died of dementia

Serge Gauthier, Pedro-Rosa Neto, Jean-Paul Soucy, and Gabriel Leonard

Clinical history – main complaint

A 30-year-old man was referred in 2001 to a neurologist because of memory complaints affecting his ability to perform at work as a cashier in a liquor store. The neurological examination was normal and the relatively mild findings on neuropsychological examination (see below) were blamed on anxiety and drug use (ectasy previously and marijuana currently).

In 2004, he was re-assessed with his wife. They concurred that his memory lapses were stable. His MMSE score was 27, the MoCA score was 28. The marriage ended in a divorce. Thereafter, he lived with a roommate who borrowed heavily from him. His father had to take care of his affairs.

In 2007 his employer had to transfer him to a less demanding position, stocking shelves and taking inventory. He had difficulty completing tasks when interrupted and was forgetting instructions by the time he needed to use them. In 2008 the MoCA had declined to 21.

General history

Thalassemia minor, with no clinical impact. Past use of ecstasy and of marijuana which ended in 2009.

Family history

His mother died at the age of 43 from a progressive dementia over 10 years confirmed at autopsy to be Gerstmann–Sträussler–Scheinker syndrome. This case was published, since both histological and neurochemical examinations were performed, demonstrating diffuse cortical neuronal loss, neuritic plaque, and status spongiosis of the neuropil, Kuru plaques in the parieto-occipital cortex and cerebellum, and reduced cortical choline-acetyl-transferase (CAT) activity in

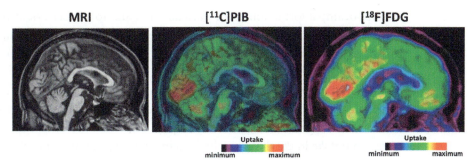

Fig. 25.1.   Sagittal PET [^{11}C]PIB (centre) and PET [^{18}F]FDG (right) uptake images superimposed on the MRI (right) images. Note increased [^{11}C]PIB uptake in the occipital cortex, pons and cerebellum (centre). Cerebellum and frontal cortex display low [^{18}F]FDG uptake (right).

the medial frontal cortex (Robitaille *et al.*, 1982). A mutation in the PRNP gene was not looked for at the time (1981), since the first observation of a heterogeneous mutation in the PRNP gene took place 8 years later (Hsiao *et al.*, 1989).

Examination

His latest assessment in 01/2010 showed some dysarthria, dragging of his left leg during ambulation, mild face bradykinesia, hyperreflexia of all four limbs, equivocal left plantar response, unsustained clonus of both ankles, and decreased foot tapping bilaterally. MMSE 26, MoCA 16.

Special studies

Blood tests showed that the plasma coeruloplasmin level was at 272 mg/L (220–480). The screen for HIV-1 and HIV-2 were both negative. Genetic studies were done in 2005, looking for alterations in the PRNP gene, which was not found.

Neuropsychological testing in 2001 showed a Full scale IQ of 116, Verbal IQ 125 and a Performance IQ of 105; learning of a list of 16 words was very poorly performed, delayed recall scores were impaired both cued and in free recall. A repeat assessment in 09/2008 and 02/2010 showed areas of significant deterioration.

FLAIR MRI of brain without enhancement in 12/2008 showed diffuse cerebral volume loss, including the cerebellum (Fig. 25.1, left). Multiplanar global imaging reformats demonstrated no particular pattern in the temporal lobes. [^{18}F]-FDG PET in 11/2008 showed mild decreased uptake in the cerebellum, especially in the right hemisphere. A repeat study in 01/2010 showed a marked deterioration of uptake in multiple cortical areas, including the temporal lobes (both laterally and the hippocampal formations), the parietal lobes and to a lesser extent the frontal lobes. The occipital cortex was relatively preserved, and the basal ganglia, thalamus and brain stem were unremarkable, but there was decreased activity in both cerebellar hemispheres.

A 11C-PIB PET scan in 02/2010 showed increased accumulation of the tracer with a cortical pattern, involving at a low level the frontal, temporal, and parietal cortices, with a much higher activity in the occipital regions. There was also significant increased uptake in the thalamus, brainstem, and cerebellum (Table 25.1).

Diagnosis

There was much hesitation in diagnosing a progressive neurodegenerative condition until 8 years into the symptoms, because of the use of marijuana and the dependant personality. The negative testing for the genetic abnormality most associated with his mother's condition was also detrimental to diagnosing his disease. The most recent findings of a mixed cerebellar, corticospinal, and dementing syndrome clearly suggest Gerstman–Sträussler syndrome.

Follow-up

It is proposed to offer the patient a trial of a cholinesterase inhibitor, considering the finding of a reduced cortical CAT activity in his mother's autopsy. The objective findings on neuroimaging allow him to obtain full medical disability for a well-defined neurological condition.

Discussion

This case illustrates the difficulties in diagnosing the presence and etiology of dementia in a young person, even when the family history is very suggestive of an autosomal dominant condition. The main confounding factors were the interpersonal relationship of the patient with his father, and the chronic use of marijuana. Only time was able to tell the neurodegenerative nature of his condition. A negative search for a mutation of the PRNP gene also delayed the diagnosis.

Gertsmann–Sträussler is a rare condition, first described in 1936 by Gerstman–Sträussler and Scheinker, characterized by dementia, amyloid deposits similar to Kuru plaques, and spongiform changes. There is heterogeneity within family members (Arata *et al.*, 2006).

Although the PIB scan showed a predominance of uptake in the occipital lobes (suggesting a high deposit of amyloid in that cortical area), there was a relative

Table 25.1. Neuropsychological test results

Test		2001	2008	2010
WAIS-3	Full Scale I.Q.	86th	16th	4th
	Verbal Scale I.Q.	95th	19th	5th
	Performance Scale I.Q.	63rd	14th	5th
	Verbal Comprehension Index		34th	25th
	Perceptual Organization Index		21st	10th
	Working Memory Index		1st	0.2
	Processing Speed Index		4th	1st
Vocabulary (WAIS-3)		95th	37th	37th
Information (WAIS-3)		90th	37th	16th
Boston Naming Test			41/60	38/60
Pyramids and Palm Trees			50/52	47/52
Phonemic Fluency (FAS)			1st	1st
Semantic Fluency			5th	0.8
Picture Completion (WAIS-3)			9th	2nd
Hooper Visual Organization Test (Score)			17.5/30	14/30
Block Design (WAIS-3)		55th	16th	16th
Rey Complex Figure – Copy			23.5/36	20/36
Immediate Memory Index (WMS-3)			4th	4th
General Memory Index (WMS-3)			0.2	0.1
Auditory Recognition Delayed Index (WMS-3)			0.4	0.4
California Verbal Learning Test–2	Total for 5 Trials	6th	2nd	0.4
	Trial 1	16th	16th	0.1
	Free Recall – Long Delay	0.1	2nd	0.1
	Recognition false positive errors	16th	30th	0.1
Digit Span			5th	0.4
Spatial Span			2nd	0.4
Digit Symbol (WAIS-3)			5th	2nd
Mental Control (WMS-3)			3rd	0.4
Mental Arithmetic (WAIS-3)			5th	2nd
Similarities (WAIS-3)		55th	37th	37th
Matrix Reasoning (WAIS-3)		73rd	63rd	50th
Wisconsin Card Sorting Test (Categories)			1	–
Tower of London -2	Total Moves		21st	0.6
	Total Time		12th	0.4
	Rule Breaks		61st	0.4
Grooved Pegboard (Seconds)	Left/Right Hand		90/79	99/96
Pinch Strength (lbs)	Left/Right Hand		23/24	22/25
Sequential Tapping (Score)	Left/Right Hand		55/58	49/47
	Both		10	13
Non-sequential Tapping (score)	Left/Right Hand		94/99	98/106

Sources: Entries refer to percentile scores unless otherwise specified; 2001 IQ scores were derived from the Wechsler Abbreviated Scale of Intelligence; ***WAIS-3:*** *Wechsler Adult Intelligence Scale*, 3rd edn; ***WMS-3:*** *Wechsler Memory Scale*, 3rd edn.

sparing of the occipital lobes on metabolic imaging using FDG-PET. This apparent dissociation has also been observed in Alzheimer's disease and is unexplained to this date.

Take home messages

Keep an open mind about the possibility of an underlying neurodegenerative disorder despite concurrent use of psychotropic substances.

Time tells the diagnosis.

Neuroimaging can help in diagnosis and management of early onset dementia.

REFERENCES AND FURTHER READING

Arata J, Takashima H, Hirano R, *et al.* (2006). Early clinical signs and imaging findings in Gerstmann–Sträussler-Scheinker syndrome (Pro102Leu). *Neurology,* **66**, 1672–8.

Hsiao K, Baker HF, Crow TJ, *et al.* (1989). Linkage of a prion protein missense variant to Gerstmann–Sträussler syndrome. *Nature,* **338**, 342–5.

Robitaille Y, Wood P, Etienne P, *et al.* (1982). Reduced cortical choline acetyltransferase activity in Gertsmann–Sträussler syndrome. *Prog NeuroPsychopharmacology,* **6**, 529–31.

University educated man with childish behavior

Ricardo Nitrini and Leonardo Caixeta

Clinical history – main complaint

A 39-year-old man, a human resource executive, was seen at the outpatient clinic of the Behavioral and Cognitive Neurology Unit of the Hospital das Clínicas, a public university hospital in São Paulo, Brazil. His wife reported that about 4 years before, she noticed that he was manifesting mild behavioral and personality changes characterized by irritability, a tendency for social withdrawal, together with a more rancorous and even mean personality trait. Progressively, he gave up drinking alcohol, which he used to consume in moderate amounts, and libido became extremely reduced. Then he started to complain of difficulties in his professional activities and to manifest obsessive-compulsive behaviors such as to demand for perfectly ironed clothes or to soap his body several times during bathing. He had an acute and rapidly reversible episode of paralysis of his legs and right arm. After a few months, he had another similar episode involving only the right side of the body, including face. He was seen by physicians and after several tests the diagnosis of probable viral meningitis was undertaken. Test for HIV-1 infection was reported to be negative.

He was dismissed from his job because he could not handle it any more. Ginkgo biloba and Hydergine[R] were prescribed. His behavior deteriorated to a more childish one with frequent cries when his demands were not immediately fulfilled. Although he had had the old habit of speaking aloud about his problems, this trait became very much increased and associated with intense gesticulations. More recently, his wife also noticed a decrease of his memory. The patient complained of lack of concentration and difficulties in organizing his activities.

General history

University educated man with no other medical problem.

Case Studies in Dementia: Common and Uncommon Presentations, ed. S. Gauthier and P. Rosa-Neto.
Published by Cambridge University Press. © Cambridge University Press 2011.

Family history

Father and mother were alive and well. A 50-year-old uncle from the maternal line has mental problems mainly characterized by apathetic behavior.

Examination

Physical examination showed a well-nourished man, with a blood pressure of 130/80 mmHg, and neurologic examination revealed only dysarthria, with normal and reactive pupils and normal reflexes. His insight about his problems seemed to be normal.

Special studies

Routine blood tests were normal. MRI showed enlargement of the sulci, fissures, and of the lateral ventricles consistent with diffuse brain atrophy. SPECT revealed slight hypoperfusion in the frontal cortex (Fig. 26.1).

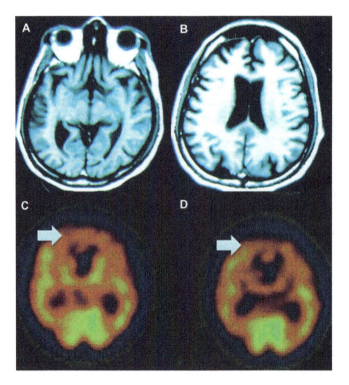

Fig. 26.1.   (a),(b) MRI shows enlargement of the sulci, fissures, and of the lateral ventricles. (c),(d) SPECT showing slight hypoperfusion in the frontal cortex (arrows).

In the initial neuropsychological evaluation he scored 29/30 in the Mini-Mental State Examination (he recalled 2 of the 3 words) (Folstein *et al.*, 1975; Brucki *et al.*, 2003). Digit-span was 4 in the forward and 3 in the backward sequence. Semantic verbal fluency (animals in one minute) was 31. In the Brief Cognitive Battery (Nitrini *et al.*, 1994, 2004), he was able to learn nine of the ten items, but free recall was low, with only five items, while he was able to recognize all ten items among 20 (with ten distractors). His performance in the clock drawing test was 10/10 (Sunderland *et al.*, 1989). In the Functional Activities Questionnaire (Pfeffer *et al.*, 1982), which is based on informant and where a score higher than 5 is common in dementia, he scored 3 when his wife informed he was unable to manage money. In a comprehensive neuropsychological evaluation he scored 136/144 in the Dementia Rating Scale (Mattis, 1988; Porto *et al.*, 2003), with more difficulties in the construction and conceptualization subscales. His performance was more severely disturbed in the copy of Rey's figure (Rey, 1970), Trail Making A and B (Reitan, 1959), and in the Wisconsin Card Sorting test (Grant and Berg, 1980). In the Logical Memory of the Wechsler Memory Scale Revised (Wechsler, 1987), his score was rated as the 10th percentile in part I and 5th percentile in part II. However, his performance was normal in the Rey Auditory Verbal Learning Test as well as in Hooper visual organization, Hooper Boston Naming test (Hooper, 1983) and in semantic and phonemic (FAS) verbal fluency tests. In conclusion, his performance revealed concentration and memory impairments together with decreased resistance to interference and response inhibition, which were indicative of frontal executive dysfunction. The cerebrospinal fluid (CSF) analysis showed pleocytosis with 45 leukocytes/mm^3, mainly lymphocytes, total protein of 70 mg/dL with 39.6% gammaglobulin (normally protein is below 40 mg/dL and gammaglobulin below 13% of the total protein), glucose of 42 mg/dL, VDRL, and *Treponema pallidum* hemagglutination assay (TPHA; 1:512) were positive.

Diagnosis

The initial diagnostic impression was a Frontotemporal Dementia (FTD), but the final diagnosis was of paretic dementia, a neuropsychiatric condition caused by neurosyphilis.

Follow-up

He was treated with intravenous aqueous crystalline penicillin G, 4 million units every 4 hours for 21 days, and with fluoxetine. Lumbar puncture performed three months after treatment showed only 2 lymphocytes/mm^3, normal protein, negative VDRL and positive TPHA with a high titer (1:1024). These CSF findings were indicative of successful treatment. One year later, CSF was normal except for a slightly elevated level of gammaglobulins (21.6%) and still positive TPHA. However, during a 8-year follow-up period, his executive dysfunction did not improve and he had episodes of depression, increased anxiety, and even delusions with persecutory ideation. Insight was well preserved, as it is possible to notice from the patient's own written report 3 years after treatment: "My reasoning is very slow. My lack of attention and anxiety are at a high level. When I receive much information at the same time, I confound them, I have difficulties in understanding. When I learn one procedure, or have an idea or planned something, and I am faced with different or adverse situations, it takes me a long time to reorganize my thoughts and to analyze the new situation. This makes me extremely angry." In a neuropsychological evaluation performed 8 years after treatment he scored 140/144 in the Dementia Rating Scale, but he still had executive dysfunctions, mainly on tasks demanding attention, response inhibition, mental flexibility, and planning.

He has been unable to go back to work or to have an independent life.

Discussion

FTD or behavioral subtype of frontotemporal lobar degeneration was the initial diagnosis in this case because the clinical picture was dominated by insidious onset of personality and behavioral changes, and neuropsychological evaluation confirmed the presence of frontal or frontotemporal involvement (Neary *et al.*, 1998). MRI and SPECT were initially interpreted as indicative of a degenerative dementia. The report that his 50-year-old uncle had cognitive and behavioral disturbances mainly characterized by mania was supportive of this initial hypothesis.

Nevertheless, there were a few pieces of evidence that did not conform to this diagnosis. The age of onset, although compatible with the diagnosis of FTD, was lower than the usual, which is around 58 years at diagnosis (Viskontas and Miller, 2009). The reports of two episodes of rapidly reversible paralysis that could be of vascular or less probably of epileptic origin, and of the diagnosis of "viral meningitis," were definitely uncommon for FTD. The relative preservation of insight was also very rare in FTD, and finally, dysarthria is not common in FTD.

Conversely, most of these events are frequent in paretic neurosyphilis, the most common cause of dementia in neurosyphilis, with most cases occurring in the 35–50-year age range (Merritt *et al.*, 1946). Although the clinical picture of paretic neurosyphilis is characterized by relatively slowly progressive personality and mood changes, together with cognitive decline, occasionally a reversible stroke or a seizure may occur as the initial manifestation or during the evolution, with the patient returning to his previous condition after the episode (Merritt *et al.*, 1946; Nitrini, 2008). Moreover, dysarthria is one of the most common neurological signs of this condition (Merritt *et al.*, 1946; Storm-Mathisen, 1978). Other neurologic signs that are common in paretic dementia include pupillary abnormalities, tremors in the lips and tongue and hyperactive deep reflexes. However, in many cases no physical signs may be disclosed even by the most thorough neurologic examination (Merritt *et al.*, 1946). The diagnosis of viral or aseptic meningitis may be wrongly done if the tests for syphilis are not performed in CSF. In this case, we could not locate the first CSF examination, but it is highly probable that tests for syphilis were not done at that time.

The diagnosis was finally confirmed by the CSF showing positive VDRL and TPHA tests together with pleocytosis, and increased concentration of protein with high percentage of gammaglobulins. Increased levels of gammaglobulin, mostly IgG, is common in paretic dementia and low glucose level may sometimes occur in this condition (Nitrini and Spina-França, 1987).

The patient was treated with high doses of penicillin and after 3 months the CSF was almost normal. After successful treatment, CSF leukocyte count should be normal 6 months after treatment. The other abnormalities may take longer to normalize, but if the CSF is not normal at 2 years, retreatment should be considered (Marra, 2009). Exceptions are the CSF–treponemal tests that may be positive many years after successful treatment.

Dementia may also occur in neurosyphilis due to multiple infarcts, but in this case this hypothesis was ruled out because the neurologic examination revealed only dysarthria and the MRI did not demonstrate infarcts. MRI showed cortical and subcortical atrophy, the usual finding in paretic neurosyphilis. The pathogenesis of the cortical and subcortical atrophy of paretic neurosyphilis, which is more severe in the frontal and temporal lobes, is attributed to the narrowing and occlusion of smaller capillaries and venules by intimal proliferation (Merritt *et al.*, 1946).

Another interesting finding in this case was his preserved insight and the normal verbal fluency together with other clear signs of frontal dysfunction. The dissociation between the presence of executive dysfunction and preserved insight corroborates the notion that different areas of the frontal cortex are responsible for these functions (Harwood *et al.*, 2005).

As paretic neurosyphilis is becoming a relatively rare disease, the likelihood of incorrect or late diagnosis tends to increase. This is regrettable because, when treatment is initiated at the beginning of the symptoms, there is a reasonable chance of complete cure. However, if treatment is postponed, as happened in this case, the progression is interrupted, but the chance of a complete recovery is small.

The American Academy of Neurology guidelines for the diagnosis of dementia propose that screening for syphilis in patients with dementia is not justified unless clinical suspicion for neurosyphilis is present (Knopman *et al.*, 2001). However, neurosyphilis has long been recognized as a "great imitator" and the clinical diagnosis may be very difficult because "pure psychiatric cases" may be found or other diagnoses may be entertained. In the developing world, neurosyphilis is a not infrequent cause of dementia (Takada *et al.*, 2003; Timermans and Carr, 2004) and screening for syphilis is still necessary in the diagnosis of dementia (Nitrini *et al.*, 2005).

To rule out the diagnosis of neurosyphilis in a case of dementia is relatively simple. Treponemal tests, such as the Fluorescent Treponemal Antibody-Absorbed (FTA-Abs), TPHA or ELISA rule out neurosyphilis when negative in blood. The non-treponemal tests, such as the VDRL or rapid plasma reagin test or the old Wassermann complement fixation, may be negative in neurosyphilis when performed in the blood test. Contrariwise, the confirmation of the diagnosis may be more difficult and is always based on the CSF examination. A positive CSF–VDRL confirms the diagnosis of neuropsyphilis but its sensibility is not too high, with cases of paretic neurosyphilis showing persistent negative CSF VDRL (Lee *et al.*, 2005). The CSF–treponemal tests have very high sensibility with low specificity because treponemal antibodies may pass through the blood-brain barrier. When the CSF–VDRL is negative and the CST–FTA-Abs or other treponemal test is positive, the diagnosis of neurosyphilis is supported by the presence of pleocytosis and elevated CSF protein in the absence of other known causes of these abnormalities (Marra, 2009).

Take home messages

Neurosyphilis may cause dementia with features that are similar to those of the degenerative diseases. To confirm this diagnosis, CSF is indispensable, but it is necessary to take into account that CSF-VDRL may be negative in cases of neurosyphilis.

REFERENCES AND FURTHER READING

Brucki SMD, Nitrini R, Caramelli P, Bertolucci PHF, Okamoto IH (2003). [Suggestions for utilization of the Mini-mental state examination in Brazil]. *Arq Neuropsiquiatr*, **61**, 777–81.

Folstein MF, Folstein SE, McHugh PR (1975). "Mini-mental state". A practical method for grading the cognitive state of patients for the clinician. *J. Psychiatr Res*, **12**, 189–98.

Grant DA, Berg E (1980). *The Wisconsin Card Sort Test Random Layout: Directions for Administration and Scoring.* Madison, Wisconsin: Wells Printing.

Harwood DG, Sultzer DL, Feil D, Monserratt L, Freedman E, Mandelkern MA (2005). Frontal lobe hypometabolism and impaired insight in Alzheimer disease. *Am J Geriatr Psychiatry,* **13,** 934–41.

Hooper H (1983). *The Hooper Visual Organization Test (VOT) Manual.* Los Angeles: Western Psychological Services.

Kaplan E, Goodglass H, Weintraub S (1983). *The Boston Naming Test.* Philadelphia: Lea and Febiger.

Knopman DS, DeKosky ST, Cummings JL, *et al.* (2001). Practice parameter: diagnosis of dementia (an evidence-based review). Report of the Quality Standards Subcommittee of the American Academy of Neurology. *Neurology,* **56,** 1143–53.

Lee JW, Wilck M, Venna N (2005). Dementia due to neurosyphilis with persistent negative CSF VDRL. *Neurology,* **65,** 1838.

Malloy-Diniz LF, Lasmar VAP, Gazinelli LZR, Fuentes D, Salgado JV (2007). The Rey Auditory–Verbal Learning Test: applicability for the Brazilian elderly population. *Rev Bras Psiquiatr,* **29,** 324–9.

Marra CM (2009). Update on neurosyphilis. *Curr Infect Dis Rep,* **11,** 127–34.

Mattis S (1988). *Dementia Rating Scale Professional Manual.* Florida: Psychological Assessment Resources.

Merritt HH, Adams RD, Solomon HC (1946). *Neurosyphilis.* New York: Oxford University Press.

Neary D, Snowden JS, Gustafson L. *et al.* (1998). Frontotemporal lobar degeneration: a consensus on clinical diagnostic criteria. *Neurology,* **51,** 1546–54.

Nitrini R, Caramelli P, Bottino CM, Damasceno BP, Brucki SM, Anghinah R (2005). [Diagnosis of Alzheimer's disease in Brazil: diagnostic criteria and auxiliary tests. Recommendations of the Scientific Department of Cognitive Neurology and Aging of the Brazilian Academy of Neurology]. *Arq Neuropsiquiatr,* **63,** 713–19.

Nitrini R, Caramelli P, Herrera E Jr, *et al.* (2004). Performance of illiterate and literate nondemented elderly subjects in two tests of long-term memory. *J Int Neuropsychol Soc,* **10,** 634–8.

Nitrini R, Lefèvre BH, Mathias SC, *et al.* (1994). [Neuropsychological tests of simple application for diagnosing dementia]. *Arq Neuropsiquiatr,* **52,** 457–65.

Nitrini R, Spina-França A (1987). [Intravenous penicillin therapy in high doses in neurosyphilis: study of 62 cases. II. Evaluation of cerebrospinal fluid]. *Arq Neuropsiquiatr,* **45,** 231–41.

Nitrini R (2008). Clinical and therapeutic aspects of dementia in syphilis and Lyme disease. In C Duyckaerts, I Litvan (eds.), *Dementias. Handbook of Clinical Neurology.* Edinburgh; Elsevier, vol. **89,** pp. 819–23.

Pfeffer RI, Kusosaki TT, Harrah CH Jr, Chance JM, Filos S (1982). Measurement of functional activities in older adults in the community. *J Gerontol,* **37,** 323–9.

Porto, CS, Charchat-Fichman, H, Caramelli, P, Bahia, VS, Nitrini, R (2003). Brazilian version of the Mattis Dementia Rating Scale: diagnosis of mild dementia in Alzheimer's disease. *Arq Neuropsiquiatr,* **61,** 339–45.

Reitan RM (1959). Correlations between the trail-making test and the Wechsler–Bellevue scale. *Percept Motor Skills,* **9**, 127–30.

Rey A (1970). *L'examen clinique en psychologie.* Paris: Presses Universitaires de France.

Storm-Mathisen A (1978). Syphilis. In PJ Vinken, GW Bruyn (eds.), *Infections of the Nervous System,* part I. *Handbook of Clinical Neurology.* Amsterdam: Elsevier, vol. **33**, pp. 337–94.

Sunderland T, Hill JL, Mellow AM, *et al.* (1989). Clock drawing in Alzheimer's disease: a novel measure of dementia severity. *J Am Geriatr Soc,* **37**, 725–9.

Takada LT, Caramelli P, Radanovic M, *et al.* (2003). Prevalence of potentially reversible dementias in a dementia outpatient clinic of a tertiary university-affiliated hospital in Brazil. *Arq Neuropsiquiatr,* **61**, 925–9.

Timermans M, Carr J (2004). Neurosyphilis in the modern era. *J Neurol Neurosurg Psychiatry,* **75**, 1727–30.

Viskontas IK, Miller BL (2009). Frontotemporal dementia. In B.L.B.F. Boeve (eds.), *The Behavioral Neurology of Dementia.* Cambridge: Cambridge University Press.

Wechsler D (1987). *Manual for the Wechsler Memory-revised.* San Antonio, Texas: The Psychological Corporation.

Workowski KA, Berman SM (2006). Sexually transmitted diseases treatment guidelines 2006. *MMWR Recomm Rep,* **55**, 1–94.

Frontotemporal lobar dementia vs. solvent intoxication: A piece that does not fit the puzzle

Louis Verret and Rémi W. Bouchard

Clinical history – main complaint

A 43-year-old male was referred to our Memory Clinic by a psychiatrist to evaluate the possibility of Frontotemporal Lobar Dementia (e.g., Frontal Dementia, Pick's Disease). He had suffered for 4 years with personality changes including attention difficulties, slowing of thoughts, apathy, loss of energy, planning difficulties, and diminished socialization. Those changes were noted by his spouse and had significant impact on his work. The symptoms had evolved rapidly at the beginning, but had been stable over the last 3 years. Structural imaging was normal. An abnormal PET-Scan prompted the psychiatrist to refer the patient to a neurologist. Adult Attention Deficit Disorder, depression, and drug abuse had been considered by previous clinicians, but ruled out after treatment trials and follow-up.

General history

The patient is highly educated, is in general good health, is married and lives with his wife and two children. He works as a mechanic and owns his own small automobile repair business; he is mainly involved in restoring antique cars and repainting them in the original color. At the time of the initial consult at the Memory Clinic, the patient was under no medication.

Family history

No family history of neuro-degenerative disorder or psychiatric ilness. His sister suffered from a brain tumor.

Case Studies in Dementia: Common and Uncommon Presentations, ed. S. Gauthier and P. Rosa-Neto. Published by Cambridge University Press. © Cambridge University Press 2011.

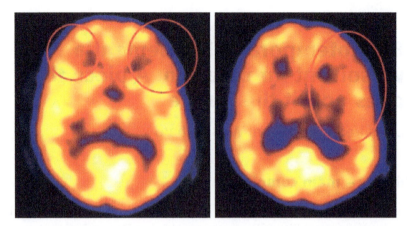

Fig. 27.1.   Two FDG PET-scan axial slices of the patient. This first PET study shows moderate hypometabolism in the left frontal lobe, and mild hypometabolism in the right. This study prompted referral to our Memory Clinic with a diagnosis of Frontotemporal Lobar Degeneration.

Examination

Normal vital signs. Normal physical and neurological examination. No frontal release sign. MMSE 29/30 (−1 for recall). MoCA 27/30 (−1 for the clock drawing, −1 in serial 7s, −1 for lexical verbal fluency). Luria motor and graphical tests were normal. Abstraction with similarities and differences were normal. 27 on the Frontal Behavioral Inventory (FBI) (Kertesz, 1997) mainly on items involving inertia and apathy. Language was normal.

Special studies

Screening blood tests were normal. Syphilis and HIV serology were negative.

MRI scan was normal; no focal atrophy.

Initial Pet-scan showed hypometabolism in the left fronto-parietal region and the right frontal region, felt to be compatible with frontal dementia by the nuclear medicine specialist (Fig. 27.1).

Neuropsychological evaluation revealed a general cognitive functioning within normal limits, but weaknesses (maximum of −1.5 SD from normal means) in some executive functions such as abstraction, attention/concentration, and working memory. No behavioral change, like the one seen in frontal cortical degeneration (disinhibition, loss of insight, loss of hygiene, familiarity, improper social conduct, modified eating habits. . .) was noted.

Diagnosis

Disease progression had been stable over the last few years before the visit to our Memory Clinic. Despite the personality changes noted by the spouse, there was an absence of behavioral and executive symptoms, and language difficulty on neurocognitive screening tests and formal neuropsychological evaluation. We felt that the patient did not fit the usual profile, or meet accepted criteria, for a diagnosis of Fronto-Temporal Lobar Dementia (Frontal Dementia or Pick's disease) of any subtype. Despite the Pet-scan result, this diagnosis was thought unlikely.

This prompted us to get back to square one, and look further at his history. This revealed that the patient had suffered from possible acute solvent intoxications many years before (acute bouts of light headedness, nausea, and headache). He claimed he then had an adequate ventilation system installed. These bouts of acute symptoms resolved afterwards.

The current symptoms had appeared a few years later. Although stable, the cognitive symptoms were such that the patient could not maintain work on a steady schedule: he and his wife mentioned they got slightly better after a few days off work. Also, the patient mentioned a mild dull headache while at work, that would resolve at home.

We felt that the most likely diagnosis was a solvent-induced chronic toxic encephalopathy. The exposure was caused by the paints used to repaint the antique cars.

Diagnosis: *Mild Chronic Toxic encephalopathy (type II)* (**WHO 1985**) **also known as** *Neurotoxic Solvent Encephalopathy type 2b* (**Cranmer and Goldberg, 1986**).

We consulted a specialist in Occupational Medicine, who agreed with our diagnostic hypothesis. No blood or urine tests are reliable for chronic solvent intoxication.

Follow-up

The patient was taken out of his job environment. On the follow-up visit 11 months later, he felt improved significantly, but still complained of lack of energy and attention difficulties. When he tried returning to his previous professional duties doing mechanics and paint, he experienced readily mild acute intoxication symptoms. This is probably caused by hypersensitivity to chemicals associated with chronic solvent intoxication. He could nevertheless return to work, but attending only to office duties.

A second Pet-Scan was performed 9 months after the first one, and the result was *normal* (Fig. 27.2).

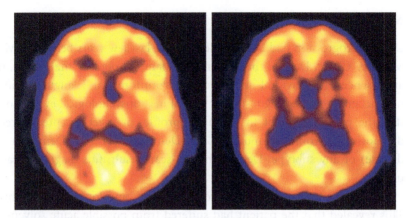

Fig. 27.2.   Two FDG PET-scan axial slices, at the same level as in Fig. 27.1. This repeat PET study, performed 9 months later, demonstrates normalization of the previously found metabolism defects, after withdrawal from the work environment where chronic solvent exposure occurred.

Repeat neuropsychological evaluation showed some improvement in the mild difficulties in executive function tests, but some results remained slightly below the norms.

Discussion

Solvents are widely used in many industrial processes in our society. Exposition may be through professional occupation or contaminated environment. Since these agents are used to dissolve fatty substances, they easily penetrate cell membranes and they cross the blood–brain barrier. They can affect the central or peripheral nervous system, either acutely or chronically, depending on the degree and length of exposure. If the central nervous system is affected, patients usually complain of fatigue, confusion or depression, and may describe memory difficulties. Patients may also describe loss of libido, increased sensitivity to alcohol and intolerance to chemical agents. Clinical evaluation should include history of exposure, which is sometimes difficult to establish with accuracy. Objective measurement at the work place is seldom available. Suggested investigation may warrant neuropsychological and imaging techniques (White and Proctor, 1997). Neuropsychological testing in case series demonstrated variable profiles of cognitive dysfunction. Structural imaging techniques revealed in some cases white matter changes. Functional imaging (SPECT scan) showed inconsistent areas of hypoperfusion (frontal and temporal lobes, thalamus, basal ganglia, and cerebellum). One case report of PET scan in a remote history of exposure to solvents reported grossly abnormal hypometabolism in frontal, hippocampal, and parietal regions. To our knowledge, there is no report in the literature of reversible functional neuroimaging in cases of chronic solvent intoxication after withdrawal of exposition. Susceptibility to chronic solvent encephalopathy is likely linked to genetic polymorphism of liver enzymes (Kesic *et al.*, 2006).

Diagnostic workout and differential diagnosis of cognitive complaints and dementia: a structured and systematic approach is mandatory. It should be performed bearing in mind to look for potentially reversible causes, even more so in young subjects where responsibilities towards family, work, income, productivity are at stake (Ridha and Josephs, 2006).

Well-performed, thorough and step-by-step history taking, preferably with a reliable informant, then general and neurological examination, including cognitive screening tests, are the first steps to investigate such complaints, and should be regarded as the first and most important "investigational" procedures.

Clinicians involved in the evaluation and care of subjects presenting cognitive complaints should have a good knowledge of the general profile and consensus criteria for the major degenerative dementia. The cognitive profile should be outlined precisely, e.g., episodic memory impairment is typical of Alzheimer's disease; visuospatial disturbances may occur early in Lewy Body Dementia. A precise outline of the cognitive deficits will help in localizing the lesion or area of dysfunction in the brain, and match with specific diagnosis.

Clinicians should also possess a wide differential diagnosis for cognitive deficits and dementia. The differential diagnosis should orient the clinical assessment as it progresses, e.g., episodic memory impairment is typical of Alzheimer's disease, but could be seen in limbic encephalitis; visuospatial disturbances can occur early in Lewy Body Dementia, but are also seen in Posterior Cortical Atrophy. Remember that, even in young subjects (30–64-year-old), "common" causes of dementia represent more than 75% of all the cases (Sampson *et al.*, 2004).

Onset and course of symptoms will aid with the pathophysiology: insidious onset and slow progression in neuro-degenerative disorders, acute onset in vascular disorders, subacute course in neoplastic diseases. . .

With the recent findings of genes involved in neurodegenerative dementias (mutations in the Amyloid Precursor Protein, Presinilin 1 and 2 for Alzheimer's disease; mutations on chromosome 17 for FTLD. . .), family history is important, particularly in young subjects.

Occupational and habits questionnaire should be thorough, and focus should be put on chemical exposure, drug use, sexually hazardous behavior . . .

A systematic review of other neurological symptoms and thorough physical examination should be performed. Extrapyramidal signs could point towards Lewy Body Dementia; chorea might suggest Huntington's disease; downward supranuclear gaze palsy may suggest Progressive Supranuclear palsy.

Other systemic illness should also be considered. For example:

- Cardiovascular system: ischemic heart disease, associated with vascular risk factors, predisposes to vascular dementia.
- Respiratory system: lung cancer could lead to a paraneoplastic encephalitis.
- Gastro-intestinal system: abdominal pain and malabsorption could raise the possibility of Whipple disease.
- Psychiatry: hallucinations are early symptoms of Lewy Body Dementia and limbic encephalitis.
- etc.

B. Ridha and K. A. Josephs, in their article (Ridha and Josephs, 2006), give us an excellent, thorough, and in-depth view of the investigation and differential diagnosis of cognitive complaints and dementia.

This meticulous "detective's work" will generate many hypotheses, guiding the rest of the investigation. Each test will then help eliminate or support diagnostic hypothesis. Sometimes, the results will be inconclusive. One should not forget that time is our ally: if treatable causes are eliminated, and degenerative etiology is contemplated, follow-up will often help in the clarification of the clinical picture, and repeated investigational procedures will become positive.

Regarding degenerative dementia, no biomarker or imaging procedure has proven to be 100% accurate. Caution should always be taken in assessing the results. When the clinical picture does not fit the result of investigational procedure, the former should prevail, and longitudinal follow-up is mandatory.

Practice parameters and consensus guidelines (*Alzheimer's and Dementia*, 2007; Knopman *et al.*, 2001) have been published to guide physicians in the investigation of dementia in the elderly. These usually include basic blood tests (vitamin B12, Thyroid function test. . .) and neuro-imaging (CT-scan), mainly to rule out potentially reversible factors contributing to the cognitive decline.

When facing an atypical and/or potentially reversible dementia, investigation should continue, eliminating the most probable causes one at a time: infectious (lumbar puncture, syphilis serology in blood and CSF, HIV, serology, . . .), genetic (FTLD and tau mutations. . .), autoimmune (paraneoplastic syndrome and anti-neuronal antibodies assay, VGKC antibodies assay. . .) (Ridha and Josephs, 2006).

Take home messages

This case shows the importance of a systematic and structured approach to cognitive complaints and dementia evaluation.

It also outlines the importance of knowing the typical profiles and consensus criteria for the major dementing illnesses. Differential diagnosis should be broad, even more so when addressing a young patient, when employment is at stake.

There is, to date, no reliable biomarker, including imaging studies that can be diagnostic of the major degenerative dementia. Their results should always be interpreted in light of the full clinical picture.

Chronic solvent encephalopathy should be included in the broad differential diagnosis of patients presenting cognitive complaints of any sort (memory, problem solving, visuospatial, personality. . .), and occupational history should always be sought.

Acknowledgments

We would like to thank Doctor Pierre Auger, Occupational Medicine, and Doctor Bernard Lefebvre, Nuclear Medicine, for their excellent clinical help.

REFERENCES AND FURTHER READING

Cranmer JM, Goldberg J (1986). Proceedings of the Workshop on Neurobehavioral Effects of Solvents. October 13–16, 1985, Raleigh, North Carolina, USA. Human aspects of solvent neurobehavioral effects. *Neurotoxicology*, **7**(4), 1–123.

Kertesz A, Davidson W, Fox H (1997). Frontal behavioral inventory: diagnostic criteria for frontal lobe dementia. *Can J Neurol Sci*, **24**(1), 29–36.

Kesic S, Calkoen F, Wenker MA, Jacobs JJ, Verberk MM (2006). Genetic polymorphism of metabolic enzymes modifies the risk of chronic solvent-induced encephalopathy. *Toxicol Ind Health*, **22**, 281–9.

Knopman DS, deKosky S, Cummings J, *et al.* (2001). Practice parameter: diagnosis of dementia (an evidence-based review). Report of the Quality Standards Subcommittee of the American Academy of Neurology. *Neurology*, **56**(9), 1143–53.

Ridha B, Josephs KA (2006). Young-onset dementia: a practical approach to diagnosis. *The Neurologist*, **12**, 2–13.

Sampson EL, Warren JD, Rossor MN (2004). Young onset dementia. *Postgrad Med J*, **80**, 125–39.

White RF, Proctor SP (1997). Solvents and neurotoxicity. *Lancet*, **349**, 1239–43.

WHO (World Health Organization)–Nordic Council of Ministers (1985). Organic Solvents and the Central Nervous System: chronic effects of organic solvents on the central nervous system and diagnostic criteria. EHS Copenhagen Denmark WHO–Nordic Council of Ministers 1985;1–39 WHO, Copenhagen.

Case 28

Man with difficulty keeping pace

Bert-Jan Kerklaan and Philip Scheltens

Clinical history

A 60-year-old man complained of stumbling for 2 years without dizziness or stiffness of the legs. One year before, he was unable to retrieve his car. Memory impairment and poor organization strategies led to mistakes in his work as an accountant in a travel agency, necessitating constant supervision. He assumed these deficits were related to emotional disturbances after the death of his mother 4 years earlier. Recently, he noticed incontinence for urine for which he started using diapers.

His spouse noticed slowness of thought and memory impairment starting 2.5 years before. She finally took over his work in the travel agency when these deficits progressed. She has recently noticed that he becomes apathetic and gets lost frequently. As he tends to fall when stumbling, she needs to keep a constant eye on him. Their relationship is under stress as he appears to be more stubborn and agitated. He refuses to use a walking aid.

Three years before he had been diagnosed with polyneuropathy elsewhere. One year later he had been re-examined because of stumbling and memory impairment. A neuropsychological examination and a MRI scan of the brain were performed and a diagnosis of vascular dementia and muscle disease of unknown origin was made. At that time his Mini-Mental State Examination (MMSE) score was 28/30. He then started taking aspirin, folic acid, and simvastatin. A year later he underwent a diagnostic procedure in our center.

General history

The patient is a highly educated man who has practiced accountancy all his life. He is married and assists his wife running a travel agency. They have no children. His previous medical history states benign prostate hyperplasia and he uses no medication besides the pills mentioned. He doesn't smoke and rarely uses alcohol.

Case Studies in Dementia: Common and Uncommon Presentations, ed. S. Gauthier and P. Rosa-Neto. Published by Cambridge University Press. © Cambridge University Press 2011.

Family history

The patient was the only child of a mother who was of Jewish descent and died when she was around 80 years old. He remembers that she developed memory impairment at an advanced age and was demented before she died. Also, he remembers she had high-arched feet, "a bit like my own." He did not know his father well, other than that he was possibly Jewish too and had been healthy.

Examination

The patient looks healthy on examination.

There is an impression of mild dementia on neurocognitive examination with obvious slowness of mental processing. The knowledge of actual events is limited and the head-turning sign is positive. On MMSE, the patient scores 27 out of 30, missing memory items. The score on the Frontal Assessment Battery is 15 out of 18 with decreased letter fluency. He just draws a circle when a clock is asked.

Neurological examination of the upper body and head is unremarkable. The legs are normotone. His feet are high-arched, and power in the flexor and extensor muscles of the feet is diminished to grade MRC 4 on the left side and grade MRC 3 on the right side with an inverse position of the right foot. Sensations of vibration and position are absent in both feet up to the ankles. There is general hyperreflexia in arms and legs except for Achilles tendon reflexes that could not be elicited. Both plantar responses are extensor. Heel-to-knee test and finger-to-nose test show no abnormalities, and Romberg sign is negative. The gait, however, has a broad base and movements appear spastic with the tendency to walk on the toes with circumduction.

Special studies

Routine laboratory testing is unremarkable with a normal level of vitamin B12. CSF studies, including amyloid-beta, tau, and tau phosphorylated at threonine 181, show no abnormalities.

EEG shows a normal background rhythm with alpha 9,5 Hz and bilateral temporal irregularities of no significance. EMG shows significant polyneuropathy of the axonal type. During extensive neuropsychological examination obvious slowness, memory impairment, and executive functioning are registered. Brain MRI shows considerable abnormalities; multifocal and confluent white matter hyperintensities are seen around the ventricles and in the deep white matter on

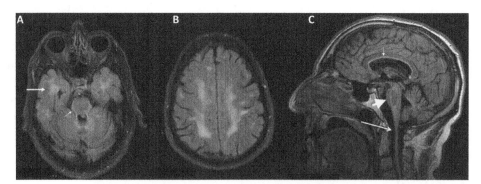

Fig. 28.1.   (a) Axial MRI FLAIR (a) showing white matter hyperintensities in the temporal lobes. (long arrow). The corticospinal tract, tegmentum, and border of the pons (short arrow) is affected, the center of the pons is not. (b) Axial MRI T2 sequence shows multifocal white matter hyperintensities with U-fibers degradation. (c) Sagittal MRI FLAIR showing a hypersignal in the lower border of the corpus callosum (short thin arrow) and the corticospinal tract in the pons (short thick arrow). The basis pontis is unaffected. The long thin arrow indicates atrophy of the cervical spinal cord.

T2-weighted images. The white matter in the temporal lobes and the lower border of the corpus callosum is affected, just like the crus posterior of the capsula interna and externa and the corticospinal tract in the pons. The tegmentum pontis including medial lemniscus is affected, but the basis pontis is spared. In combination with white matter abnormalities in the medulla oblongata a characteristic pattern is seen on sagittal T2-weighted and Fluid-Attenuated Inversion-Recovery (FLAIR) images. The cervical spinal cord appears atrophic without white matter involvement. Clinical findings in combination with the typical pattern of white matter involvement on the MRI scan prompted us to measure the activity of Glycogen Branching Enzyme (GBE) in leukocytes. With 25nmol/min per mg, this activity is deficient as the normal range extends from 149–347 nmol/min/mg. Next, DNA of the patient is examined looking for specific mutations. Our patient is found to be homozygous for Y329S, a mutation on chromosome 3.

Diagnosis

Adult Polyglucosan Body Disease (APBD). This is a rare hereditary metabolic disorder. Features of this disease are the combination of slowly progressive cognitive deficits, bipyramidal disorder with incontinence for urine and polyneuropathy. The clue to his diagnosis is the typical pattern of cerebral white matter involvement on MRI (Fig. 28.1).

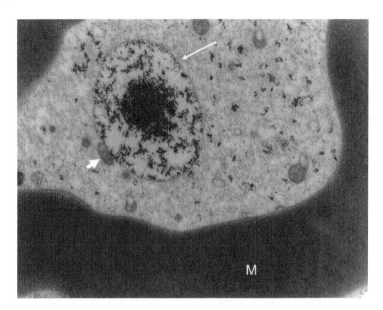

Fig. 28.2.   Electronmicroscopic image of the biopsy of the sural nerve from a APBD patient not described, showing a polyglucosan body (long thin arrow) in an axon. Short thick arrow: mitochondrion. M = myelin sheath.

Follow-up

One-and-a-half years after the initial visit, the patient finally agreed to use a walking stick. The course of the cognitive deficits is slowly progressive, and he visits a day care center twice a week. The other 2 days he is in the travel agency, where his wife can keep an eye on him. Keeping the books has become impossible and his wife notices a deterioration in his short-term memory as he keeps repeating himself. His health is declining after a urinary tract infection and deep vein thrombosis. On examination, the patient talks in stereotypical sentences and grammatical mistakes are noted. The score on MMSE is now 24/30.

Discussion

Taking the information from history, neurological, and neurocognitive examination together, we can conclude that our 60-year-old patient suffers from slowly progressive cognitive impairments in combination with a bipyramidal syndrome with polyneuropathy and urine incontinence. It appears that the cognitive impairment leads to a presenile form of dementia, characterized not only by memory deficits but also by mental slowness and executive dysfunction. These deficits correspond to a more global neurodegenerative process. The differential diagnosis at this point is broad and comprises hereditary, infectious, metabolic, inflammatory, and neoplastic disorders.

The family history seems to point towards a hereditary disorder with either a dominant or recessive mode of transmission. Although a disorder with a recessive mode of transmission seems unlikely, given the fact that only one parent appears to have been affected, the Jewish descent may increase this possibility, as carriership of certain recessive disorders has a high prevalence in the Ashkenazi population.

The negative results of EEG, blood, and CSF studies help us to exclude most of the metabolic, inflammatory and infectious disorders. Finally, we are able to diagnose the patient with APBD by recognizing the typical pattern of white matter involvement on MRI scan of the brain.

APBD is a rare hereditary metabolic disorder. Only about 50 cases have been reported worldwide. As with most recessive disorders, most patients are sporadic. They present themselves between their fifth and seventh decade with walking difficulties. By then, mild cognitive impairment and a voiding disorder is present or develops within a short time period. There is a gradual progression with decline of intellectual abilities and gait, and reported survival ranges from 2 to 25 years (Gray *et al.*, 1988).

On examination, a bipyramidal syndrome with sensorimotor polyneuropathy is found (Cavanagh, 1999). On neurocognitive and extensive neuropsychological examination, the cognitive impairment appears to relate to the diffuse degradation of brain parenchyma: problems in language and memory are reported, and patients generally are slow with impaired attention (Rifai *et al.*, 1994). Both the type of cognitive impairment at presentation and the speed of cognitive decline vary (Savage *et al.*, 2007) Often, a diagnosis of vascular dementia is made when imaging reveals high signal in the white matter (Bigio *et al.*, 1997).

In APBD, T2-weighted and FLAIR sequences show non-enhancing high signal in the white matter. Initially, these lesions are focal and localized in the deep white matter in the center semi-ovale and around the ventricles, extending into the temporal lobes. The capsula interna and externa as well as the cervicomedullar region are involved, with rostral extension to medulla and pons. The basis pontis is spared with the exception of the corticospinal tract. This pattern can be particularly well observed with sagittal T2 and FLAIR images, so these are crucial. There is generalized atrophy of both cerebrum, particularly the corpus callosum, cerebellum, and myelum. No white matter involvement is seen in the latter. Progression is characterized by confluent high signal extending into the gray matter with involvement of the U fibers (Berkhoff *et al.*, 2001; van der Knaap and Valk, 2005).

Over the last few decades, extensive research has shed some light on the pathophysiology of APBD. Particularly, similarities with Glycogen Storage Disorder type IV (GSD), a fatal glycogen storage disorder at very young age, have stimulated research. It is now generally accepted that APBD is a late onset variant of GSD, affecting mainly the central and peripheral nervous system. In both disorders numerous Polyglucosan Bodies (PB) are found. PB are inclusion bodies measuring up to 70 μm that contain mostly abnormally branched glycogen. The finding of PB is related to degradation of nervous tissue (Milde *et al.*, 2001; Peress *et al.*, 1979). Parallel to GSD, a deficiency of GBE was demonstrated in leukocytes in some, but not all, APBD patients. Subsequently, several mutations have been described in both Jewish and non-Jewish patients with APBD and GBE deficiency, with Y329S being the most prevalent mutation (Klein *et al.*, 2004; Lossos *et al.*, 1998). No mutations were discovered in patients with APBD without GBE deficiency, although numerous PB were present. In these patients, the diagnosis of APBD is based upon clinical features, the specific pattern of white matter involvement on cerebral MRI and the demonstration of PB under the microscope.

When a diagnosis of APBD is suspected and results of imaging support this diagnosis, the next step is to measure the activity of GBE in leucocytes. When a deficiency is identified DNA analysis should follow, particularly in the case of a positive family history or Jewish descent. Other than for research, DNA analysis may lead to proper genetic counseling. In the case of a normal level of GBE, sural nerve or skin biopsy is advised, even when no symptoms or signs of polyneuropathy are present. When PB are found in young patients, or when they are numerous, large in size or extraneuronally located, a disorder is highly probable. In APBD PB are found in axons or in myo-epithelial cells in sweat glands (Fig. 28.2) (Klein *et al.*, 2004; Milde *et al.*, 2001). From our experience it may be worthwhile to ask for a second look through the microscope in case of a high suspicion but a negative result of the first examination of the biopsy.

This patient is a typical case of APBD. He is the first patient in the Netherlands in whom genetic analysis has confirmed the Y329S mutation. Because this mutation is inherited in a recessive mode, it is uncertain whether his mother was affected too. He has no children who may benefit from genetic counseling. Unfortunately, no therapy other than symptomatic treatment is available, although a clinical trial examining the effect of supplementation with a triglyceride on neurological functions has recently started in the US.

Take home messages

When a patient suffers from a cognitive disorder, bipyramidal syndrome with a voiding disorder and polyneuropathy, consider the possibility of APBD.

On cerebral MRI with midsagittal and transversal FLAIR sections, a typical pattern of white matter involvement is seen: from the cervico-medullar junction rostral to the pons with sparing of the basis pontis and involvement of the temporal lobes and capsula externa bilaterally.

In case of these findings, measure the activity of Glycogen Branching Enzyme in leukocytes. A nerve or skin biopsy, looking for Polyglucosan Bodies, should be planned when this activity is within normal range.

REFERENCES AND FURTHER READING

Berkhoff M, Weis J, Schroth G, Sturzenegger M (2001). Extensive white-matter changes in case of adult polyglucosan body disease. *Neuroradiology*, **3**, 234–6.

Bigio EH, Weiner MF, Bonte FJ, White CL (1997). Familial dementia due to adult polyglucosan body disease. *Clin Neuropathol*, **4**, 227–34.

Cavanagh JB (1999). Corpora-amylacea and the family of polyglucosan diseases. *Brain Res Rev*, **2–3**, 265–95.

Gray F, Gherardi R, Marshall A, Janota I, Poirier J (1988). Adult polyglucosan body disease (APBD). *J Neuropathol Exp Neurol*, **4**, 459–74.

Klein CJ, Boes CJ, Chapin JE, *et al.* (2004). Adult polyglucosan body disease: case description of an expanding genetic and clinical syndrome. *Muscle Nerve*, **2**, 323–8.

Lossos A, Meiner Z, Barash V, *et al.* (1998). Adult polyglucosan body disease in Ashkenazi Jewish patients carrying the Tyr329Ser mutation in the glycogen-branching enzyme gene. *Ann Neurol*, **6**, 867–72.

Milde P, Guccion JG, Kelly J, Locatelli E, Jones RV (2001). Adult polyglucosan body disease. *Arch Pathol Lab Med*, **4**, 519–22.

Peress NS, Dimauro S, Roxburgh VA (1979). Adult polysaccharidosis. Clinicopathological, ultrastructural, and biochemical features. *Arch Neurol*, **13**, 840–5.

Rifai Z, Klitzke M, Tawil R, *et al.* (1994). Dementia of adult polyglucosan body disease. Evidence of cortical and subcortical dysfunction. *Arch Neurol*, **1**, 90–4.

Savage G, Ray F, Halmagyi M, Blazely A, Harper C (2007). Stable neuropsychological deficits in adult polyglucosan body disease. *J Clin Neurosci*, **5**, 473–7.

van der Knaap MS, Valk J (2005). *Magnetic Resonance of Myelination and Myelin Disorders*. New York: Springer.

Case 29

Young woman with abnormal movements but no family history

Ryan V. V. Evans and Kevin M. Biglan

Clinical history – main complaint

A 45-year-old right-handed woman presents to the Neurology clinic with several years of cognitive difficulty. She denies any significant problems with memory or thinking, but admits that it takes her longer to complete tasks than it used to. Her husband reports that she has trouble maintaining attention and concentration. For example, 1 year ago she had stopped working as an executive secretary because she could not longer keep up with the pace and variety of tasks assigned to her. She also has difficulty learning new tasks and is inflexible to change. Additionally, her husband reports a change in personality over the last 10 years or so. Previously cheerful and easy-going, she has become more irritable. She tends to follow a specific daily routine and gets upset when that pattern is altered.

General history

She has a long-standing history of depression, which has been fairly well-controlled on sertraline 100 mg daily. There are no other chronic medical problems or regular medications. She is married with two children, aged 17 and 14. Having completed high school and attended 1 year of college, she had been working as an executive secretary until being fired 1 year ago for poor work performance. She drinks alcohol on occasion, but denies tobacco or recreational drug use.

Family history

Her father had depression and committed suicide at age 50. Her mother has hypertension, but is otherwise healthy at age 71. A paternal uncle has been diagnosed with tremor and anxiety. Several other people on her father's side have had trouble with alcoholism.

Case Studies in Dementia: Common and Uncommon Presentations, ed. S. Gauthier and P. Rosa-Neto. Published by Cambridge University Press. © Cambridge University Press 2011.

Examination

Vital signs: BP 128/72; pulse 76 and regular; weight 132 pounds.

General examination: Thin, but well developed and well nourished. Lungs are clear and heart is regular without murmurs or gallops. No carotid bruits.

Mental status: Alert and interactive, fully oriented. Speech is fluent and prosodic, and naming and repetition are intact. Affect is full. She scores 20/30 on the MoCA, losing points for visuospatial processing, attention, verbal fluency, abstraction, and delayed recall.

Cranial nerves: Versions are full, but have some saccadic intrusions. She has difficulty initiating saccades, which often require an eye blink to start. Other cranial nerves are normal.

Motor: Bulk and strength are normal. There is slight rigidity in the arms, as well as mild bradykinesia with finger tapping and rapid alternating movements. There is mild motor impersistence when asked to hold her eyes closed or extend her tongue. There are frequent choreiform movements affecting all limbs, the trunk, and the face.

Sensory: Normal.

Co-ordination: Normal.

Reflexes: Normal.

Gait: Slightly wide-based, with good arm swing and stride length. Choreiform movements of the trunk and limbs occasionally intrude upon normal walking, causing loss of balance from which she is able to recover without falling. She has difficulty with tandem gait.

Special studies

CT of the head demonstrated very mild generalized atrophy with more pronounced atrophy of the head of the caudate nucleus (Fig. 29.1).

Diagnosis

The initial diagnostic impression was Huntington disease, despite the lack of a clear family history.

Follow-up

Genetic testing was performed, which demonstrated an expansion of the CAG repeat region in the *huntingtin* gene on chromosome 4 (42 repeats on one allele,

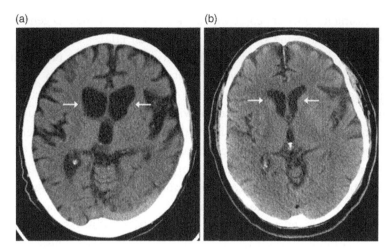

Fig. 29.1. (a) Head CT showing marked atrophy of the caudate nuclei (arrows) and moderate generalized atrophy in a patient with manifest Huntington Disease (HD). (b) For comparison, Head CT of an age-matched patient without HD showing mild generalized atrophy without atrophy of the caudate nuclei (arrows).

15 repeats on the other). Additionally, a more thorough family history revealed that her father and several of his relatives had involuntary movements.

Discussion

Huntington disease (HD) is a neurodegenerative disease characterized clinically by the triad of a movement disorder, dementia, and behavioral disturbances. Grossly, the pathological hallmark is atrophy of the caudate nuclei (see Fig. 29.1), while microscopically it is loss of medium spiny neurons in the striatum. The exact pathophysiologic mechanisms that lead to these changes are unknown, but there is evidence that impaired mitochondrial function and oxidative stress play a role. The prevalence of HD worldwide is estimated at 3–10 per 100 000. Approximately 30 000 people in the US have clinical manifestations of HD with an additional 150 000 healthy people at risk of developing HD.

HD is inherited in an autosomal dominant fashion and is caused by the expansion of a CAG repeat in Exon 1 of the *huntingtin* gene on chromosome 4. The CAG expansion is unstable and may increase in length from one generation to the next, resulting in anticipation, whereby children may have earlier onset of HD symptoms than their affected parents. Following isolation of the HD gene in 1993, we now have a readily available genetic test that can determine with certainty which at-risk individuals will develop the disease. Therefore, there are an increasing number of people who are known to carry the HD genetic mutation but are not yet showing symptoms (pre-manifest HD).

Following clinical onset of HD, disability accrues over a period of 15 to 20 years, and the disease is universally fatal in individuals who do not die of competing causes of death. Because the onset of HD typically occurs in midlife, at approximately age 40, affected individuals may lose a significant portion of their productive adult life. Classically, the diagnosis of HD has been defined by the appearance of clear motor abnormalities, most notably chorea. Other motor abnormalities include bradykinesia, impaired fine motor control, oculomotor deficits, balance difficulty, dysarthria, and dysphagia. Over time, almost all individuals with HD develop dementia and behavioral disturbances. Behavioral disturbances may take the form of psychiatric diseases such as depression, obsessive-compulsive disorder, or anxiety. Psychosis (with delusions more commonly than hallucinations) occurs rarely. Affected individuals may also have more complex personality changes, frequently with features of apathy and irritability, rather than with overt psychiatric disease.

The dementia associated with HD is often described as a *subcortical* dementia (Zakzanis, 1998). Rather than exhibiting significant cortical deficits (aphasia, agnosia, apraxia), individuals with HD typically have impairments in executive function (planning, organizing, and executing sequential tasks), attention and concentration, working memory, visuospatial processing, and mental flexibility. These deficits are thought to derive from abnormalities in frontal-subcortical circuits, in which the basal ganglia play an important role. Attention, concentration, and executive dysfunction are among the cognitive functions impaired earliest in HD, and they track well with the progression of motor features (Bamford *et al.*, 1995; Lemiere *et al.*, 2004). Patients may complain of disorganization or difficulty following tasks (recipes, computer programs, etc.) that used to be easy for them. Performances on neuropsychological tests such as the Trail Making and Stroop Tests reveal impairment compared with healthy controls. Mental inflexibility involves concreteness of thought, resistance to change, limited perspective in problem solving, a narrow range of interests and difficulty generalizing information. This may lead to anxiety with change, difficulty with transitions, irritability, and other behavioral problems. Mental flexibility can be objectively assessed using the Wisconsin Card Sorting Test (WCST) and tests of abstraction. Difficulty with visuospatial processing may be harder to identify in a clinical context, but individuals with HD have clear impairments on a number of neuropsychological tests that evaluate this domain of cognition.

Disorientation and semantic memory loss of the type seen in Alzheimer's disease (AD) are not common in HD. While people with HD may have memory deficits, those deficits involve difficulty with tasks that require retrieval and synthesis of known facts. In HD dementia, there is dissociation between the ability to complete tasks of recall and recognition, generally defined by performance on the Hopkins Verbal Learning Test (HVLT). People with AD have significant impairments of both recall of learned verbal information and recognition of that information when prompted from a list. However, while individuals with HD demonstrate impaired delayed recall, they are accurate with recognition tasks. Memory loss is not time dependent in HD as it is in AD, where recent knowledge is lost more easily than distant knowledge. Additionally, in tasks such as category fluency, people with HD show the ability to improve with cuing, whereas people with AD do not.

Importantly, cognitive decline and behavioral dysfunction in HD are highly correlated with overall functional impairment. This correlation is independent of the level of motor function. One recent study demonstrated that cognitive dysfunction, motor dysfunction, and a combined measure of apathy and executive dysfunction accounted for over 90% of the variance in functional capacity for a group of individuals with HD (Hamilton et al., 2003). Furthermore, apathy and executive dysfunction contributed significantly more to the level of functional capacity than did motor dysfunction. In practice, patients with HD may complain of difficulty following complex directions, multitasking, making decisions, remembering important information or learning new information. These impairments may manifest as functional problems ranging from decreased work performance and trouble managing finances to an inability to complete all the activities of daily living. As a result, affected individuals often lose the ability to work, live, and function independently at a relatively young age.

More recent evidence demonstrates that cognitive changes and neuropsychiatric symptoms often precede the classical motor onset of HD by as long as several decades. TRACK-HD is a multinational longitudinal observational study following roughly 120 individuals each with HD, pre-manifest HD, and healthy controls. Baseline data from this study demonstrated impairments in working memory, recognition of negative facial emotions, and smell identification in both HD and pre-manifest HD (Tabrizi et al., 2009). Other studies have found that people with pre-manifest HD have problems with attention, working memory, and executive function when compared with normal controls (Lemiere et al., 2004). The Neurobiological Markers of Huntington Disease (Predict-HD) is the largest ongoing study of largely expansion positive pre-manifest individuals. Predict-HD is currently following over 1000 participants from HD families with approximately 3/4 positive for the CAG expansion for HD (Paulsen et al., 2008). To date, Predict-HD has demonstrated that episodic memory and recognition of negative emotions are sensitive markers of cognitive impairment in pre-manifest HD. Interestingly, while cognitive tests can distinguish pre-manifest HD and early HD from late HD, there is not a clear relationship between the onset of dementia and CAG repeat length.

Treatment for HD is exclusively symptomatic at present. We do not yet have a cure for HD, or any proven therapies that slow progression of the disease. Even from a purely symptomatic standpoint, cognitive impairment in HD can be difficult to treat. While several small, open-label studies of cholinesterase inhibitors in HD have shown trends towards improvement in cognition, a recent randomized trial of donepezil failed to demonstrate any cognitive benefit (Cubo *et al.*, 2006). Similarly, a 16-week open-label study of the NMDA-antagonist memantine showed an improvement in chorea, but failed to show any cognitive improvement (Ondo *et al.*, 2007). A recent pilot study of atomoxetine (a non-stimulant norepinephrine reuptake inhibitor used in ADHD) demonstrated mild improvement in cognitive function in HD, but this result will need to be replicated in larger randomized trials (Beglinger *et al.*, 2009). Chorea is typically treated with dopamine-blocking medications, such as the atypical neuroleptics (e.g., risperidone, quetiapine), or the dopamine-depleting medication tetrabenazine. Tetrabenazine is currently the only FDA-approved medication for the treatment of chorea in HD. It leads to clinically-meaningful reduction in chorea – about 25%, on average (Huntington Study Group 2006). Tetrabenazine does not appear to carry the same risks of typical extrapyramidal side effects (parkinsonism, akathisia, acute dystonic reactions, tardive dyskinesia, blunting of affect) as do the atypical neuroleptics. However, there are lingering concerns that tetrabenazine may worsen depression and increase the risk of suicidal behaviors. Additionally, because atypical neuroleptics can treat both chorea and behavioral disturbances in HD, they continue to be the treatment of choice for some physicians. Mood disorders in HD are typically treated with serotonin reuptake inhibitors (SSRIs), though tricyclic antidepressants and monoamine oxidase inhibitors are also effective for depression. Psychological counseling is also an important part of the comprehensive care plan for many patients with HD.

Cognitive impairment is a common and functionally disabling problem in HD. In recent years we have clarified many details about the domains of cognition affected in HD and the progression of those impairments. Current large observational studies in manifest and pre-manifest HD, TRACK-HD and Predict-HD, will help identify the earliest cognitive and behavioral changes and may help elucidate treatment decisions. Future research aimed at identifying therapies that delay or slow cognitive decline or improve cognitive symptoms are essential.

Take home messages

Dementia in HD is characterized by difficulties with executive function, working memory and attention rather than by memory loss and aphasia. Cognitive decline in HD is highly correlated with functional impairment. Effective treatments for cognitive impairment in HD are lacking, and should be a focus of future research.

REFERENCES AND FURTHER READING

Bamford KA, Caine ED, Kido DK, *et al.* (1995). A prospective evaluation of cognitive decline in early Huntington's disease: Functional and radiographic correlates. *Neurology*, **45**, 1867–73.

Beglinger LJ, Adams WH, Paulson H, *et al.* (2009). Randomized controlled trial of atomoxetine for cognitive dysfunction in early Huntington disease. *J Clin Psychopharmacol*, **29**, 484–7.

Cubo E, Shannon KM, Tracy D, *et al.* (2006). Effect of donepezil on motor and cognitive function in Huntington disease. *Neurology*, **67**, 1268–71.

Hamilton JM, Salmon DP, Corey-Bloom J, *et al.* (2003). Behavioural abnormalities contribute to functional decline in Huntington's disease. *J Neurol Neurosurg Psychiatry*, **74**, 120–2.

Huntington Study Group (2006). Tetrabenazine as antichorea therapy in Huntington disease: A randomized controlled trial. *Neurology*, **66**, 366–72.

Lemiere J, Decruyenaere M, Evers-Kiebooms G, *et al.* (2004). Cognitive changes in patients with Huntington's disease (HD) and asymptomatic carriers of the HD mutation: a longitudinal follow-up study. *J Neurol*, **251**, 935–42.

Ondo WG, Mejia NI, Hunter CB (2007). A pilot study of the clinical efficacy and safety of memantine for Huntington's disease. *Parkinsonism Relat Disord*, **13**, 453–4.

Paulsen JS, Langbehn DR, Stout JC, *et al.* (2008). Detection of Huntington's disease decades before diagnosis: the Predict-HD study. *J Neurol Neurosurg Psychiatry*, **79**, 874–80.

Tabrizi SJ, Langbehn DR, Leavitt BR, *et al.* (2009). Biological and clinical manifestations of Huntington's disease in the longitudinal TRACK-HD study: cross-sectional analysis of baseline data. *Lancet Neurology*, **8**, 791–801.

Zakzanis K (1998). The subcortical dementia of Huntington's disease. *J Clin Exp Neuropsychol*, **20**, 565–78.

Elderly lady with right-sided visual hallucinations

Will Guest, Gerald Pfeffer, and Neil Cashman

Clinical history – main complaint

This 82-year-old woman presented with apparently sudden-onset neurological symptoms. She noticed a homonymous visual field defect in the right lower quadrant with simple visual hallucinations in that region including blue–violet flashes and wire-mesh patterns. She also provided a history of oscillopsia, with mild dysarthria and dysphagia. Coincident with this were difficulties reaching for objects with her right hand and slightly off-balance gait. She presented to hospital 2 days after the onset of her symptoms. Cognition and language were intact at presentation, and she was constitutionally well. She had not had other symptoms such as headache, sleep disturbance, nor any other dysfunction in motor or sensory abilities. She did report persistent vertigo for the last 3 weeks, which had been assessed by a neurologist and otolaryngologist and investigated with CT scans of the head and vestibular apparatus without reaching a diagnosis. Otherwise review of systems did not reveal abnormalities suggestive of connective tissue disease, metabolic/endocrine dysfunction, or other medical illness.

Family history

Medical history and family history was unremarkable, except that the patient was on ranitidine for gastric reflux. She did not abuse drugs, cigarettes, or alcohol.

Examination

On examination, this patient appeared well and comfortable. Vital signs were normal except for blood pressure of 160/90 mmHg. There was no lymphadenopathy; cardiovascular and respiratory examination was normal. The abdomen was soft and there was no organomegaly. Dermatologic exam was normal and no active joints were demonstrated. Neurological examination revealed normal cognitive function including language and memory. Cranial nerve examination

Case Studies in Dementia: Common and Uncommon Presentations, ed. S. Gauthier and P. Rosa-Neto. Published by Cambridge University Press. © Cambridge University Press 2011.

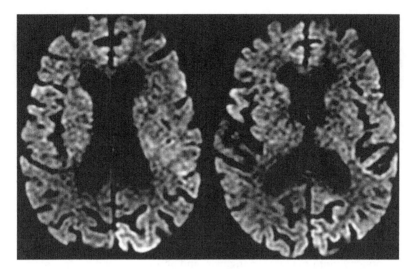

Fig. 30.1. Transverse axial DWI images demonstrating signal abnormality in the left occipital cortex. The basal ganglia (not shown) were normal.

demonstrated the homonymous visual field defect in the right lower quadrant. Eye movements exhibited broken smooth pursuit and hypometric saccades. Mild dysarthria was present. Motor examination was normal except for an action tremor in both hands and wide-based gait. Optic ataxia was present when reaching for objects with the right hand. Sensory examination was normal.

Special studies

Standard CBC, liver/renal panel, and expanded electrolyte panel were normal. TSH was in range, and ANA was weakly positive with titer 1:160. VDRL and Lyme serology were negative. Paraneoplastic antibody panel on blood and CSF were negative. CSF analysis revealed normal cell counts and protein, with no organisms, although 14–3–3 protein was positive. EEG initially demonstrated mild diffuse theta-range slowing. On subsequent records diffuse encephalopathy gradually became more apparent, and periodic sharp elements resembling periodic sharp wave complexes began to appear. On MRI, volume loss was apparent bilaterally in the occipito-parietal regions, and there was DWI cortical signal abnormality most apparent in the left occipital pole (Fig. 30.1). No other abnormalities were detected on the other sequences, including post-gadolinium images.

Diagnosis

Creutzfeldt–Jakob disease (CJD).

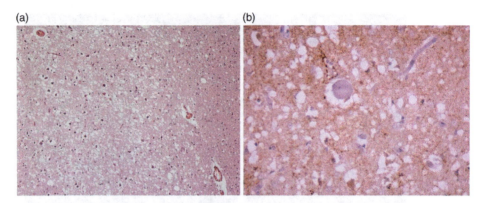

Fig. 30.2.   (a) Low-magnification haematoxylin-eosin section of neocortex with a margin of white matter at right. The cortex demonstrates spongiosis. (b) High-magnification haematoxylin-eosin section of neocortex with prion protein stain. There is pronounced neuronal loss, spongiosis, and abnormal prion protein staining in a synaptic (stippled) pattern.

Follow-up

The patient's clinical evolution was characterized by a relentlessly progressive course over several weeks. The visual field defect expanded into a right homonymous hemianopia, and optic ataxia also developed on the left. Dysarthria and dysphagia worsened until she was dependent on tube feeding. Cognitive changes ensued rapidly, with memory loss, paranoid ideation, and emotional lability. Within weeks she became akinetic and mute. Startle myoclonus was prominent 3 weeks after initial presentation. Death occurred within 3 months of admission.

Neuropathology: autopsy was performed, which revealed cortical spongiosis and neuronal loss (Fig. 30.2(a)). Prion protein stains demonstrated accumulation of prion protein in the cortex, in a stippled pattern (Fig. 30.2(b)). These findings confirmed the clinical diagnosis of CJD.

Discussion

Overview: the human prion diseases are a comparatively rare cause of dementia, with an estimated incidence of 1 case per million people per year, although some uncorroborated reports would place the true incidence much higher (Manuelidis and Manuelidis, 1989). Sporadic CJD (sCJD) accounts for 85% of cases, with most of the remainder due to autosomal dominantly-inherited mutations of the PRNP gene on chromosome 20 that codes for human prion protein. Depending on the site of the mutation and polymorphic codon 129 status, the illness may manifest as familial CJD (fCJD), Gerstmann–Sträussler–Scheinker Syndrome (GSS), or Fatal Familial Insomnia (FFI). Prion-contaminated dura mater grafts, cadaveric pituitary hormones, corneal transplants, and depth electrodes have led to iatrogenic CJD in over 400 people (Hamaguchi *et al.*, 2009), while there have been 178 cases to date of new variant CJD (vCJD) from consumption of bovine spongiform encephalopathy prions. vCJD transmission has also been observed through blood and blood products (Peden *et al.*, 2004).

Differential diagnosis: the differential diagnosis for a patient presenting with signs suggestive of CJD is broad, as it encompasses most causes of dementia. The conventional clinical picture of possible CJD involves a rapidly progressive dementia and two of the following signs: myoclonus, cerebellar and/or visual symptoms, extrapyramidal and/or pyramidal signs, and akinetic mutism. In fact, this description belies considerable heterogeneity in the presentation of the prion diseases. There are many atypical presentations of prion disease that resemble more common dementing conditions. The Oppenheimer–Brownell variant of CJD, for example, accounts for roughly 10% of cases and manifests exclusively with ataxia and cerebellar deficits (Appleby *et al.*, 2009). It is particularly important to differentiate CJD from Alzheimer's disease (AD), which is often the presumed etiology for symptoms of cognitive decline in the elderly. AD is associated with loss of memory and executive function, but motor deficits are rare. Furthermore, prion disease is generally more rapidly progressive than AD, although patients with GSS may exhibit a more gradual deterioration spanning 2–7 years that resembles Alzheimer's-type dementia (Novakovic *et al.*, 2005). In at least one family with GSS, the disease mimicked an atypical frontotemporal dementia (Giovagnoli *et al.*, 2008). Neuropsychiatric symptoms are common in the early stages of vCJD and sCJD and may point toward an incorrect diagnosis; patients with cognitive and affective variants of CJD have a longer delay in receiving diagnostic testing for CJD (Appleby *et al.*, 2009).

Diffuse Lewy body disease, like CJD, is characterized by motor signs but follows the classic Parkinsonian pattern of tremors, rigidity, and bradykinesia rather than ataxia and myoclonus. In vascular dementia, the changes in cognitive function are usually abrupt rather than progressive, but with multi-infarct dementia (including CADASIL, cerebral autosomal-dominant arteriopathy with subcortical infarcts, and leukoencephalopathy) damage from each accumulated lesion may be incremental and produce an apparently continuous decline. Structural abnormalities like normal pressure hydrocephalus, may present with the classic triad of ataxia followed by dementia and urinary incontinence that much resembles CJD. Imaging studies showing enlarged ventricles out of proportion to cortical atrophy suggest this diagnosis, which can be confirmed by large-volume lumbar puncture. Treatable possibilities include vitamin B12 deficiency, vasculitis, hypothyroidism, or Hashimoto's encephalopathy. Progressive multifocal leukoencephalopathy, AIDS dementia complex, and tertiary neurosyphilis may seem similar to CJD and would be suggested by exposure history and HIV and VDRL testing.

New variant vCJD is phenotypically distinct from sCJD, with a younger average age of onset (28 vs. 68 for sCJD) and a longer average disease course (14 months vs. 8 months). Psychiatric disturbances including depression or a schizophrenia-like psychosis often precede dementia by several months (Spencer *et al.*, 2002), and an unusual sensory symptom, a feeling of "stickiness" of the skin, has been reported in half of cases. In younger patients with suspected vCJD, the differential diagnosis also includes inherited conditions like Huntington's disease or adult-type neuronal ceroid lipofuscinosis (Kufs' disease) that can be explored by genetic testing.

Heidenhain variant CJD accounts for approximately 20% of sCJD cases and is characterized by presentation with visual symptoms, including visual field defects, hallucinations, disturbed color perception, optical anosognosia, and cortical blindness (Kropp *et al.*, 1999). Clinical signs of limbic system involvement (like aggressiveness) or basal ganglia deterioration (like rigidity, tremor, athetosis, or limb hypertonicity) are seen less often in the Heidenhain variant than in classic CJD. The clinical course is typically more rapid than other CJD variants, with death occurring an average of 6 months after presentation. MRI findings unique to this variant include cortical signal abnormality predominantly affecting the occipital lobes and occipital volume loss, although findings typical to other variants of CJD may also be present. EEG classically demonstrates periodic sharp wave complexes but may reveal intermittent non-specific changes depending on the stage of disease. Neuropathological changes include neuronal loss and cortical spongiosis which predominantly affects the occipital lobes. The majority of patients have the M/M type 1 PrP genotype at codon 129 of PRNP (Parchi *et al.*, 1999).

Clinical suspicion for a cortically based neurodegenerative illness such as CJD was elevated in this patient on the basis of the clinical picture. Her presentation with a homonymous right lower visual field defect, hallucinations, and optic ataxia localize the lesion to the upper bank of the calcarine sulcus in the left occipital lobe, extending up to the association area in the superior parietal lobule (the so-called dorsal visual perceptual stream) (Battaglia-Mayer and Caminiti, 2002). Optic ataxia typically is caused by a cortical lesion, although reports of subcortical lesions causing this deficit have been published. The patient initially reported sudden onset of symptoms, which raised suspicion for a vascular etiology. However, in the context of her progressive cognitive and psychiatric symptoms, with the known cortically based localization described above, the clinical diagnosis of CJD became apparent. Support for this diagnosis was eventually obtained in the MRI, CSF, EEG, and neuropathological findings.

It is unclear whether this patient's vertigo was related to her disease. Vertigo would be expected to arise from brainstem pathology, but the brainstem is usually unaffected in the M/M or M/V type 1 genotype that strongly predominates for this variant. However, a recent series found that vertigo was a presenting symptom in 2% of CJD patients.

Testing: given the phenotypic variability of CJD and the risk of mistaking it for other conditions, diagnostic tests are useful to investigate the possibility of CJD. According to a study of 364 patients with suspected CJD (Poser *et al.*, 1999), a positive 14–3–3 CSF protein test is 95% sensitive and 93% specific for CJD, although caution should be exercised when interpreting this test as virtually any syndrome accompanied by neuronal injury can occasion "false positives." Bilateral hyperintensity of the striatum on long repetition time MRI images is 67% sensitive and 93% specific. Periodic sharp wave complexes on EEG are 65% sensitive and 93% specific, but are more prominent in the late phases of disease; frontal intermittent rhythmical delta activity may be more suggestive of the initial phases of disease (Wieser *et al.*, 2004). Positive findings on these tests do not exclude other causes of disease but do make them much less likely and elevate a possible diagnosis of CJD based on clinical findings to a probable diagnosis; definite diagnosis requires neuropathological studies, except in the case of subjects satisfying probable criteria of CJD with pathogenic PRNP mutations. Although there are no curative treatments for CJD available, rapid arrival at a correct diagnosis is important to exclude treatable causes of dementia and aid in end-of-life planning in consultation with family members.

Treatment: therapeutic options for all the human prion diseases are currently limited to palliation, as there are no agents capable of reliably causing a sustained improvement in clinical course. A large and diverse selection of drugs have been tried with limited success (Stewart *et al.*, 2008), including antivirals, antifungals, antibiotics, antimalarials, antidepressants, antioxidants, and analgesics. A small double-blind placebo-controlled study of the analgesic flupirtine on 26 sCJD patients demonstrated reduced deterioration in cognitive function, but it did not affect survival. Clinical trials of doxycycline, quinacrine, pentosan polysulfate, and simvastatin are currently ongoing. Other approaches, including active vaccination with prion protein and specific fragments, or passive antibody infusion directed toward the prion protein, have been validated in animal disease models (Li *et al.*, 2010) but have not yet reached human trials.

Take home messages

Prion diseases exhibit considerable phenotypic variability and may represent the underlying cause of dementia in patients diagnosed with more common neurologic diseases.

Ante-mortem diagnostic tests, including CSF 14–3–3 protein analysis, MRI, and EEG, can confirm or exclude a suspected diagnosis of CJD with a relatively high sensitivity and specificity.

The Heidenhain variant of sCJD is associated with visual symptoms like optic ataxia, hallucinations, and cortical blindness.

REFERENCES AND FURTHER READING

Appleby BS, Appleby KK, Crain BJ, *et al.* (2009). Characteristics of established and proposed sporadic Creutzfeldt–Jakob disease variants. *Arch Neurol,* **66**, 208–15.

Battaglia-Mayer A, Caminiti R (2002). Optic ataxia as a result of the breakdown of the global tuning fields of parietal neurones. *Brain,* **125**, 225–37.

Giovagnoli AR, Di Fede G, Aresi A, *et al.* (2008). Atypical frontotemporal dementia as a new clinical phenotype of Gerstmann-Straussler-Scheinker disease with the PrP-P102L mutation. Description of a previously unreported Italian family. *Neurol Sci,* **29**, 405–10.

Hamaguchi T, Noguchi-Shinohara M, Nozaki I, *et al.* (2009). The risk of iatrogenic Creutzfeldt–Jakob disease through medical and surgical procedures. *Neuropathology* **29**, 625–31.

Kropp S, Schulz-Schaeffer WJ, Finkenstaet M, *et al.* (1999). The Heidenhain variant of Creutzfeldt–Jakob disease. *Arch Neurol,* **56**, 55–61.

Li L, Napper S, Cashman N (2010). Immunotherapy for prion diseases: opportunities and obstacles. *Immunotherapy,* **2**, 137–40.

Manuelidis EE, Manuelidis L (1989). Suspected links between different types of dementias: Creutzfeldt–Jakob disease, Alzheimer disease, and retroviral CNS infections. *Alzheimer Dis Assoc Disord,* **3**, 100–9.

Novakovic KE, Villemagne VL, Rowe CC, *et al.* (2005). Rare genetically defined causes of dementia. *Int Psychogeriat,* **17**, S149–94.

Parchi, P., Giese, A., Capellari, S., *et al.* (1999). Classification of sporadic Creutzfeldt–Jakob disease based on molecular and phenotypic analysis of 300 subjects. *Ann Neurol,* **46**, 224–33.

Peden AH, Head MW, Ritchie, *et al.* (2004). Preclinical vCJD after blood transfusion in a PRNP codon 129 heterozygous patient. *Lancet,* **264**, 527–9.

Poser S, Mollenhauer B, Krauss A, *et al.* (1999). How to improve the clinical diagnosis of Creutzfeldt–Jakob disease. *Brain,* **12**, 2345–51.

Spencer MD, Knight RSG, Will RG (2002). First hundred cases of variant Creutzfeldt–Jakob disease: retrospective case note review of early psychiatric and neurological features. *BMJ,* **324**, 1479–82.

Stewart LA, Rydzewska LHM, Keogh GF, *et al.* (2008). Systematic review of therapeutic interventions in human prion disease. *Neurology,* **70**, 1272–81.

Wieser HG, Schwarz U, Blaettler T, *et al.* (2004). Serial EEG findings in sporadic and iatrogenic Creutzfeldt–Jakob disease. *Clin Neurophysiol,* **115**, 2467–78.

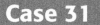

Woman with gait impairment and difficulty reading

Joseph M. Ferrara and Irene Litvan

Clinical history – main complaint

A 75-year-old woman presented with a 4-year history of progressive social withdrawal, decreased fluency, and difficulty handling complex tasks, such as planning trips and parties. Approximately 1 year after symptom onset, her gait developed a stiff appearance, and she began to suffer occasional falls. Additional symptoms soon followed, including impaired manual dexterity; fleeting tremor in the left leg; slow, harsh, monotonous speech; and dysphagia, necessitating a soft diet. Despite normal visual acuity, the patient developed difficulty reading, which she attributed to dry eyes and "trouble following the lines" of print.

General history

Her medical history was notable for hypertension, treated with hydrochlorothiazide, but no additional vascular risk factors, apart from her age. She reported constipation, controlled with a stool softener, but denied urinary incontinence and orthostatic lightheadedness. She had occasional insomnia, but no symptoms of REM behavior disorder. She was married, had a master's degree, and was working fulltime as an administrator prior to her neurological illness. She had no known neurotoxin exposures.

Family history

The patient's brother had a mild hand tremor, which manifested during activities, but there was no additional family history of neurological disease, including dementia or parkinsonism.

Case Studies in Dementia: Common and Uncommon Presentations, ed. S. Gauthier and P. Rosa-Neto. Published by Cambridge University Press. © Cambridge University Press 2011.

Examination

The patient's blood pressure was 145/86 mmHg without orthostatic hypotension. The remainder of her vital signs and general examination were normal.

On neurological examination, there was bradyphrenia and diminished spontaneous speech. Her score on the Folstein Mini-Mental State Examination (MMSE) was 28/30 with deductions for misidentification of the year (stated as 1907, rather than 2007) and one error in delayed recall. Because of her history of apathy and impaired mental flexibility, the Frontal Assessment Battery (FAB) was performed; the patient scored 14/18; z-score: −1.9 (see Discussion section below).

Upward and downward vertical saccades were absent, and horizontal saccades were slow and hypometric. Vertical pursuit movements were essentially absent, with preservation of the oculocephalic reflex. Horizontal pursuit movements showed normal range, but there was convergence insufficiency. Cranial nerve examination also revealed hypomimia with diminished rate of eyelid blinking and hypokinetic spastic dysarthria. Motor examination showed mild, symmetrical rigidity in the distal extremities and more pronounced proximal limb and cervical rigidity, which limited range of motion in the neck. Alternating limb movements showed mild to moderate bradykinesia, slightly worse in the left hand. There was no weakness, atrophy or tremor. Sensation, including cortical sensory function, was normal and there were no cerebellar signs. Deep tendon reflexes were diffusely brisk but plantar responses were mute. The patient was able to arise from the seated position independently but only with the use of her hands. Upon standing, she had mild anterocollis. She required a walker to ambulate, and her gait had a lurching appearance with an irregular stride length. With the "pull test," in which the examiner stands behind the patient and asks her to maintain her balance when pulled backwards, she was unable to shift her feet to recover.

Special studies

Magnetic Resonance Imaging (MRI) of the brain showed prominent mesencephalic atrophy, dilation of the third ventricle, and mild cerebral atrophy. Formal neuropsychological testing was performed, including the Mattis Dementia Rating Scale-2 (Rosser and Hodges, 1994), California Verbal Learning Test (Delis et al., 1987), Boston Naming Test, Neuropsychiatric Inventory, and Hamilton psychiatric rating scale for depression. On the Mattis Dementia Rating Scale, the patient scored 118/144 (first percentile), due to deficits in attention, initiation-perseveration, construction, and conceptualization, with only a mild impairment on the memory subscale. On the California Verbal Learning Test, there was a severe impairment in free recall, but lesser deficits in cued recall, and relatively intact word recognition. The Hamilton psychiatric rating scale did not reveal evidence of depression.

Diagnosis

Based upon her history and examination, the patient met National Institute of Neurological Disorders and Stroke – Society for Progressive Supranuclear Palsy (NINDS-SPSP) diagnostic criteria for "probable" Progressive Supranuclear Palsy (PSP). Available data show that the diagnosis of PSP will be pathologically confirmed in essentially 100% of patients who meet these criteria (Litvan *et al.*, 1996).

Follow-up

The patient's motor function progressively worsened, and she died from respiratory complications, approximately 6 years following symptom onset. A neuropathological examination of her brain revealed neuronal and glial tau pathology typical of PSP in the substantia nigra, subthalamic nucleus, and globus pallidus, as well as the motor and pre-motor cortices, ventral thalamus, corpus striatum, and olivopontocerebellar system.

Discussion

Progressive supranuclear palsy is a sporadic neurodegenerative disease, which is defined clinicopathologically by the constellation of atypical parkinsonism, supranuclear vertical gaze palsy, and a characteristic pattern of tau accumulation within the brainstem and basal ganglia. The age-adjusted prevalence of PSP is estimated to be about 5 per 100 000 persons (Nath *et al.*, 2001), making it one of the more common atypical parkinsonian syndromes. Symptom onset is typically in the sixth or seventh decade of life, and survival averages 5 to 8 years, with death often resulting from pulmonary complications (Litvan *et al.*, 1996; O'Sullivan *et al.*, 2008). The cause of PSP is not known. Genetic factors play a role, as a common variant in the gene encoding microtubule-associated protein tau confers an increased risk (Rademakers *et al.*, 2005), but a causal gene or defined familial inheritance pattern is not apparent. No environmental risk factors have been pinpointed, and the rarity of PSP encumbers epidemiological studies, though research in this area is in progress. Atypical parkinsonism with tau pathology and clinical features quite similar to PSP is endemic to specific tropical regions, for example Guadeloupe. Plant-derived mitochondrial toxins are suspected to contribute to Guadeloupean parkinsonism and similar disorders, but it is uncertain what extent disease mechanisms overlap with sporadic PSP (Caparros-Lefebvre *et al.*, 2006).

Classically, patients with PSP present with insidious onset of bradykinesia, associated with postural instability and falls; however, approximately 20% of patients have a cognitive or behavioral presentation (Kaat *et al.*, 2007). Indeed, J.C. Steele, J.C. Richardson and J. Olszewski noted cognitive and behavioral dysfunction in their seminal description of PSP nearly fifty years ago (Steele *et al.*, 1964), and PSP later served as the archetype disease in Martin Alberts' influential characterization of "subcortical dementia" (Albert *et al.*, 1974). The description of PSP as a subcortical dementia is somewhat flawed, since PSP pathology affects the frontal lobes directly (not merely the subcortical targets of striatothalamocortical circuits), and the degree of cognitive dysfunction parallels frontal atrophy (Paviour *et al.*, 2006). Nonetheless, regardless of whether the clinical deficits of PSP better reflect frontal pathology or frontal deafferentation, the pattern of cognitive dysfunction in PSP is unquestionably distinct from that of more common "cortical dementias," such as Alzheimer's disease.

The most immediately apparent cognitive deficit in patients with PSP is slowed information processing, which manifests as a delayed response time, particularly when completing complex tasks, and is often evident before formal mental status testing is performed. Bradyphrenia is distinct from bradykinesia, as delayed response times in PSP persist after controlling for slowed execution of movement and can be quantified using event-related brain potential measures that do not require a motor response (e.g., an increased latency of the P300) (Litvan, 1994; Dubois *et al.*, 1996). Patients with PSP also exhibit executive dysfunction, i.e. impairments in various frontal domains responsible for cognitive flexibility and problem-solving. Difficulties are evident in tests that require abstract thinking (i.e., distinguishing relevant commonalities) or those in which feedback is used to shift conceptual sets. In such tasks, patients are often unable to inhibit contextually inappropriate actions, resulting in perseverative errors. Other repetitive phenomenon seen in PSP patients may also be akin to perseveration; these include palilalia (involuntary repetition of one's own spoken words) and the "applause sign" (a tendency to initiate an automatic program of sustained applause when one is asked to initiate a voluntary program of three claps) (Dubois *et al.*, 2005).

As seen in the case that was presented above, individuals with PSP perform relatively normally on tests of short-term memory (e.g., digit span retention); indeed, memory is less impaired in patients with PSP than in those with Parkinson disease with dementia, dementia with Lewy bodies or Alzheimer's disease (Litvan, 1994; Dubois *et al.*, 1996; Aarsland *et al.*, 2003). On verbal learning tasks, patients demonstrate deficits in free recall with lesser impairments in word recognition. This pattern suggests that impaired information retrieval, rather than impaired information storage, accounts for the forgetfulness seen in PSP patients. On attentional tasks (e.g., target detection using finger tapping), PSP patients show only modestly reduced vigilance (Litvan, 1994). Progressive non-fluent aphasia is a known phenotypic variant of PSP (Williams and Lees, 2009), but language deficits are otherwise usually subtle, with impaired verbal fluency being the most consistent abnormality, as was observed in our patient (Albert *et al.*, 1974; Lange *et al.*, 2003). Like most chronic neurological diseases, PSP may result in dysphoric mood; however, unlike many, apathy is a prominent problem independent of depression, and affects up to 90% of patients. In the patient presented above, her family initially attributed her progressive social withdrawal to depression; however, clinical testing did not confirm a mood disorder, and apathy was prominent. Following apathy, disinhibition is the most common behavioral correlate in PSP, affecting about one-third to one-half of patients. Agitation is less evident (affecting 20% or fewer patients), and psychosis is unusual (Millar *et al.*, 2006).

Comprehensive psychometric testing readily illuminates the spectrum of cognitive deficits associated with PSP but is not feasible at the "bedside." Because the Folstein MMSE, a widely used screening tool for dementia, is insensitive for the dysexecutive syndrome of PSP (Folstein *et al.*, 1975; Millar *et al.*, 2006), other screening instruments are needed in this population. The FAB and Addenbrooke's cognitive examination have been studied for this purpose and demonstrate superior psychometric properties (Bak *et al.*, 2005; Dubois *et al.*, 2000). In the patient presented above, the FAB was performed, which is a six-part bedside scale designed to evaluate executive function. FAB tasks include the following: (1) the similarities test which assesses conceptualization (the patient is asked the abstract concept linking items); (2) a lexical fluency test, which assesses mental flexibility (the patient is asked to recite as many words as possible beginning with a given letter within 1 minute); (3) Luria's "fist-edge-palm" sequence, which assesses motor programming (the patient is asked to place her hand in three successive positions – a fist resting horizontally, a palm resting vertically, and a palm resting horizontally); (4) the conflicting instruction test, which assesses sensitivity to interference (the patient is asked to tap her hand once when the examiner taps twice, and the examiner performs a series of interspersed single and double taps); (5) the Go–No Go test, which assesses inhibitory control (the patient is asked to tap her hand once when the examiner taps once, and the examiner performs a series of interspersed single and double taps); and (6) the prehension behavior test which assesses environmental autonomy (the examiner instructs the patient not to take his hands, then with the patient's hands palm up upon her knees, the examiner brings his hands close to the patient's hands and touches the patient's palms to see if she will spontaneously take them). Each item of the FAB is scored from 0 to 3, with higher scores indicating better performance. Another brief screening test of cognition, which we routinely use in our movement disorder clinic, is the Montreal Cognitive Assessment (MoCA). For most patients, the MoCA takes less than 10 minutes to administer and contains executive function testing (phonemic fluency, a modified Trail-making B, and verbal abstraction tasks), as well as measures of orientation, attention, short-term memory, language, and visuospatial functions (Nasreddine *et al.*, 2005).

Apart from bradykinesia and postural instability, other common motor symptoms of PSP include muscular rigidity, neck dystonia, spastic dysarthria, dysphagia, and a characteristic astonished facial appearance. Parkinsonian symptoms are usually bilateral and symmetrical in onset, more pronounced in proximal muscles, and minimally responsive to levodopa. As its name suggests, the most distinctive feature of PSP is restriction of gaze, which is accompanied by preservation of the oculocephalic reflex. Vertical eye movements are affected preferentially, but not exclusively. Supranuclear gaze palsy is not, however, a consistent finding early in the course PSP, and abnormal (slow or hypometric) volitional saccades are a more sensitive sign in patients with a shorter disease duration. Patients with PSP may develop other deficits in oculomotor function, such as saccadic pursuit, excessive square-wave jerks during fixation, impaired convergence, so-called "apraxia" of eyelid opening, blepharospasm, and inability to suppress the vestibulo-ocular reflex (Litvan *et al.*, 1996). Additional, less common features of PSP include pyramidal tract signs and involuntary monotonous vocalizations.

Recently, a systematic chart review of consecutive patients with pathologically diagnosed PSP confirmed the presence of an alternate clinical phenotype with features reminiscent of idiopathic Parkinson disease (Williams *et al.*, 2005). This variant, termed PSP-Parkinsonism (PSP-P), accounts for approximately one-third of cases and is characterized by asymmetric onset, tremor, early bradykinesia, and non-axial dystonia. Patients with PSP-P respond more favorably to dopamine-replacement therapies, at least initially, and a minority (4%) develop levodopa-induced dyskinesias. In patients with PSP-P, gaze palsy and frontal dementia occur late in the course of the disease, if at all, and on average, survival for PSP-P exceeds the classical variant of PSP (now termed Richardson's syndrome) by 3 years (Williams and Lees, 2009). Less often, patients with PSP pathology may present with a progressive non-fluent aphasia, pure akinesia, or symptoms of corticobasal syndrome (Imai *et al.*, 1987; Williams and Lees, 2009).

The clinical diagnosis of PSP can be difficult, especially before the onset of overt oculomotor dysfunction, and only about 70% of patients with PSP pathology receive a correct ante-mortem diagnosis (Williams *et al.*, 2005). Accordingly, several studies have sought to establish an accurate biomarker through imaging and laboratory tests. In patients with clinically diagnosed PSP, magnetic resonance imaging shows atrophy of the brainstem, which is present in the dorsal midbrain out of proportion to the pons. This pattern of atrophy alters brainstem contours, creating a hummingbird or penguin-shaped silhouette on mid-sagittal views and the shape of a morning glory flower on axial imaging. Atrophy also affects the superior cerebellar peduncle and cortical regions, particularly the frontal lobes (Sitburana and Ondo, 2009). Recently, the ratio of different tau proteolytic products (55 verus 33 kDa forms) in the CSF was noted to distinguish patients with PSP from other neurodegenerative disorders, including other tauopathies such as corticobasal degeneration and frontotemporal dementia (Borroni *et al.*, 2008). Imaging and laboratory markers have not, however, been validated in patients with pathologically confirmed disease, and their utility in patients with short symptom duration or subtle symptoms is not established. At present, a histopathological examination of the brain is needed to diagnose PSP with certitude.

Neuropathologically, PSP is characterized by neuronal loss and gliosis associated with the deposition of filamentous, abnormally hyperphosphorylated tau protein in neurons and glia (Dickson *et al.*, 2007). Tau is important for the assembly and stabilization of microtubules, and the microtubule-binding domain of the protein contains a 31 amino acid region that is repeated either three (3R) or four (4R) times, depending upon alternative mRNA splicing. The 4R isoform predominates within the pathological lesions of PSP, as is the case in most tauopathies, though the imbalance seems less pronounced in individuals with the PSP-P variant (Williams and Lees, 2009). In patients with PSP, tau immunohistochemistry typically demonstrates neurofibrillary tangles (often globose in shape), neuropil threads, tuft-shaped astrocytes, and oligodendrial coiled bodies, as were evident in the case presented above. Topographically, pathological changes are first evident within the subthalamic nucleus, the zona compacta of the substantia nigra, and the internal segment of the globus pallidus. With more advanced disease other regions are involved, such as the dentate nucleus, pontine nuclei, caudate, cerebellar white matter, and frontal cortex (Williams *et al.*, 2007).

Treatment of PSP is challenging. There are no therapies that slow the progression of disease, and symptomatic therapies are generally disappointing. Despite a profound loss of dopaminergic neurons and a relative sparing of striatal dopamine receptors, levodopa provides little if any benefit, perhaps due to pathology in "downstream" basal ganglia structures such as the globus pallidus. Because PSP affects cholinergic neurons of the pedunculopontine nucleus, striatum, and other brain regions, centrally acting acetylcholinesterase inhibitors have been explored as a potential treatment for motor and cognitive symptoms. Unlike patients with Alzheimer's disease, for whom acetylcholinesterase inhibitors produce modest improvements in cognition and functional status, PSP patients treated with donepezil show little if any cognitive benefit and suffer a decline in motor function (Litvan *et al.*, 2001). Given the neuropathological complexity of PSP, it seems unlikely that a treatment strategy based upon neurotransmitter replacement will provide meaningful symptomatic effects; however, potential disease-modifying therapies that retard tau pathology are now in human trials.

Take home messages

Progressive supranuclear palsy is a sporadic neurodegenerative disease within the tauopathy family.

Patients with PSP may present with a dysexecutive syndrome secondary to pathology of the frontal lobes and/or striatothalamocortical circuits.

The Folstein mini-mental state examination is insensitive to the cognitive deficits that are present in patients with PSP, and other bedside tests, such as the Frontal Assessment Battery and Montreal Cognitive Assessment, are more suitable screening instruments for this patient population.

REFERENCES AND FURTHER READING

Aarsland D, Litvan I, Salmon D, *et al.* (2003). Performance on the dementia rating scale in Parkinson's disease with dementia and dementia with Lewy bodies: comparison with progressive supranuclear palsy and Alzheimer's disease. *J Neurol Neurosurg Psychiatry*, **74**, 1215–20.

Albert ML, Feldman RG, Willis AL (1974). The "subcortical dementia" of progressive supranuclear palsy. *J Neurol Neurosurg Psychiatry*, **37**, 121–30.

Bak TH, Rogers TT, Crawford LM, *et al.* (2005). Cognitive bedside assessment in atypical parkinsonian syndromes. *J Neurol Neurosurg Psychiatry*, **76**, 420–2.

Borroni B, Malinverno M, Gardoni F, *et al.* (2008). Tau forms in CSF as a reliable biomarker for progressive supranuclear palsy. *Neurology*, **71**, 1796–803.

Caparros-Lefebvre D, Steele J, Kotake Y, *et al.* (2006). Geographic isolates of atypical Parkinsonism and tauopathy in the tropics: possible synergy of neurotoxins. *Mov Disord*, **21**, 1769–71.

Delis DC, Kramer JH, Kaplan E, *et al.* (1987). *California Verbal Learning Test: Research Edition.* New York, NY: Psychological Corporation.

Dickson DW, Rademakers R, Hutton ML (2007). Progressive supranuclear palsy: pathology and genetics. *Brain Pathol*, **17**, 74–82.

Dubois B, Deweer B Pillon B (1996). The cognitive syndrome of progressive palsy. *Adv Neurol*, **69**, 399–403.

Dubois B, Slachevsky A, Litvan I, *et al.* (2000). The FAB: a frontal assessment battery at bedside. *Neurology*, **55**, 1621–6.

Dubois B, Slachevsky A, Pillon B, *et al.* (2005). "Applause sign" helps to discriminate PSP from FTD and PD. *Neurology*, **64**, 2132–3.

Folstein MF, Folstein SE, McHugh PR (1975). "Mini-mental state." A practical method for grading the cognitive state of patients for the clinician. *J Psychiatr Res*, **12**, 189–98.

Imai H, Narabayashi H, Sakata E (1987). Pure akinesia and the later added supranuclear ophthalmoplegia. *Adv Neurol*, **45**, 207–12.

Kaat LD, Boon AJ, Kamphorst W, *et al.* (2007). Frontal presentation in progressive supranuclear palsy. *Neurology*, **69**, 723–9.

Lange KW, Tucha O, Alders GL, *et al.* (2003). Differentiation of parkinsonian syndromes according to differences in executive functions. *J Neural Transm*, **110**, 983–95.

Litvan I (1994). Cognitive disturbances in progressive supranuclear palsy. *J Neural Transm*, **42**, 69–78.

Litvan I, Agid Y, Calne D, *et al.* (1996). Clinical research criteria for the diagnosis of progressive supranuclear palsy (Steele-Richardson-Olszewski syndrome): report of the NINDS-SPSP international workshop. *Neurology*, **47**, 1–9.

Litvan I, Phipps M, Pharr VL, *et al.* (2001). Randomized placebo-controlled trial of donepezil in patients with progressive supranuclear palsy. *Neurology*, **57**, 467–73.

Millar D, Griffiths P, Zermansky AJ (2006). Characterizing behavioral and cognitive dysexecutive changes in progressive supranuclear palsy. *Mov Disord*, **21**, 199–207.

Nasreddine ZS, Phillips NA, Bedirian V, *et al.* (2005). The Montreal Cognitive Assessment, MoCA: a brief screening tool for mild cognitive impairment. *J Am Geriatr Soc*, **53**, 695–9.

Nath U, Ben-Shlomo Y, Thompson RG, *et al.* (2001). The prevalence of progressive supranuclear palsy (Steele–Richardson–Olszewski syndrome) in the UK. *Brain*, **124**, 1438–49.

O'Sullivan SS, Massey LA, Williams DR, *et al.* (2008). Clinical outcomes of progressive supranuclear palsy and multiple system atrophy. *Brain*, **131**, 1362–72.

Paviour DC, Price SL, Jahanshahi M, *et al.* (2006). Longitudinal MRI in progressive supranuclear palsy and multiple system atrophy: rates and regions of atrophy. *Brain*, **129**,1040–9.

Rademakers R, Melquist S, Cruts M, *et al.* (2005). High-density SNP haplotyping suggests altered regulation of tau gene expression in progressive supranuclear palsy. *Hum Mol Genet*, **14**, 3281–92.

Rosser A, Hodges J (1994). The dementia rating scale in Alzheimer's disease, Huntington's disease and progressive supranuclear palsy. *J Neurol*, **241**:531–6.

Sitburana O, Ondo WG (2009). Brain magnetic resonance imaging (MRI) in parkinsonian disorders. *Parkinsonism Relat Disord*, **15**, 165–74.

Steele JC, Richardson JC, Olszewski J (1964). Progressive supranuclear palsy. *Arch Neurol*, **10**, 333–59.

Williams DR, de Silva R, Paviour DC, *et al.* (2005). Characteristics of two distinct clinical phenotypes in pathologically proven progressive supranuclear palsy: Richardson's syndrome and PSP-parkinsonism. *Brain*, **128**, 1247–58.

Williams DR, Holton JL, Strand C, *et al.* (2007). Pathological tau burden and distribution distinguishes progressive supranuclear palsy-parkinsonism from Richardson's syndrome. *Brain*, **130**, 1566–76.

Williams DR, Lees AJ (2009). Progressive supranuclear palsy: clinicopathological concepts and diagnostic challenges. *Lancet Neurol*, **8**, 270–9.

Man with problems with reading and calculating

Paulo Caramelli and Mirna Lie Hosogi-Senaha

Clinical history – main complaint

OO is a 69-year-old right-handed man, retired economist, who presented in June 2006 with a 1-year history of progressive word finding difficulties and mild phonoarticulatory problems.

General history

Despite the language problem, OO was responsible for providing care to his wife, who had advanced Alzheimer's disease, as well as managing the routine home activities and also managing his financial and bank account affairs. Moreover, he was able to drive safely around the city on his own, with good orientation both for time and space. In the last 6 months his daughter also reported some minor difficulties with calculations, together with occasional oral comprehension problems. In addition, mild depressive symptoms were recorded.

The patient had systemic arterial hypertension and diabetes mellitus, both under regular drug treatment. There was no history of previous head trauma. No report of learning disabilities or dyslexia during his childhood was recorded.

Family history

Family history for cognitive impairment was unremarkable.

Examination

OO scored 28 out of 30 points at the Mini-Mental State Examination (MMSE). In a simple delayed recall test, he was able to remember five out of ten figures, which is considered slightly impaired. However, his autobiographic memory was judged to be normal, since during conversation, he was able to correctly recall

Case Studies in Dementia: Common and Uncommon Presentations, ed. S. Gauthier and P. Rosa-Neto.
Published by Cambridge University Press. © Cambridge University Press 2011.

events within a 2-week period before the consultation. On a category fluency task (animals) his performance was markedly impaired, since he was able to generate only four items in 1 minute. His functional performance was preserved, with independence for instrumental activities of daily living, except for tasks demanding more complex linguistic abilities.

Special studies

Language and speech evaluation

Spontaneous speech and buccofacial praxis: OO's oral output was significantly reduced. His speech was slow, with articulatory simplification and marked changes in prosody. He was able to communicate through short and simple sentences and had difficulties in maintaining a longer dialog. Omissions of verbs and grammatical elements were evident in some instances, together with hesitations, word-finding problems (word repetitions, categorizations, and absence of words) and some semantic and phonemic paraphasias. As for buccofacial praxis, he was able to perform single and complex oral movements.

Language testing: on comprehensions tests, OO did not present errors in sentences with single words and simple syntactic structures, but failed in understanding more complex syntactic constructions. Repetition of single words was normal, but he showed some difficulties on repetition of phrases from the Boston Diagnostic Aphasia Examination. In the Boston Naming Test, OO was able to name only 35 out of 60 items and verbal fluency tests showed a disproportionate impairment of letter fluency in comparison to category fluency (Table 32.1).

On oral reading tests, OO was able to read irregular words and non-words. On the other hand, on writing to dictation, he experienced difficulties in writing irregular words rather than regular and non-words, suggesting surface dysgraphia. Table 32.1 displays the results of the main language tests employed.

Neuropsychological examination

OO scored 107 out of 144 points at the Mattis Dementia Rating Scale (DRS), which is below the Brazilian norms for this test (123/144). His performance was impaired in the subscales Initiation/Perseveration (24 out of 37) and Memory (15 out of 25) of the DRS. Further testing yielded mild impairment in executive functions and in verbal episodic memory tasks, probably due to interference by the language deficits (see Table 32.1).

Laboratory tests and neuroimaging results

Laboratory blood tests, namely complete blood cell count, thyroid, renal, and liver function tests, liver transaminases, Syphilis serology, vitamin B12 serum

Table 32.1. Performance of patient OO in language tests

Tasks	Performance
Oral comprehension	
Words	30/30
Simple sentences (Beta MT-86)	18/18
Complex sentences (Beta MT-86)	11/20
Written comprehension (Beta MT-86)	
Words	5/5
Simple sentences	4/4
Complex sentences	0/4
Repetition	
Words and non-words (Beta MT-86)	30/30
Repetition of sentences with high-frequency words (Boston)	5/8
Repetition of sentences with low-frequency words (Boston)	5/8
Confrontation naming	
Boston Naming Test	35/60
Fluency	
Living things	
Animals	3
Birds	4
Aquatic animals	1
Total	8
Artifacts	
Domestic utensils	5
Transportation	3
Musical instruments	4
Total	12
Letter fluency	
F	2
A	1
S	1
Total	4
Oral reading	
Words and non-words	30/30
Writing to dictation	
Words and non-words (HFSP protocol)	55/79

levels, and anti-thyroid antibodies were unremarkable. Magnetic resonance imaging (MRI) of the brain showed mild left frontotemporal lobe atrophy and a SPECT scan displayed hypoperfusion on left frontal and temporal areas (Fig. 32.1). Quantitative analysis of the SPECT images with Statistical Parametric Mapping (SPM) indicated significant perfusion deficits on the left anterior cingulate gyrus.

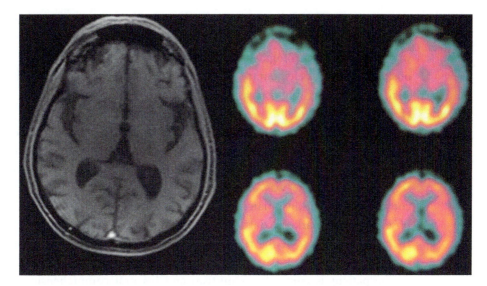

Fig. 32.1. T1-weighted, MRI (right side, axial view) shows very mild left perisylvian atrophy; SPECT images (left side, 4 axial views) show hypoperfusion on left frontal and temporal areas.

Initial diagnosis

Based on the overall clinical, neuropsychological, language, and neuroimaging data, a diagnosis of Progressive Non-Fluent Aphasia (PNFA) was made.

Follow-up

Duloxetine was started for the depressive symptoms with good clinical response. Six months later (December 2006), OO was re-examined. He scored 27 out of 30 points in the MMSE. His speech output worsened, with frequent pauses and hesitations, besides more impairment in naming abilities. He presented mild ideomotor apraxia. A slight limitation in vertical gaze was also noticed, especially upwards.

A trial with memantine (10 mg bid) was undertaken in an attempt to improve oral communication (off-label indication), but no benefits were recorded either by the patient or by his family or also on objective clinical evaluation. The drug was discontinued after 4 months of initiation.

In October 2007, his speech output was markedly reduced and oral comprehension was more impaired. He was unable to use money; spatial orientation was still unimpaired. Six months later, in April 2008, he was severely aphasic, with the speech output being limited to single words and to short simple sentences. His daughter reported the occurrence of falls (five in the previous four months), always backwards, secondary to balance and gait difficulties. Postural instability was evident on neurological examination. Supranuclear vertical gaze palsy was observed as well as elementary motor perseveration, with the so-called "applause sign." A diagnosis of possible progressive supranuclear palsy (PSP) was made (Litvan *et al.*, 1996).

By the end of 2008, OO began to present dysphagia, mainly for liquids. The daughter also reported the emergence of hyperorality behaviors, such as compulsive eating and bringing objects to his mouth. In June 2009, his speech output was severely reduced (he was able to produce only two words during the entire consultation). Parkinsonian signs, namely bradykinesia and rigidity, were observed, with marked axial involvement and an asymmetric limb distribution (being more intense at the right side). Oral levodopa treatment was started, at increasing doses, but no significant clinical benefits were documented.

The patient is currently in mutism and his oral comprehension is severely impaired. He is restricted to a wheelchair, due to severe balance and gait impairment. Dysphagia worsened significantly, making placing a feeding tube necessary (gastrostomy). He presents marked bradykinesia and rigidity, which are still more evident in axial muscles and at the right side of the body.

Diagnosis

Possible progressive supranuclear palsy.

Discussion

Primary progressive aphasia (PPA) is a clinical syndrome characterized by progressive dissolution of language with relative preservation of other cognitive abilities for at least 1 to 2 years (Mesulam, 1982, 2003; Rogalski and Mesulam, 2007). Mesulam in 1982 was the first who described in detail patients with the clinical syndrome of PPA and after the publication of his seminal paper, hundreds of cases have been reported and different patterns of language impairment have been described (Westbury and Bub, 1997; Clark *et al.*, 2005).

Recent studies have classified the clinical presentations of PPA into three main subtypes: agrammatic, logopenic, and semantic variant (Gorno Tempini *et al.*, 2004; Rogalski and Mesulam, 2007). The neuroimaging and pathological correlates of each PPA subtype have also been investigated (Gorno-Tempini *et al.*, 2004; Knibb *et al.*, 2006).

The agrammatic variant (progressive non-fluent aphasia – PNFA) is characterized by non-fluent speech output, labored articulation, agrammatism, anomia, complex syntactic comprehension impairment, and preserved semantic comprehension.

Patients with logopenic progressive aphasia (LPA) have marked word finding pauses, slow speech and relative intact syntax in output. Furthermore, logopenic patients present preserved single-word comprehension, but can have difficulties in syntactic comprehension. Gorno-Tempini *et al.* (2004) suggest that a short-term phonological memory deficit could be the core mechanism underlying the clinical presentation of LPA. In some instances the logopenic and agrammatic subtypes are grouped together as PNFA.

Semantic dementia (semantic variant of PPA or temporal lobe variant of frontotemporal dementia) is characterized by fluent speech, preservation of phonologic and syntactic aspects of language, and anomia with single-word comprehension deficits. Despite the impairment of semantic knowledge, syntactic comprehension is preserved. In written language examination, surface dyslexia and dysgraphia are found. Furthermore, the patients have impairment on tests of non-verbal associative knowledge to unfamiliar stimuli (Senaha *et al.*, 2007).

We report the case of a 69-year-old man with initial clinical presentation compatible with the diagnosis of PNFA, who later developed classic symptoms and signs of PSP. The clinical course was rapidly progressive and less than 4 years after the onset of symptoms the patient is in mutism, restricted to a wheelchair, and totally dependent for basic activities of daily living.

Features of PNFA as the initial manifestation of PSP have already been described before (Mochizuki *et al.*, 2003; Karnik *et al.*, 2006). Moreover, a recent clinico-pathological study conducted in France, which evaluated 18 patients with primary progressive language and speech disorders, found that two out of five patients with progressive anarthria had tau pathology on neuropathological examination, consistent with the diagnosis of PSP (Deramecourt *et al.*, 2010).

The diagnosis of PPA has a dynamic nature, since there is commonly a progression from the initial language syndrome to another clinical condition. In fact, PPA may be viewed as part of the spectrum of the frontotemporal lobe degeneration syndromes, which includes frontotemporal dementia, semantic dementia, and also PSP and corticobasal degeneration. Hence, the case of patient OO illustrates the overlap of linguistic and motor manifestations over time in PSP and corroborates the previous observations that the disease may present initially as a non-motor disorder. This observation reinforces the recommendation that cognitive evaluation, including careful language and speech examination, should be part of the routine clinical assessment of patients with atypical parkinsonian syndromes. Similarly, a full neurologic examination, with special attention to motor functions, balance/gait and ocular movements, should also be regularly performed during the follow-up of PPA patients, especially in PNFA.

Take home messages

PNFA may be the initial clinical presentation of PSP.

Cognitive, language, and speech evaluation should be part of the routine clinical assessment of patients with atypical parkinsonian syndromes.

REFERENCES AND FURTHER READING

Clark DG, Charuvastra A, Miller BL, Shapira JS, Mendez MF (2005). Fluent versus nonfluent primary progressive aphasia: a comparison of clinical and functional neuroimaging features. *Brain Language*, **94**, 54–60.

Deramecourt V, Lebert F, Debachy B, *et al.* (2010). Prediction of pathology in primary progressive language and speech disorders. *Neurology*, **74**, 42–9.

Gorno-Tempini ML, Dronkers NF, Rankin KP, *et al.* (2004). Cognition and anatomy of three variants of primary progressive aphasia. *Ann Neurol*, **55**, 335–46.

Karnik NS, D'Apuzzo M, Greicius M (2006). Non-fluent progressive aphasia, depression, and OCD in a woman with progressive supranuclear palsy: neuroanatomical and neuropathological correlations. *Neurocase*, **12**, 332–8.

Knibb JA, Xuereb JH, Patterson K, Hodges JR (2006). Clinical and pathological characterization of progressive aphasia. *Ann Neurol*, **59**, 156–65.

Litvan I, Agid Y, Calne D, *et al.* (1996). Clinical research criteria for the diagnosis of progressive supranuclear palsy (Steele-Richardson-Olszewski syndrome): report of the NINDS-SPSP international workshop. *Neurology*, **47**, 1–9.

Mesulam MM (1982). Slowly progressive aphasia without generalized dementia. *Ann Neurol*, **11**, 592–8.

Mesulam MM (2003). Primary progressive aphasia – a language-based dementia. *N Engl J Med*, **349**, 1535–42.

Mochizuki A, Ueda Y, Komatsuzaki Y, Tsuchiya K, Arai T, Shoji S (2003). Progressive supranuclear palsy presenting with primary progressive aphasia – clinicopathological report of an autopsy case. *Acta Neuropathol*, **105**, 610–14.

Rogalski E, Mesulam M (2007). An update on primary progressive aphasia. *Curr Neurol Neurosci Rep*, **7**, 388–92.

Senaha MLH, Caramelli P, Porto CS, Nitrini R (2007). Semantic dementia: Brazilian study of 19 cases. *Dementia Neuropsych*, **1**, 366–73.

Westbury C, Bub D (1997). Primary progressive aphasia: a review of 112 cases. *Brain Language*, **60**, 381–406.

Man with gait impairment and urine incontinence

Eric Schmidt and Maxime Ros

Clinical history – main complaint

The clinical history started 4 years ago with a rather slow decline, mainly movement difficulties and a right bradykinesia. The patient progressively complains of urinary incontinence requiring protective undergarments. He also presents postural hypotension. Initially, there was no cognitive decline. The patient was referred to a neurological department.

General history

Retired engineer in good general health. Lives with his wife. No medical problem and no medications. Right handed.

After extensive examination, the patient was diagnosed with Multiple System Atrophy (MSA) due to the co-existence of autonomic failure with orthostatic hypotension and Parkinsonism. The MRI showed no white matter disease, enlarged ventricles but a flow void in the cerebral aqueduct suggesting a normal CSF dynamics. The hypothesis of hydrocephalus was waived. Levodopa was introduced up to 1 g per day, but the patient did not respond; the Levodopa unresponsiveness was declared. The MSA diagnosis was explained to the patient and the family.

Within the last months the patient's condition worsened: his hypokinetic gait deteriorated requiring walking aids. A cognitive decline was noted. The burden for the caregiver was clearly increased.

The patient was referred to our hydrocephalus clinic to address the potential benefit of a ventricular shunt.

Family history

Father and mother died, respectively, at age 80 of lung cancer and 84 of stroke. No family disease has been identified.

Case Studies in Dementia: Common and Uncommon Presentations, ed. S. Gauthier and P. Rosa-Neto. Published by Cambridge University Press. © Cambridge University Press 2011.

Examination

BP 160/85; pulse 65 regular. The gait velocity was reduced with a highly variable stride length and a broad based pattern. External cues only mildly improve the gait. There was a postural instability and clear bradykinesia with rest tremor and rigidity of the right upper limb. Deep tendons reflexes were present, no Babinski's sign. The discussion with the patient was limited to simple answers to our questions. He was sitting in the chair without complaining. MMSE was 21/30. The neuropsychological examination confirmed memory and learning difficulties. The dementia diagnosis was assigned using the *Diagnostic and Statistical Manual*, fourth edition.

Special studies

The MRI showed enlarged ventricles with an Evan's ratio of 0.43. The fourth ventricle was also enlarged. Diffuse cortical atrophy with large sulci. There was no transependymal edema on the FLAIR-weighted images.

We performed a computerized lumbar infusion study to measure cerebrospinal fluid (CSF) dynamics.

The patient was awake, lay on the left side on a flat bed, the head at the level of the heart. Particular attention was paid to the tranquillity of the patient during the test. A lumbar puncture was performed with a 20-gauge needle (Fig. 33.1(a) No.1), which was connected *via* a three-way tap to an infusion pump (Fig. 33.1(a) No.2) and to a pressure transducer (Fig. 33.1(a) No.3). Signal was recorded and analyzed with a computer (Fig. 33.1(a) No.4). The CSF pressure, once zeroed at the level of the heart, yields a measure of the intracranial pressure (ICP). ICP was measured at baseline for a few minutes. Then the subarachnoid space was infused with normal saline solution (0.9%) at room temperature (20 °C) with a rate of 1.5 ml/min.

Subsequently, ICP rose until a steady-state plateau had been achieved. This "plateau" ICP corresponded to the equilibrium at which the mock CSF infusion flow was re-absorbed by the arachnoid villi.

An example of normal CSF infusion test was displayed Fig. 33.1(b). Mean ICP at baseline was normal (9.1 mmHg) with a low pulsatility amplitude (AMP = 1.3 mmHg). During the infusion, ICP rose until a steady plateau was reached (25 mmHg). The resistance to CSF outflow was normal: (25–9.1)/1.5 = 10.6 mmHg/ml/min.

The patient's infusion test was reproduced Fig. 33.2(a). The pressure was normal at baseline with normal ICP (ICP = 15 mmHg) and amplitude (AMP = 1.82 mmHg). However the CSF dynamics was clearly altered: infusion had to be stopped as ICP went higher than the accepted threshold (40 mmHg). ICP pulse amplitude increased *pari passu*, suggesting that the system did not tolerate an extra CSF volume, that is an altered compliance. The resistance to

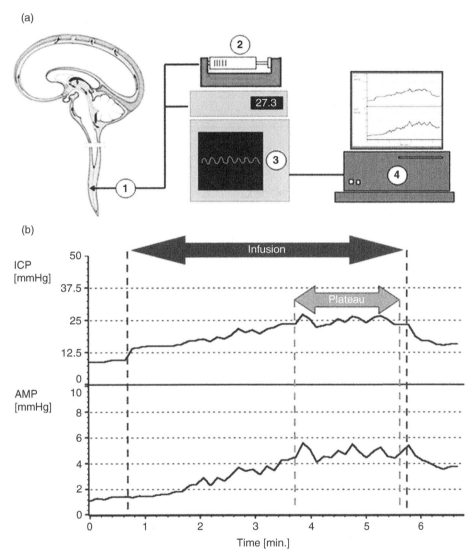

Fig. 33.1. (a) Infusion study setting: needle (No. 1), infusion pump (No. 2), pressure transducer (No. 3), computer (No. 4). (b) Normal infusion study.

CSF outflow was estimated superior to 18 mmHg/ml/min, which is undoubtedly pathological (Boon *et al.*, 1997).

Diagnosis

The diagnosis of MSA was not incorrect, in that the patient actually presents the signs and patterns of this disease. But we also identified an hydrocephalic

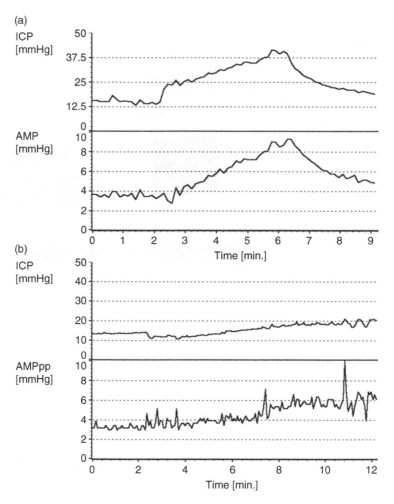

Fig. 33.2.   (a) Patient's infusion study prior to the shunt. (b) Infusion study to check the function of the shunt.

pattern: the clinical signs, enlarged ventricles, and deranged CSF dynamics strongly suggest the diagnosis of normal pressure hydrocephalus.

The probabilistic diagnosis of a syndrome combining MSA and NPH.

As part of the symptoms, especially hypokinetic gait and urinary problems, are deemed to be partially reversible after shunt inversion (Marmarou et al., 2005), we proposed a neurosurgical procedure. After gauging the pros and cons with the patient and his family, the insertion of a shunt was accepted and the patient was operated on. A ventriculo-peritoneal shunt was inserted.

Follow-up

The patient improved quickly after the surgery, not only in terms of gait, but also neuropsychologically.

One month after the shunt insertion, the patient was able to walk without aid. The gait velocity improved, the patient was more stable. There was a strong positive effect for the caregiver. The urinary incontinence also partially improved, requiring only night protective underwear.

Psychologically, the patient was more awake and active. He was interested in reading and watching the television. His wife was fully satisfied with the surgical procedure. However, the autonomic dysfunction and Parkinsonism were still present. MSA was lurking.

At 6 months, the benefit of the shunt reached a plateau.

At 1 year, the patient's wife noted a decline, not only in terms of gait but also in general status. The patient shuffled, his walking capacities slightly deteriorated. He fell several times at home and was less interested in his family life. No other sign of Parkinsonism.

Eighteen months after the surgery, the decline was obvious. The patient was more apraxic and the memory loss was prominent. We performed a head CT scan, which was normal excluding any subdural hematoma. The ventricular catheter was in place.

We finally checked the shunt to be sure that it was functioning optimally. We performed an infusion study in the pre-chamber of the shunt (*cf.* Fig. 33.2(b)). The baseline pressure was normal (13 mmHg) and pulsatile. The opening pressure of the valve was in accordance with its setting. We drew the conclusion that the shunt was working properly.

The benefit of the shunt has been outweighed by the neurodegenerative disease.

Discussion

Gait disorders and dementia

Gait disorders are common in elderly populations and their prevalence increases with age. At the age of 60 years, 85% of people have a normal gait, but at the age of 85 years or older this proportion has dropped to 18% (Sudarsky, 2001). These gait disturbances can also reflect an early pre-clinical neurodegenerative disease (Snijders *et al.*, 2007). On one hand, quantitative gait measures predict future risk of cognitive decline and dementia in initially non-demented older adults (Verghese *et al.*, 2007). But on the other hand, hypokinetic gait disorders occur in many different neurological diseases, such as NPH, Parkinson's disease, subcortical arteriosclerotic encephalopathy, Alzheimer's disease, and other rare disorders. It has been shown that about 35% of the gait disorders in a neurological referral practice are hypokinetic; of these, about 55% are related to Parkinson's disease and NPH (Sudarsky, 1997).

Dementia and gait disorders are frequently associated symptoms, and this issue has to be addressed in the daily clinical practice. Ask this simple question: do I underestimate the gait difficulties of this demented patient?

NPH and prognostic tests

In front of a patient with clinical symptoms of NPH, it is important to estimate the probability of improvement after shunt insertion. In that respect, evidence-based guidelines for use in supplementary tests have been developed (Marmarou *et al.*, 2005).

A positive response to a 40 ml tap test has a higher degree of certainty for a favorable response to shunt placement than can be obtained by clinical examination. However, the tap test cannot be used as an exclusionary test because of its low sensitivity (26%–61%). Determination of the CSF outflow resistance via an infusion test carries a higher sensitivity (57%–100%) compared with the tap test and a similar positive predictive value of 75% to 92%. Prolonged external lumbar drainage in excess of 300 ml is associated with high sensitivity (50%–100%) and high positive predictive value (80%–100%) but its complication rate is rather high (meningitis 10%, root irritation 10%). To date, a single standard for the prognostic evaluation of NPH patients is lacking; however, supplemental tests can increase predictive accuracy for prognosis.

A 40 ml tap test is still a relevant approach to explore the potential benefit of a shunt in a patient suspected of hydrocephalus. More sophisticated tests, especially dynamic tests, are sometimes needed, but require the expertise and *armamentarium* of an hydrocephalus unit.

NPH and comorbidities

The main question for the clinician is not whether the patient suffers from NPH or a concurrent irreversible disorder, but whether the hydrocephalus or the presence of a non-shunt responsive comorbidity are the major contributors to the symptomatology. In patients not responding to shunt surgery, cerebrovascular disease and Alzheimer's disease are the predominant disorders thought to mimic the NPH syndrome. This presumption is based on the fact that Alzheimer's disease and cerebrovascular disease are the most frequent causes of dementia, including cases improving after shunt operation (Golomb *et al.*, 2000; Bech-Azeddine *et al.*, 2007). It has also been hypothesized that NPH share common pathophysiology with Alzheimer's disease (Silverberg *et al.*, 2003) and/or cerebrovascular disease (Krauss *et al.*, 1996), which further confounds the clinical picture.

Extrapyramidal motor signs in NPH have been described in the literature (Curran and Lang, 1994). Recent studies suggest that clinical motor signs of NPH subjects extend beyond gait deficits and include extrapyramidal manifestations such as bradykinesia, akinesia, or rigidity. Objective improvement of some but not all of these features was seen following temporary or permanent CSF diversion (Mandir *et al.*, 2007).

The findings support the perception of NPH as a multi-etiological clinical entity, possibly overlapping various neurodegenerative conditions (Bech-Azeddine *et al.*, 2007).

Take home messages

Patients with Normal Pressure Hydrocephalus (NPH) syndrome are traditionally described as presenting a clinical triad of progressing hypokinetic gait, dementia, urinary incontinence, and radiologically defined hydrocephalus, i.e., enlarged ventricles on CT or MRI.

However, the clinical picture of NPH is frequently confounding. We report an uncommon case of neurodegenerative disorder with Parkinsonism, orthostatic hypotension, hypokinetic gait, cognitive decline, and hydrocephalus that partially improved after shunt insertion, bridging NPH and Multiple System Atrophy (MSA).

Tap test and infusion tests help to identify patients that might benefit from a shunt.

REFERENCES AND FURTHER READING

Bech-Azeddine R, Høgh P, Juhler M, Gjerris F, Waldemar G (2007). Idiopathic normal pressure hydrocephalus: clinical comorbidity correlated to cerebral biopsy findings and outcome of CSF shunting. *J Neurol Neurosurg Psychiatry*, **78**(2), 157–61.

Boon AJ, Tans JT, Delwel EJ, *et al.* (1997). Dutch normal-pressure hydrocephalus study: prediction of outcome after shunting by resistance to outflow of cerebrospinal fluid. *J Neurosurg*, **87**(5), 687–93.

Curran T, Lang AE (1994). Parkinsonian syndromes associated with hydrocephalus: case reports, a review of the literature, and pathophysiological hypotheses. *Mov Disord*, **9**, 508–20.

Golomb J, Wisoff J, Miller DC, *et al.* (2000). Alzheimer's disease comorbidity in normal pressure hydrocephalus: prevalence and shunt response. *J Neurol Neurosurg Psychiatry*, **68**, 778–81.

Krauss JK, Regel JP, Vach W, Droste DW, Borremans JJ, Mergner T (1996). Vascular risk factors and arteriosclerotic disease in idiopathic normal-pressure hydrocephalus of the elderly. *Stroke*, **27**, 24–9.

Mandir AS, Hilfiker J, Thomas G, *et al.* (2007). Extrapyramidal signs in normal pressure hydrocephalus: an objective assessment. *Cerebrospinal Fluid Res*, **13**, 4–7.

Marmarou A, Bergsneider M, Relkin N, Klinge P, Black PM (2005). Development of guidelines for idiopathic normal-pressure hydrocephalus: introduction. *Neurosurgery*, **57**(3 Suppl), S40–52.

Silverberg GD, Mayo M, Saul T, Rubenstein E, McGuire D (2003). Alzheimer's disease, normal-pressure hydrocephalus, and senescent changes in CSF circulatory physiology: a hypothesis. *Lancet Neurol*, **2**, 506–11.

Snijders AH, van de Warrenburg BP, Giladi N, Bloem BR (2007). Neurological gait disorders in elderly people: clinical approach and classification. *Lancet Neurol*, **6**(1), 63–74.

Sudarsky L (1997). *Clinical Approach to Gait Disorders of Aging: an Overview.* Philadelphia: Lippincott-Raven.

Sudarsky L (2001). Gait disorders prevalence, morbidity, and etiology. *Adv Neurol*, **87**, 111–17.

Verghese J, Cuiling W, Lipton RB, Holtzer R, Xiaonan X (2007). Quantitative gait dysfunction and risk of cognitive decline and dementia. *J Neurol Neurosurg Psychiatry*, **78**, 929–35.

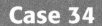

Case 34

Falling before forgetting

Vesna Jelic, Inger Nennesmo, Sven-Eric Pålhagen,
and Bengt Winblad

Clinical history – main complaint

A 67-year-old man was admitted to the Movement Disorders Clinic with a history of unstable gait with frequent falls, intermittent blurred vision with diplopia while reading or watching television, personality changes with social withdrawal, lack of initiative, and reduced spontaneous speech. The patient's wife reported that, during the past 2 years she had observed him exhibiting balance problems and generally slowed movements, noting that he would sit in the same position in front of the TV for a couple of hours without moving.

Neither subject nor informant confirmed memory difficulties were noted to be major presenting problems on admission.

General history

The patient was a retired engineer, residing with his wife. The couple had no biological children, but had adopted a daughter and a son. The patient had no history of smoking or of alcohol or drug abuse. Hypertension was diagnosed 2 years before admission and was managed using a beta-blocker. He had recently been diagnosed with benign prostatic hyperplasia and was treated for that with alpha-blocker (doxazosin).

Family history

The patient's mother died at the age of 84, a few years after being diagnosed with Alzheimer's disease. However, this clinical diagnosis was not confirmed by a post-mortem pathological examination. During her life she had also suffered from cardiovascular problems and diabetes. The patient's father died in his 40s of tuberculosis.

Case Studies in Dementia: Common and Uncommon Presentations, ed. S. Gauthier and P. Rosa-Neto.
Published by Cambridge University Press. © Cambridge University Press 2011.

The patient had three brothers, one of whom was subject to a coronary bypass due to angina and underlying coronary artery disease.

Examination

General examination was unremarkable. Blood pressure (BP) in flat-lying position was 160/80 mmHg, the pulse was regular, 68/min. Standing BP obtained after 5 minutes was 160/85, with pulse 70/min. Carotid pulses were without bruits.

Neurological examination revealed hypomimia with reduced blink frequency, reduced spontaneous speech with monotonous prosody, and bilaterally reduced hearing. Vertical ocular movements for voluntary gaze as well as smooth pursuit ocular movements were slow and limited toward an upward direction to two-thirds of normal range. Volitional horizontal gaze and smooth pursuit of a visual target were also slowed and saccadicaly fragmented. Convergence eye movements were limited, but the patient did not report diplopia during examination. He had symmetrical bradykinesia without rigidity. Muscle strength was preserved, deep tendon reflexes were brisk and symmetric, plantar responses were flexor. Palmo-mental reflex was positive bilaterally. No resting or action tremor was observed and there was no dysmetria during coordination tests. He walked steadily with normal-based gait, had reduced arm swing and performed turning with an en bloc movement, altogether markedly unstable.

Neither aphasia nor apraxia signs were elicited. He could not perform whole sequence of Luria's fist-palm-edge test and showed a tendency to perseverate.

MMSE score was 23/30. He gave the date incorrectly by one day, could not subtract backwards and had difficulty in recalling two of three words. He could not perform the Clock Test due to dysexecutive problems.

Neuropsychological testing revealed difficulties in word fluency, working memory (digit span forward and backwards), visuospatial episodic memory (retention of a complex figure), attention and executive function (Trial Making B), and showed slowed information processing speed. He performed within the low average range on a test of verbal episodic memory (free recall and recognition of twelve random words test, FRR12RWT).

Special studies

Routine laboratory tests were normal. Cerebral spinal fluid (CSF) total-tau, phosphorylated tau, and beta42-amyloid were within reference intervals. CSF-neurofilament light chain (NFL) was increased (870 ng/L, ref < 380 ng/L).

EEG showed normal background activity within range of alpha band, 9–10 Hz and blocking on eyes opening.

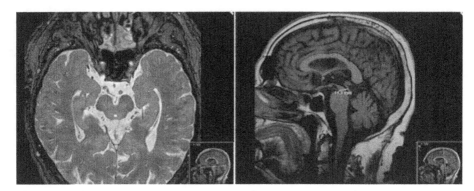

Fig. 34.1. Sagittal T1 weighted MRI shows the "Penguin sign" (right),caused by the reduction of midbrain diameter (11 mm). Axial T2 weighted MRI shows the "Mickey Mouse sign" (left) caused by the the thinning of the mesencephalon with prominent interpeduncular cisterns.

MRI examination of the brain showed the sagittal diameter of the mesencephalon (midbrain) reduced to 11 mm (the "Penguin sign," Fig. 34.1) and thinning of the mesencephalon tegmentum with prominent interpeduncular cisterns (the "Mickey Mouse sign," Fig. 34.1).

Diagnosis

The initial clinical diagnosis was based on the patient's history and neurological examination. Symptom debut with gait instability, frequent falls, and incomplete parkinsonism with postural instability, symmetric bradykinesia without rigidity or tremor, disturbance in ocular motility and early occurrence of subcortical dementia with frontal-dysexecutive problems, and relatively preserved memory made Progressive Supranuclear Palsy (PSP) the most likely diagnosis. Absence of pyramidal or cerebellar signs or dysautonomia and early occurrence of dementia ruled out Multiple System Atrophy (MSA) as an alternative diagnosis. Absence of asymmetric apraxia or alien-hand syndrome did not speak in favor of Cortico-basal Degeneration (CBD). Diagnosis of Lewy body dementia was less likely due to absence of hallucinations, fluctuations, notable visuospatial dysfunction with features of cortical-dementia, dysautonomia, or generalized EEG slowing.

Follow-up

The patient did not respond to levodopa treatment (daily dose up to 300 mg/d) and did not tolerate memantine administered *ex-juvantibus* (daily dose of 20 mg/d).

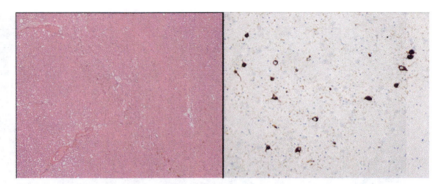

Fig. 34.2.   Hematoxilin eosin micrographs show loss of pigmented cells in substantia nigra (left). Cells positive for tau pathology in the pons (dark colored; right side).

During the following year the frequency of falls increased. There was a tendency to lean backwards, which determined the direction of falls. He developed vertical gaze palsy with staring gaze, axial rigidity with retrocolis, affective lability, as well as bulbar symptoms including swallowing difficulty and dysarthria. He demonstrated no spontaneous speech, but could answer with short and often stereotyped sentences. According to the family, further memory deterioration was notable in daily life and the patient appeared to lack insight into his problems which additionally increased the frequency of his falling. One year after initial admission the patient was newly admitted to long-term care, where he died at the end of the following year due to complications of bronchopneumonia.

The neuropathological examination of the brain revealed prominent changes especially in the basal ganglia, midbrain, and brainstem. Using silver impregnation, numerous neurofibrillary tangles were identified in these regions.

A reduced number of pigmented cells were found in substantia nigra. Immunohistochemistry showed widespread tau-pathology both intraneurally and in oligodendrocytes (Fig. 34.2), and an occasional tufted astrocyte was also present. The nature and distribution of the pathologic changes implicated the diagnosis of PSP.

Discussion

The patient had a prototypical Progressive Supranuclear Palsy (PSP), a neurological disorder characterized by postural instability and falls within a year of disease onset, as well as reduced vertical eye movements. Supportive features are symmetrical bradykinesia, axial rigidity, no response to levodopa treatment, early onset of cognitive impairment with features of mild forgetfulness, but with marked impairment in verbal fluency and executive functions, including working memory (Litvan *et al.*, 1996; Burn and Lees, 2002). This is an uncommon disease with an estimated prevalence of 6.4/100 000 in the general population

(Golbe, 2001). Three clinical phenotypes have been described, including: (1) classical Steele–Richardson–Olszewski syndrome with vertical gaze palsy and early onset of dementia; (2) PSP-Parkinsonism (PSP-P) with asymmetric bradykinesia and rigidity early during the course of the disease; and (3) Pure Akinesia with Gait Freezing (PAGF) and absence of dementia during the first 5 years after onset of symptoms (Litvan *et al.*, 1996; Williams and Lees, 2010; Williams *et al.*, 2007). The variety of clinical presentations make difficult early differential diagnosis from other Parkinson-plus variants such as MSA and CBD or from multi-infarct state or diffuse Lewy body disease. There are no specific markers for the disease and MRI finding of midbrain atrophy is a diagnostically supportive neuroradiological feature (Schrag *et al.*, 2000). Typical CSF biomarkers are not helpful to differentiate among atypical Parkinsonian disorders due to lack of specificity. A common observation in PSP is increased CSF-Neurofilament (NFL) in the presence of normal tau and phosphorylated-tau, which is useful in differentiation from idiopathic Parkinson's disease (Constantinescu *et al.*, 2010). Definitive diagnosis is established by *post-mortem* pathological examination findings in the brain, including: loss of pigment in substantia nigra corresponding to nigrostriatal dopaminergic degeneration and tau-positive inclusions in several subcortical structures such as basal ganglia, especially the pallidum, subthalamic nucleus, brainstem, and dentate nucleus.

Take home messages

Early symptoms of gait instability with frequent falls, oculomotor disturbances, and additional neurological signs of symmetric incomplete parkinsonism without tremor can precede cognitive impairment in some dementing diseases.

In patients presenting with an atypical Parkinsonian disorder and postural instability, cognitive testing should be performed.

Dementia in such cases is of a subcortical type characterized by a frontal-dysexecutive syndrome.

REFERENCES AND FURTHER READING

Burn DJ, Lees AJ (2002). Progressive supranuclear palsy: Where are we now? *Lancet Neurology*, 1, 359–69.

Constantinescu, R, Rosengren L, Johnels B, Zetterberg H, Holberg B (2010). Consecutive analyses of cerebrospinal fluid axonal and glial markers in Parkinson's disease and atypical Parkinsonian disorders. *Parkinsonism Rel Disord*, 16, 142–5.

Dickson DW, Rademakers R, Hutton ML (2007). Progressive supranuclear palsy: pathology and genetics. *Brain Pathol*, **17**, 74–82.

Golbe LI (2001). Progressive supranuclear palsy. *Curr Treat Options Neurol*, **3**, 473–7.

Golbe LI, Ohman-Strickland PA (2007). A clinical rating scale for progressive supranuclear palsy. *Brain*, **130**, 1552–65.

Litvan I, Agid Y, Calne D, *et al.* (1996). Clinical research criteria for the diagnosis of progressive supranuclear palsy (Steele Richardson–Olszewski syndrome): report of the NINDS-SPSP International Workshop. *Neurology*, **47**, 1–9.

Schrag A, Good CD, Miszkiel K, *et al.* (2000). Differentiation of atypical parkinsonian syndromes with routine MRI. *Neurology*, **54**, 697–702.

Williams DR, Holton JL, Strand K, Revesz T, Lees AJ (2007). Pure akinesia with gait freezing: a third clinical phenotype of progressive supranuclear palsy. *Mov Disord*, **22**, 2235–41.

Williams DR, Lees AJ (2010). What features improve the accuracy of the clinical diagnosis of progressive supranuclear palsy–parkinsonism (PSP–P)? *Mov Disord* **00**, 000–000.

Man who stopped drinking

Mary M. Kenan and Rachel S. Doody

Clinical history – main complaint

Mr. M is an 81-year-old, left-handed, Caucasian man referred by his internist for evaluation of cognitive change. By his niece's report, the patient was alcoholic for more than 50 years, but became abstinent with full, sustained remission three years prior to the first visit. After he stopped drinking, there was no evidence of cognitive difficulty. He was ambulatory at the time he discontinued drinking, but had difficulty going up and down stairs due to unsteadiness of gait. At the time of his wife's death 2 years before the first visit, the family noticed mild forgetfulness for recent events or details, and gait difficulty that progressed over time. He began using a walker or wheelchair for longer distances. During this time, he also experienced several falls and/or syncopal episodes.

One month before the first visit, over the course of a few days, his chronic difficulties with cognition and gait worsened significantly. He became unable to express himself coherently and had difficulty comprehending language. He could no longer walk, even with assistive devices, and became wheelchair bound. His caregiver noticed that he had increased difficulty using his left hand and that he tended to lean to the left. His primary care doctor did an MRI, which showed atrophy and non-specific white matter changes, and referred the patient to us.

At the time of the initial assessment, he was forgetful and tended to repeat back phrases that were said to him or questions asked of him (echolalia). His expressive speech was sometimes nonsensical. He had trouble reading, writing, and following instructions. His complex activities of daily living, as well as dressing and toileting were impaired and he had episodes of incontinence. He displayed anxiety and apathy, but his mood was generally euthymic. He has no delusions, hallucinations, or other evidence of psychosis.

Case Studies in Dementia: Common and Uncommon Presentations, ed. S. Gauthier and P. Rosa-Neto. Published by Cambridge University Press. © Cambridge University Press 2011.

General history

Mr. M obtained 16 years of education. He had been a widower for 2 years and lived in his own home with round-the-clock caregivers. Recently, he required the assistance of two caregivers at a time due to his inability to perform transfers. He was accompanied to the visit by a paid caregiver and his niece who held his medical and financial powers of attorney. He had no major medical illnesses and had experienced no seizures, loss of consciousness, psychiatric history, or blood transfusions between 1977 and 1985. In addition to his 50-year history of alcohol dependence (now in remission), he was addicted in the past to prescription drugs including valium, sleeping aids, and pain killers.

Family history

Positive for dementia in his mother, which started at age 92 and progressed to the time of her death at age 94. His maternal grandmother also developed dementia in her late 80s or early 90s, which progressed until the time of her death in her late 90s. The patient's father died of bone cancer in his 40s. He is an only child.

Examination

Vital signs: H = 5 feet, 7 inches, W = 170, BP = 130/80, P = 80 sitting, unable to stand for standing assessment. The patient was alert and oriented to his name, but not to personal details or to time or place. He initially introduced his niece as his doctor and his caregiver as "half a nurse." He later identified the doctor as his granddaughter. He could name the city and state. He could name high frequency words and repeat a phrase. He was otherwise disoriented to time and place, could not register words for verbal recall testing, nor recall any words after a 10-minute delay. He could add 3 plus 2, but could not calculate serial 7s. He could spell "world" forward but not in reverse. He could not read and follow a command, write a sentence, or copy intersecting pentagons. His score on the Mini-Mental Status Examination (Folstein *et al.*, 1975) was 5/30. He was unable to engage in paired associate learning. He could respond with a simple social statement and gave his first name. His comprehension of verbal one- and two-step commands was inconsistent. Repetition for words or a brief passage was intact, as was attention to the examiner. He was able to draw a circle, but could not sign his name. His score on the Baylor Profound Mental Status Examination (Doody *et al.*, 1999) was 17/25. Cranial Nerves: 1. – Not tested. II. – Pupils equal, round, and reactive to light and accommodation. Disks appeared normal with normal cup to disc ratios and sharp disk margins. II., IV., VI. – He had ocular dysmetria and intermittent ophthalmoplegia with a few beats of nystagmus on lateral gaze. V. – Normal facial sensation and corneal responses. VII. – Normal strength of facial musculature. VIII.– Hearing intact to finger rub bilaterally. IX., X. – Palate elevated symmetrically. XI. – Normal sternocleidomastoid strength. XII. – Tongue protrudes in the midline. Motor Examination: He had mildly hypophonic speech. His motor testing was complicated by severe ataxia that was primarily appendicular. He also had spontaneous and action-induced myoclonus in all extremities. Formal strength testing established a pattern of mild proximal muscle weakness in the upper and lower extremities with relative preservation of distal strength. Reflexes: 2+ and symmetric at biceps, brachioradialis, triceps, knee jerks, and absent ankle jerks. Plantar responses were downgoing. He also had glabellar and snout reflexes. Cerebellar: there is extreme limb ataxia affecting all extremities. Sensory examination: unreliable, but he clearly attended to stimulation of all extremities. Gait: he was unable to stand or to walk.

Diagnosis

Initial impression was that of an acute-on-chronic change of cognition and gait, which occurred about a month before the first visit, most likely due to Wernicke's encephalopathy, plus underlying dementia. Potentially contributing factors in the differential diagnosis of the dementia were alcoholism in the past, suspected nutritional insufficiency, possible multi-infarct dementia, and possible Alzheimer's disease.

Follow-up

The patient was treated emergently for Wernicke's encephalopathy with intravenous thiamine hydrochloride immediately following the new patient visit. There is no universal consensus regarding the dosing level or duration of supplementation for Wernicke's encephalopathy secondary to alcohol abuse, but studies support empirically treating the condition with a minimum of 500 mg of parenteral thiamine hydrochloride (dissolved in 100 ml of normal saline), given by infusion over a period of 30 minutes, three times per day for 2 to 3 days. If clinical improvement occurs, treatment is continued at 250 mg thiamine intravenously or intramuscularly daily for 3–5 days or until improvement ceases (Sechi and Serra, 2007).

According to his niece, after receiving 2 days of intravenous treatment in the first week, and 3 days of treatment in the second week, he improved to his level of function prior to the acute deterioration. He became more alert and attentive with clear, expressive speech. He regained the ability to walk using a walker within

2 weeks. At a follow-up visit 3 weeks after the initial visit, his MMSE had improved from 5 to 12 and he could perform paired associate learning, learning 1/4 paired associates on each of two trials. He could also answer simple questions about similarities and differences.

Laboratory evaluation: the patient's serum chemistries were normal except for a very slight elevation of glucose at 104 mg/dL on a non-fasting sample, and slight elevation of triglycerides at 165 mg/dL. ANA was non-specifically elevated at 1:40 in a non-specific speckled pattern. His CBC, sedentary rate, thyroid function test, serum protein electrophoresis, B12, folate, homocysteine, and methylmalonic acid were normal as were his chest X-ray and EKG. His MRI showed atrophy and non-specific white matter changes. Apolipoprotein E (ApoE) genotype was E2/E3. He was diagnosed with mild Alzheimer's disease and resolved Wernicke's encephalopathy.

Cholinesterase inhibitor treatment and high dose vitamin E and C were prescribed, but he decided not to take the cholinesterase inhibitor. He returned for a follow-up visit 7 months after his initial visit and showed continued improvement in cognition. He was alert and oriented to himself and the medical situation. He knew all aspects of time and place except for the exact date. He registered information well and recalled 3/3 words after a brief delay. He could spell world forwards and in reverse, but did not attempt serial 7s. He could read a command, write a sentence, and copy intersecting pentagons. On the MMSE, he scored 24/30 with serial 7s and 29/30 with the version requiring him to spell "world" backward. He completed three of four elements correctly on a clock drawing test. He learned 3/4 paired associates on each trial. But, despite these cognitive improvements, there was clearly still a concurrent dementia based on the patient's performance on comprehensive neuropsychological testing. Delayed verbal and visual memory performance was impaired on the Wechsler Memory Scale-Revised (WMS-R), visual perception was impaired on the Rey Complex Figure Copy (Osterrieth, 1944), attention and concentration were defective on the Verbal Series Attention Test (VSAT) and the Wisconsin Card Sorting Test (WCST; Berg, 1948), and he made several motor programming errors and a few praxis errors. The patient and family agreed to start treatment with a cholinesterase inhibitor.

Discussion

The patient's history suggested both an insidious dementia and an acute change due to some other factor. Given this patient's protracted period of alcoholism, it is possible that he had experienced previous episodes of acute Wernicke's encephalopathy, which went clinically undetected or unreported. The clinical diagnosis of Wernicke's encephalopathy is complicated by a sometimes non-specific clinical presentation or unrecognized neurological signs of the disease (Sechi and Serra, 2007). Charness *et al.* (1989) reported that an accurate clinical diagnosis of acute Wernicke's encephalopathy prior to death is made as infrequently as 1 in 22 patients based upon post-mortem studies. In our clinical experience, the effects of cerebral degeneration resulting from aging, combined with poor nutrition and a compromised cholinergic system due to Alzheimer's disease can acutely precipitate or reactivate Wernicke's encephalopathy in former alcoholics who have successfully reduced or abstained from alcohol use. Once treated with thiamine, the patient improved greatly, from severe dementia with an MMSE of 5 to mild dementia with an MMSE of 29. Even though the acute cognitive decline and cerebellar signs improved, formal psychometric testing documented the underlying dementia as suspected, 7 months after the initial evaluation. This case illustrates the importance of obtaining a careful chronology of symptoms in the history, and of entertaining the possibility of both acute and chronic processes.

Take home messages

In the context of progressive neurocognitive decline due to Alzheimer's disease, acute Wernicke's encephalopathy can present, even after a period of sustained abstinence from alcohol.

A dual diagnosis of acute Wernicke's encephalopathy and Alzheimer's disease should be considered for patients in full or partial remission from alcoholism who experience sudden decline. Acute confusion, gait ataxia, myoclonus, ophthalmoplegias or other ocular changes, and impaired expressive speech and comprehension can all be part of the clinical presentation.

Patients with suspected Wernicke's encephalopathy should be urgently and empirically treated with an infusion of at least 500 mg thiamine hydrochloride (dissolved in 100 ml of normal saline), administered over a 30-minute period, three times per day for 2–3 days. If clinically improved, treatment should continue with 250 mg thiamine intravenously or intramuscularly daily for 3–5 days or until there is no further improvement (Sechi and Serra, 2007). Such treatment can produce significant functional and cognitive improvements even in patients with underlying Alzheimer's disease.

Treatment for mild to moderate Alzheimer's disease co-existing with Wernicke's encephalopathy consists of a cholinesterase inhibitor, once symptoms of acute Wernicke's encephalopathy are resolved.

REFERENCES AND FURTHER READING

Berg EA (1948). A simple objective treatment for measuring flexibility in thinking. *J Gen Psychol*, **39**, 15–22.

Charness ME, Simon RP, Greenberg DA (1989). Ethanol and the nervous system. *N Engl J Med*, **321** (7), 442–53.

Doody RS, Strehlow SL, Massman PJ, Feher EP, Clark C, Roy JR (1999). Baylor Profound Mental Status Examination: a brief staging measure for profoundly demented Alzheimer disease patients. *Alz Dis Assoc Dis*, **13**(1), 53–9.

Folstein MF, Folstein SE, McHugh PR (1975). "Mini Mental State": a practical method for grading the cognitive state of patients for the clinician. *J Psychiatr Res*, **12**(3), 189–98.

Mahurin R, Cooke N (1996). The Verbal Series Attention Test: Clinical utility in the assessment of dementia. *Clin Neuropsychol*, 1043–52.

Osterrieth PA (1944). Le test de copie d'une figure complexe. *Archives de Psychologie*, **30**, 206–356; translated by J. Corwin and F.W. Bylsma (1993), *The Clinical Neuropsychologist*, **7**, 9–15.

Sechi GP, Serra A (2007). Wenicke's encephalopathy: new clinical settings and recent advances in diagnosis and management. *Lancet Neurol*, **6**, 442–55.

Wechsler D (1997). *Wechsler Memory Scale-Revised*. San Antonio: Psychological Corporation.

Woman with dementia and hepatic disease

Benjamin Lam, Mario Masellis, and Sandra E. Black

Clinical history – main complaint

A 59-year-old woman presents with gradual onset of cognitive symptoms including deficits in memory, attention, spatial orientation, and difficulties with task planning and execution. Marked confabulation was also noted by her family in the two years leading up to her presentation.

Three years prior to these symptoms, she was diagnosed with liver cirrhosis of unknown cause. Because confabulation is often seen in the setting of alcoholism, she was extensively investigated for alcoholic liver disease and alcohol abuse. Her family kept close surveillance as well, but despite both pathological investigations and observation, there was no evidence of alcohol use. The patient was, in fact, abstinent.

Around the time of diagnosis, there was increasing difficulty with reasoning and grasping complex situations. As her course progressed over 5 years, she developed word-finding difficulties, increasingly poor memory, aggressive and narcissistic behaviors, and profound functional decline. Memory retrieval did not benefit from cueing.

Liver function continued to decline as well and 6 years into her course she experienced two bouts of acute encephalopathy. These required hospitalization along with protein restriction and treatment with lactulose. She responded, but despite therapy remained significantly cognitively impaired, with the greatest deficits observed in short-term memory.

Although she and her family initially believed that her cognitive symptoms started after the onset of her cirrhosis, it became apparent in retrospect that she had very mild impairments prior to this. Because of the insidious and extremely slow progression, this detail had escaped their notice. Of note, memory was again the most affected cognitive domain.

Case Studies in Dementia: Common and Uncommon Presentations, ed. S. Gauthier and P. Rosa-Neto. Published by Cambridge University Press. © Cambridge University Press 2011.

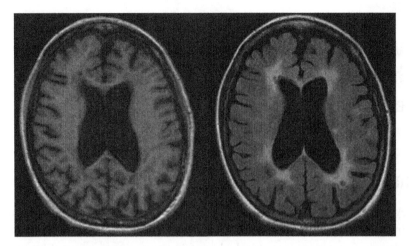

Fig. 36.1. Axial T1 weighted MRI shows general atrophy on T1 (left) with confluent periventricular white matter disease as seen on the FLAIR sequence (right).

Special studies

Brain imaging showed generalized atrophy and subcortical white matter disease (Fig. 36.1). EEG showed bilateral generalized slowing consistent with a toxic metabolic etiology, although this may also be seen in AD and Lewy body dementia.

Neuropsychological testing was limited because of poor patient cooperation. Within these limitations she showed poor encoding, visuospatial disorientation, and borderline performance on tests of working memory. She had poor visual memory (3 of 30 items on immediate and delayed recall). On word list recall, she retained only 5/12 items after four learning trials. She did not improve with repetition. The results were consistent with moderate to severe decline in cognitive function.

Diagnosis

The diagnosis was hepatic encephalopathy with a secondary diagnosis of incipient Alzheimer's dementia, with the former exacerbating and/or unmasking the latter. The likelihood of an underlying neurodegeneration was supported by her apparent cognitive decline prior to the onset of the liver disease, the prominent short term memory deficit, and a family history of dementia (Fig. 36.2).

Follow-up

Following investigations by general surgery and the liver transplant team, it was felt that this lady was suffering from significant and progressive liver pathology

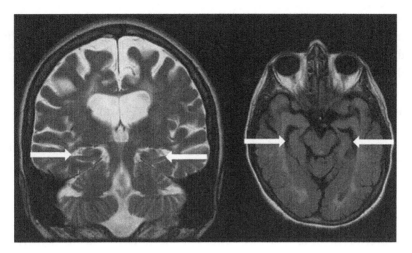

Fig. 36.2.   Bilateral hippocampal atrophy (arrows) seen on sagittal T2 weighted MRI (left) and axial FLAIR sequence (right).

sufficient to cause her hepatic encephalopathy. The liver damage and symptoms were considered severe enough for her to be placed on a waiting list for liver transplantation.

However, as it emerged that she might have a non-reversible neurodegenerative condition, her candidacy for the procedure was brought into question. There was much debate as to whether such a course of action was appropriate, because she was deemed to be at an early stage of AD and the hepatic encephalopathy was thought to be the major contributor to her cognitive and functional decline.

Caution was also raised as the diagnosis of AD, being based purely on clinical grounds, was not at all certain. Furthermore, with the presence of a co-existing medical condition to explain her cognitive decline, the patient's findings, at best, would support only a diagnosis of possible AD.

This troubling uncertainty is highlighted by a case report of an elderly gentleman who was believed to have AD, only later to be discovered to have portal systemic shunting which, when corrected, resulted in resolution of his cognitive symptoms (Miyata *et al.*, 2009).

On these grounds, her cognitive neurology team supported her remaining on the transplant waiting list. In the meantime she is being followed with regard to her cognitive course to see if it is consistent with Alzheimer's disease.

Discussion

This lady clearly demonstrates many of the features of hepatic encephalopathy, including quantified liver disease and response to protein restriction and lactulose therapy. However, she also has features of Alzheimer's disease, with memory and language deficits, family history, and imaging supportive of this diagnosis. Hence, she was thought to have two mutually exacerbating disorders.

Typical hepatic encephalopathy

Hepatic Encephalopathy (HE) is a neuropsychiatric disorder characterized by the insidious onset of impaired attention, altered personality, and irregular sleep patterns. Progression proceeds along a continuum of disorientation, increasing psychomotor slowing, and eventual stupor and coma. Cognitive and behavioral symptoms are often accompanied by motor incoordination and intermittent loss of tone (asterixis). Pathologically, HE is characterized by astrocytic swelling and rarefaction of the nucleus (Alzheimer type II astrocytes), indicating that astrocytes may be the primary site of cellular damage in HE. The exact etiology of HE remains unclear but seems to be a combination of toxicity by ammonia and manganese, and alterations in neurotransmitter systems, particularly glutamate (Hazell and Butterworth, 1999; Eroglu and Bryne, 2009).

This patient not only shared many of these clinical features, but also had liver enzyme elevation and her cognitive symptoms responded to standard treatments of HE – namely protein restriction and lactulose.

The parsimonious answer is not always the correct one

It is one of the cardinal rules of clinical diagnosis that the simplest and most common explanation is usually the correct one. This case, however, illustrates that this diagnostic axiom needs to be tempered by the understanding that brain pathologies can often co-exist. This can make it difficult at times to definitively confirm one of the suspected diagnoses, such as AD in this case. It is possible that this patient was in the early stages of AD which was exacerbated by the hepatic insult. This is similar to the relationship between Cerebrovascular Disease (CVD) and AD in which concomitant CVD may act in concert with AD pathology to accelerate the onset of dementia (Black, 2007). In fact, this lady also had moderate subcortical ischemic vasculopathy as a further exacerbating factor.

The duty to care

Another issue raised is that of the ethical duty to provide the best appropriate care. For a scarce and resource-intensive procedure, such as organ transplantation, what should be the policy on allocation? Who should receive precious organs? Who should be excluded? In this case, should the patient's possible

Alzheimer's disease preclude her from even being considered for a liver transplant, even though the procedure may dramatically improve her quality of life?

Considerations relating to offering transplantation in this case are

(1) Post-transplant success requires an individual who is highly motivated and compliant, both by choice and ability, in following a complicated regimen of anti-rejection medications and personal care. This woman's behavioral symptoms bring the feasibility of this into question. For example, she had trouble complying with a two hour cognitive test as a result of her behaviors and cognitive problems. Would she be able and willing to stay on the necessary medications?

Although not without merit, one rebuttal to this argument is that, in the presence of a supportive caregiver, this may not be an issue as many patients with AD depend on the assistance of their caregivers to take medications and perform other instrumental activities of daily living. Patients with Alzheimer's disease already often contend with polypharmacy that is sustainable through such support.

(2) A second potential argument against transplantation is that, given the eventuality that this patient may well succumb to her Alzheimer's disease within 10 years, an available liver should be given to someone who might benefit longer from the treatment.

A counter-argument arises from the inherent danger in the implied nihilism of this position. Alzheimer's patients are capable of having a reasonable quality of life. Even in severe stage disease, for instance, social interaction is relatively spared (Gillioz *et al.*, 2009). Furthermore, it implies a double standard whereby the welfare of someone with a neurodegenerative condition is somehow considered less important than that of a young, middle-aged, economically productive individual. Similar issues were encountered in the early days of renal dialysis, when scarcity made the issue of who should receive treatment an acute one (Rothenberg, 1992).

In the end, one is faced with a difficult balance of considerations, which must be approached with all the more caution in these very complex situations involving issues of cognitive capacity and mental ability. While one does not wish to preclude a person's access to life-saving or life-altering treatment, one must also consider whether it is justifiable to give such a scarce and precious resource to an individual who will have an uncertain number of years of reasonable quality of life remaining, especially, since doing so may deny treatment to an individual with more potential years of benefit.

Take home messages

Alzheimer's disease can co-occur in the setting of reversible causes of cognitive impairment. As in the case of vascular disease, the two etiologies can combine to produce significant impairment.

The presence of a co-morbid neurodegenerative condition can create ethical dilemmas regarding the allocation of scarce, resource-intensive treatments. While one should try to avoid precluding someone from life-saving or life-altering therapy, one must also consider the cost and potential futility of giving such therapy when doing so may deprive another individual of such treatment, who may ultimately derive greater benefit. This balance of considerations yields no easy solution.

Acknowledgments

We would like to thank Dr. Gary Levy for his initial referral of this patient, as well as Dr. Ron Keren for his assessment and advice on the case. We would also like to acknowledge funding support provided by the Brill Chair of Neurology, Department of Medicine and the Brain Sciences Research Program, Sunnybrook Health Sciences Centre, University of Toronto.

REFERENCES AND FURTHER READING

Black SE (2007). Therapeutic issues in vascular dementia: studies, designs, and approaches. *Can J Neurol Sci*, **34** (Suppl 1), S125–30.

Darvesh S, Leach L, Black SE, Kaplan E, Freedman M (2005). The behavioural neurology assessment. *Can J Neurol Sci*, **32**, 167–77.

Eroglu Y, Bryne WJ (2009). Hepatic encephalopathy. *Emerg Med Clin North Am*, **27**, 401–14.

Freedman M, Leach L, Kaplan E, *et al.* (1994). *Clock Drawing: A Neuropsychological Analysis.* New York: Oxford University Press.

Fridman V, Galetta SL, Pruitt AA, Levine JM (2009). MRI findings associated with acute liver failure. *Neurology*, **72**, 2130–3.

Gillioz AS, Villars H, Voisin T, *et al.* (2009). Spared and impaired abilities in community-dwelling patterns entering the severe stage of Alzheimer's disease. *Dement Geriatr Cogn Disord*, **28**(5), 427–32.

Hazell AS, Butterworth RF (1999). Hepatic encephalopathy: an update of pathophysiologic mechanisms. *Proc Soc Exp Biol Med*, **222**(2), 99–112.

Miyata K, Tamai H, Uno A, *et al*. (2009). Congenital portal systemic encephalopathy misdiagnosed as senile dementia. *Intern Med*, **48**(5), 321–4.

Rothenberg LS (1992). Withholding and withdrawing dialysis from elderly ESRD patients: part 1 – a historical view of the clinical experience. *Geriatr Nephrol Urol*, **2**(2), 109–17.

Case 37

Young woman with recurrent "stroke" attacks

Masamichi Ikawa and Makoto Yoneda

Clinical history – main complaint

A 44-year-old right-handed woman developed impairment of cognitive function, aphasia and muscle weakness after three "stroke" attacks at the ages of 40, 42, and 43, respectively. She initially presented with easy fatigability and weight loss at the age of 27, and developed sensorineural deafness at the age of 40. She developed dementia as the result of recurrent "stroke" attacks, and requires assistance for activities of daily living.

General history

The patient had shown normal birth and developmental milestones. She received a high-school education and currently lives with her husband and a son. She was transiently affected by congestive heart failure at the age of 27.

Family history

The patient has non-consanguineous parents. Her mother has a history of renal disease and small stature, and her brother has diabetes mellitus and deafness.

Examination

Height 158 cm; Weight 48 kg; BMI 19.2. Blood pressure 108/72 mmHg, Pulse 75/min, regular. She was alert, but apathetic. She presented with moderate aphasia and disturbance of writing. Orientation and short-term memory were moderately impaired. She requires assistance in activities of daily living such as dressing and hygiene. She presented with mild muscular weakness and atrophy in

Case Studies in Dementia: Common and Uncommon Presentations, ed. S. Gauthier and P. Rosa-Neto. Published by Cambridge University Press. © Cambridge University Press 2011.

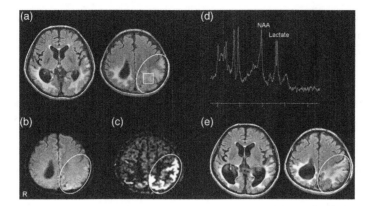

Fig. 37.1.   (a)–(d) Brain MR images obtained at the most recent stroke-like attack (at age 43). (a) Diffusion-weighted images (DWI) and (b) fluid-attenuated inversion recovery (FLAIR) images demonstrated hyperintensity and swelling in the left parietal lobe (the acute lesion, indicated by circle), and atrophy in the right temporo-parietal lobes due to previous attacks. The square on FLAIR images indicates the volume of interest on MR spectroscopy (MRS). (c) Continuous arterial spin labeling (CASL) perfusion images showed hyperperfusion in the acute lesion (circle). (d) MRS obtained from the acute lesion demonstrated a remarkably increased lactate peak and decreased N-acetyl-aspartate (NAA) peak. (e) Brain MR images performed 2 years after this attack. FLAIR images showed hyperintensity and atrophy in the subcortical white matter of the left temporal lobe (circle).

the extremities, but was able to walk unaided. Deep tendon reflexes in the extremities were diminished without pathological reflex.

Special studies

All routine laboratory data were normal, except for a high serum lactate level (24.8 mg/dl) and lactate/pyruvate ratio (22.1). Brain MRI performed at the most recent stroke-like attack (at age 43) demonstrated hyperintensity and swelling on both Fluid-Attenuated Inversion Recovery (FLAIR) images and Diffusion-Weighted Images (DWI), hyperperfusion on Continuous Arterial Spin Labeling (CASL) perfusion images, and a remarkably increased lactate peak and decreased N-Acetyl-Aspartate (NAA) peak on MR Spectroscopy (MRS) in the left parietal lobe (Fig. 37.1(a)–(d)). The right temporo-parietal lobes were atrophic due to previous attacks.

These MRI findings corresponded to stroke-like episodes in mitochondrial myopathy, encephalopathy, lactic acidosis, and stroke-like episodes (MELAS). Gene analysis demonstrated an A-to-G transition at nucleotide position 3243 (A3243G) in mitochondrial DNA (mtDNA). The brain MRI performed two years after the most recent attack demonstrated atrophy in the left parietal lobe and dilation of the ventricles (Fig. 37.1(e)).

Diagnosis

The patient was diagnosed as having MELAS due to stroke-like episodes and A3243G.

Follow-up

The patient has been treated by oral administration of L-arginine after the latest stroke-like attack. L-arginine has prevented stroke-like attacks and mildly improved cognitive function.

Discussion

MELAS is the most common type of mitochondrial disease, and is mainly caused by A3243G (Goto *et al.*, 1990). The clinical features of MELAS syndrome consist of stroke-like episodes, myopathy, lactic acidosis, diabetes mellitus, and cardiomyopathy (Pavlakis *et al.*, 1984). Particularly, stroke-like episodes are diagnostic symptoms of MELAS. Stroke-like episodes occur repeatedly and provoke acute neurological symptoms (e.g., headache, epilepsy, hemiparesis, and aphasia) due to "stroke-like" brain lesions (Pavlakis *et al.*, 1984). Therefore, stroke-like episodes are frequently misdiagnosed as ischemic cerebral infarction in adult patients.

Stroke-like episodes affect various brain functions and leave sequelae, particularly inducing impaired cognitive function after each relapse. Moreover, stroke-like episodes not only involve radiologically demonstrable lesions, but also influence the whole brain. MRS has demonstrated decline of neuronal density indicated by NAA concentration in an apparently-normal region during the prolonged course in a patient with MELAS (Tsujikawa *et al.*, 2010). Therefore, stroke-like episodes progressively impair cognitive functions, leading to dementia. Indeed, cognitive impairment and dementia are frequent findings in patients with MELAS (Amemiya *et al.*, 2000; Kaufmann *et al.*, 2004). Although only focal deficits of cognitive performance (e.g., impairments of visual construction, attention, abstraction, flexibility) appear at onset, general intellectual deterioration becomes gradually distinguished (Finsterer, 2008). Psychosis or personality change as well as dementia often develop with progression (Amemiya *et al.*, 2000; Koller *et al.*, 2003).

The pathogenesis of stroke-like episodes remains obscure. However, recent studies have shown that mitochondrial angiopathy (neural damage due to impaired mitochondria in the blood vessels and inappropriate intracranial hemodynamics) and cytopathy (neural damage due to mitochondrial dysfunction itself), neuronal hyperexcitability (neural damage due to imbalance between energy supply and demand) and oxidative stress participate in the process of stroke-like episodes (Ohama *et al.*, 1987; Yoneda *et al.*, 1999; Iizuka *et al.*, 2002; Ikawa *et al.*, 2009).

To confirm the diagnosis of MELAS, pathological gene mutation and histological or biochemical abnormality of mitochondria as well as clinical features represented by stroke-like episodes are fundamental (Pavlakis *et al.*, 1984). Recently, functional imaging has been useful for not only detecting stroke-like lesions, but also evaluating mitochondrial dysfunction and contributing to diagnosis. In acute stroke-like lesions, conventional CT or MRI images have shown the lesions spreading beyond the vascular territories (Kuriyama *et al.*, 1984). Additionally, MRA and CASL images demonstrate vasodilatation and hyperperfusion, DWI or Apparent Diffusion Coefficient (ADC) maps show vasogenic edema, and MRS indicates increased lactate concentrations (Yoneda *et al.*, 1999; Moller *et al.*, 2005; Tsujikawa *et al.*, 2010). These findings indicate anerobic metabolism and endothelial dysfunction caused by mitochondrial dysfunction, and are pathognomonical.

Although there are no radical therapeutic strategies focusing on MELAS, the therapeutic effects of L-arginine for stroke-like episodes have been demonstrated recently. L-arginine infusions in the acute phase of attacks has significantly improved symptoms, and oral administration in the remitting phase has significantly decreased the frequency and severity of stroke-like episodes (Koga *et al.*, 2005, 2006).

In this case, the patient developed dementia due to recurrent "stroke" attacks. Dementia caused by stroke-like episodes is apt to be misdiagnosed as vascular dementia. For juvenile patients with recurrent atypical "stroke" attacks, evaluation of mitochondrial dysfunction using functional imaging and gene analysis should be recommended.

Take home messages

Patients with dementia and recurrent atypical "stroke" attacks should be suspected of MELAS.

Functional imaging can be useful in cases showing atypical presentation of dementia.

REFERENCES AND FURTHER READING

Amemiya S, Hamamoto M, Goto Y, *et al.* (2000). Psychosis and progressing dementia: presenting features of a mitochondriopathy. *Neurology*, **55**, 600–1.

Finsterer J (2008). Cognitive decline as a manifestation of mitochondrial disorders (mitochondrial dementia). *J Neurol Sci*, **272**, 20–33.

Goto Y, Nonaka I, Horai S (1990). A mutation in the tRNA (Leu) (UUR) gene associated with the MELAS subgroup of mitochondrial encephalomyopathies. *Nature*, **348**, 651–3.

Iizuka T, Sakai F, Suzuki N, *et al.* (2002). Neuronal hyperexcitability in stroke-like episodes of MELAS syndrome. *Neurology*, **59**, 816–24.

Ikawa M, Okazawa H, Arakawa K, *et al.* (2009). PET imaging of redox and energy states in stroke-like episodes of MELAS. *Mitochondrion*, **9**, 144–8.

Kaufmann P, Shungu DC, Sano MC, *et al.* (2004). Cerebral lactic acidosis correlates with neurological impairment in MELAS. *Neurology*, **62**, 1297–302.

Koga Y, Akita Y, Nishioka J, *et al.* (2005). L-arginine improves the symptoms of stroke-like episodes in MELAS. *Neurology*, **64**, 710–12.

Koga Y, Akita Y, Nishioka J, *et al.* (2006). Endothelial dysfunction in MELAS was improved by L-arginine supplementation. *Neurology*, **66**, 1766–9.

Koller H, Kornischka J, Neuen-Jacob E, *et al.* (2003). Persistent organic personality change as rare psychiatric manifestation of MELAS syndrome. *J Neurol*, **250**, 1501–2.

Kuriyama M, Umezaki H, Fukuda Y, *et al.* (1984). Mitochondrial encephalomyopathy with lactate-pyruvate elevation and brain infarctions. *Neurology*, **34**, 72–7.

Moller HE, Kurlemann G, Putzler M, *et al.* (2005). Magnetic resonance spectroscopy in patients with MELAS. *J Neurol Sci*, **229–230**, 131–9.

Ohama E, Ohara S, Ikuta F, *et al.* (1987). Mitochondrial angiopathy in cerebral blood vessels of mitochondrial encephalomyopathy. *Acta Neuropathol*, **74**, 226–33.

Pavlakis SG, Phillips PC, DiMauro S, *et al.* (1984). Mitochondrial myopathy, encephalopathy, lactic acidosis, and strokelike episodes: a distinctive clinical syndrome. *Ann Neurol*, **16**, 481–8.

Tsujikawa T, Yoneda M, Shimizu Y, *et al.* (2010). Pathophysiologic evaluation of MELAS strokes by serially quantified MRS and CASL perfusion images. *Brain Dev*, **32**, 143–9.

Yoneda M, Maeda M, Kimura H, *et al.* (1999). Vasogenic edema on MELAS: a serial study with diffusion-weighted MR imaging. *Neurology*, **53**, 2182–4.

Young man with slow cognitive decline

Marie Christine Guiot and Pedro Rosa-Neto

Clinical history – main complaint

A 31-year-old right-handed man (patient FA) was referred for clinical evaluation due to a 3-year history of progressive deterioration of memory and academic performance.

FA was previously healthy, with a successful academic history and active social life. At age 29, family members noticed progressive difficulty with his university courses, which was initially attributed to fatigue and stress. Such difficulties were exacerbated during the preceding months, to the point FA had to quit his studies. There was a clear decline in communication skills and a personality change. FA got involved in multiple car accidents and often would not find his way back home. Patient and family members denied recent sensory symptoms (including auditory and visual hallucinations), pain, headache, motor deficits, tremors, gate unsteadiness, or dizziness.

General history

Previous medical history was negative for neurological or systemic diseases.

Family history

Negative for neurological diseases or other relevant systemic diseases.

Examination

Mental status: patient presented alert and disoriented in place and time. MMSE score was 15/30. Speech was slightly slurred with normal comprehension and repetition. Impairment was observed for simple calculations, reading, naming,

Case Studies in Dementia: Common and Uncommon Presentations, ed. S. Gauthier and P. Rosa-Neto. Published by Cambridge University Press. © Cambridge University Press 2011.

writing, and drawing. Finger gnosis and right-left orientation were intact. Clear perseveration was observed on alternating sequences.

Cranial nerves: PERL, visual fields, and fundoscopic exam were normal. Difficulty was observed on vertical ocular movements; nystagmus could not be elicited. Facial sensation and strength were normal. Hearing was intact. Tongue protrusion was in midline without atrophy or fibrillations; palatal elevation was symmetric. Strength in sternocleidomastoids and trapezius was 4+/5.

Motor: trophism was globally reduced and upper limb paratonia was noted. No fasciculations were noted. Strength was 4+/5 throughout. Reflexes: deep tendon reflexes were bilaterally brisk. Plantar responses were bilaterally flexor. Frontal release signs such as snout, glabellar, or palmomental reflex were present. Sensory: Normal assessment at light touch, pinprick, vibration and proprioception. Intact finger to nose, heel to shin, and rapid alternating movements. Romberg was negative. Gate and stand: Discrete truncal ataxia was observed. Gait was slow, cautious, with slightly wide base, but without postural instability. Romberg test was negative.

Special studies

Tox, autoimmune, malignancy, hormonal, and complete metabolic work-up were normal. CSF studies revealed normal cell counts and proteins levels (14–3–3 protein was negative). MRI revealed diffuse atrophy predominantly in posterior regions and cerebellum, with unspecific T2 lesions. Electroencephalogram showed background activity consisting of diffuse slow waves, without epileptiform discharges. Neuropsychological testing revealed dysfunction in verbal and visuospatial memory, language, and fine motor abilities. Verbal IQ was 71, performance IQ was 56 and global IQ was 61. Left hemisphere dominance for language. Sequencing of the PRPN gene revealed no nucleotide substitution, insertion, or deletion mutations. PRPN genotyping revealed homozygosis for methionine at codon 129.

Diagnosis

Prion-related syndrome was part of the differential diagnosis.

Follow-up

FA's gait became progressively unsteady in following years, which caused numerous falls and minor head injuries. Global degeneration occurred during the course of 4 years. He developed myoclonic jerks and generalized tonic–clonic seizures.

FA died 7 years after disease onset, due to uncal herniation secondary to a chronic subdural hematoma.

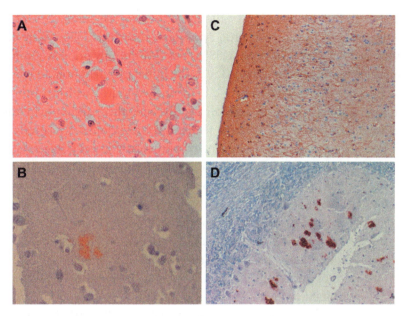

Fig. 38.1. (a) Pathological evaluation revealed numerous plaques in the cerebellum and cortex stained by congo red and birefringent on polarization. (b) These plaque-like structures display strong reactivity for the antibody against the prion protein (PrP) in the cortex and (d) throughout most of cerebellar molecular layer. (c) Important astrocytic reactivity is indicated by high immumoreactivity to GFAP. Minimal spongiform changes were observed in cortical and subcortical structures.

Brain necropsy revealed (1) bilateral uncal herniation and hemorrhages in midbrain and pons; (2) cerebral edema; (3) recent cerebral infarction involving the occipital cortex and the left parahippocampal cortex; (4) presence of amyloid plaques with immunohistochemistry positive for prion (with marked involvement of the cerebellum) and (5) extensive cortical gliosis but no spongiform changes; (6) cerebellar atrophy predominant in the superior vermis (Fig. 38.1).

Discussion

Gerstmann–Straussler–Scheinker Syndrome (GSSS) was originally described in 1936 in a family carrying the P102L mutation in the PrP gene. In fact, GSS occurs almost exclusively as an inheritable disease associated with a PrP gene mutation, the P102L being the most frequent.

Clinical picture is highly dependent on mutation type and onset usually occurs in the third or fourth decade. The clinical course is the slowest among all human prion syndromes and may progress over several years (average of 5 years). The typical clinical presentation of the most frequent mutation, P102L, consists of progressive ataxia, upper neuron symptoms, dysarthria followed by dementia in advanced stages of the disease. GSSS is possibly the only prion syndrome in which supranuclear gaze palsy can feature as the initial manifestation. In contrast, GSSS carriers of A117V mutation have dementia associated with dysarthria, rigidity, tremor, and hyper-reflexia. Tremor, rigidity, and other parkinsonian features were also described in A117V carriers. Unlike CJD, myoclonus is relatively infrequent in GSSS. Due to clinical heterogeneity, particularly in early stages, GSSS may be misdiagnosed as spinocerebellar ataxias, olivopontocerebellar atrophy, early-onset Parkinson's disease, dystonia or progressive supranuclear palsy. Because many of these conditions can also be inherited, the definitive diagnosis of GSS requires molecular studies for mutations in the *PRNP* gene.

Interestingly, FA had a typical clinical presentation suggestive of GSSS, but the diagnosis could not be confirmed (absence of PRPN mutations).

One-third of carriers of *PRNP* mutations have negative family history. P102L is a missense mutation that substitutes a lysine for a proline at codon 102. Other mutations associated with GSSS are P105L, A117V, Q187H, F198S, D202N, Q212P, Q217R, Y145STOP as well as insertion of eight octapeptide repeats. Although homozygosis for methionine at codon 129, like observed in the patient FA, confers vulnerability to prion diseases, the molecular pathology of this case remains unknown since PRPN genotype did not reveal a known PRPN GSSS mutation.

Brain necropsy in our patient revealed typical GSSS neuropathological features, with amyloid plaques immunoreactive for PrP displaying multicentric morphology. Amyloid plaques predominate in the cerebellar molecular layer. In addition, there was important diffuse inflammatory reaction. The spongiform transformation, which was almost absent in FA, present variably in patients with GSSS.

Amyloid plaques consisting of proteinase-resistant prion protein constitutes a neuropathological feature also present in other prion syndromes including PrP-cerebral amyloid, sporadic, or variant form of Creutzfeldt–Jakob Disease (CJD).

Take home messages

Consider GSSS in patients presenting with dementia and supranuclear palsy.
Consider GSSS in young patients with progressively cognitive deline.
Consider GSSS in individuals without family history and CSF negative for 14–3–3.

FURTHER READING

Arata J, Takashima H, Hirano R, *et al.* (2006). Early clinical signs and imaging findings in Gerstmann–Sträussler–Scheinker syndrome (Pro102Leu). *Neurology*, **66**, 1672–8.

Hsiao K, Baker HF, Crow TJ, *et al.* (1989). Linkage of a prion protein missense variant to Gerstmann–Sträussler syndrome. *Nature* **338**, 342–5.

Ironside JW, Head MW (2004). Neuropathology and molecular biology of variant Creutzfeldt–Jakob disease. *Curr Top Microbiol Immunol*, **284**, 133–59.

Kovacs GG, Puopolo M, Ladogana A, *et al.* (2005). Genetic prion disease: the EUROCJD experience. *Hum Genet*, **118**, 166–74.

Rossor MN, Fox NC, Mummery CJ, Schott JM, Warren JD (2010). The diagnosis of young-onset dementia. *Lancet Neurol*, **9**(8), 793–806.

Wadsworth JD, Collinge J (2010). Molecular pathology of human prion disease. *Acta Neuropathol*, in press.

Case 39

Young woman with lateralized motor symptoms

Taim Muayqil, Richard Camicioli, Lothar Resch, Rajive Jassal, and Edward S. Johnson

Clinical history – main complaint

A 40-year-old woman of Vietnamese origin was referred with a history of progressive short-term memory decline for 12 months. She had become repetitive and experienced difficulty in completing simple tasks, such as signing a cheque, operating a stove or dialing a phone. Her driving also suffered, and she could no longer reliably go out shopping due to family concerns about her getting lost. There was also a history of becoming physically slower, particularly when dressing or bathing, speech limitation, and feeling depressed and generally weak.

She also gave a history of poor sleep with occasional headaches. Her appetite had increased and sometimes she would wake up during the night to snack. There was no history of abnormal or involuntary movements.

General history

Review of her past history showed that she was hepatitis B virus (HBV) carrier and had dermatitis. She also had an old right frontal parietal lesion with mild left hand weakness. This lesion was discovered 10 years prior by a CT scan with a history of a simple focal seizure of the left hand when she was 13 years old. She did not have recurrent seizures. She had a left facial injury from an old motor vehicle accident. She was not on any medication upon presentation. The patient had 11 years of formal schooling and was working as a parking attendant.

Family history

The family history revealed she had an uncle who had behavioral difficulties when in his fourth decade.

Case Studies in Dementia: Common and Uncommon Presentations, ed. S. Gauthier and P. Rosa-Neto. Published by Cambridge University Press. © Cambridge University Press 2011.

Examination

Her vital signs were normal. On cognitive assessment she scored 15/30 on the Mini Mental State Exam (MMSE), points were mainly lost in domains of memory, calculation, language, and visual spatial function. Her best forward digit span was four numbers in length. She could not copy the examiner during the Luria task and was not able to correctly perform tests of inhibitory control or conflicting instructions. There was no grasp reflex. She was not able to write her name and she had a decrease in speech production. There was also naming difficulty.

Further neurological examination showed intact cranial nerves. On the motor exam she had generalized bradykinesia, rigidity of the right upper extremity, and a right pronator drift. The reflexes were symmetrical and graded +3, plantar responses, coordination, gait, postural stability and sensory functions were normal.

Special studies

CBC and differential, urea, electrolytes including calcium and magnesium, liver function tests, as well as B12, and TSH were normal. Angiotensin Converting Enzyme (ACE) was slightly elevated on two occasions. Cerebrospinal fluid (CSF) analysis for cells, gram stain, bacterial culture, AFB, fungal culture, herpes viruses PCR, protein, glucose and lactate was also normal. In addition to the old right frontal parietal lesion, a cranial MRI revealed bilateral periventricular non-enhancing white matter signal change that also extended into the anterior temporal poles and was sparing the U fibers (Fig. 39.1). A conventional four-vessel angiogram was normal. Serology was negative for syphilis, HIV, and autoimmune or hypercoagulable markers. Screening for paraneoplastic anti-bodies (anti-Hu, Yo, and Ri) was negative. Skin biopsy of the dermatitis did not show any deposited material in the vascular media. Arylsulphatase A and B, Very Long Chain Fatty Acids (VLCFA), urine organic acids and amino acid quantification were either negative or normal. A CT scan of the chest and abdomen did not reveal any malignant or inflammatory disease. An electro-encephalogram (EEG) showed mild generalized slowing of the background with no focal abnormalities.

Diagnosis

The initial diagnostic impression was of a progressive dementia of subacute onset in a young individual. Given the extensive white matter changes on the MRI the differential included inflammatory disorders such as multiple sclerosis, systemic

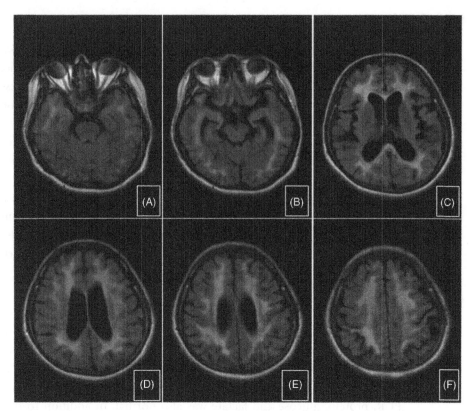

Fig. 39.1.   FLAIR MRI demonstrating ventricular enlargement and diffuse cerebral atrophy, including the mesial temporal regions. Extensive white matter hyperintensity is noted involving the temporal lobes up to the anterior poles (A), occipital (B), fronto-parietal regions (C, D, E, F). Signal change is also appreciated in the corpus callosum (C), periventricular white matter (B, C, D, E, & F) and centrum semi-ovale (F).

lupus erythematosis, rheumatoid arthritis, Sjogren's syndrome, sarcoidosis, Behçet's disease, primary CNS angiitis, or a non-vasculitic autoimmune meningoencephalitis (NAIM). However the complete clinical picture and/or the necessary investigative tests were not supportive. An infectious disorder such as progressive multifocal leukoencephalopathy was considered less likely because of the prolonged course and the absence of an immune compromising illness. The normal CSF and the inability to identify an infectious etiology by other investigative methods argued against an infectious cause. A vascular etiology like Cerebral Autosomal Dominant Arteriopathy with Subcortical Infarcts and leukoencephalopathy (CADASIL) was also considered however the skin biopsy was negative. The imaging changes were less likely to be microangiopathic disease given the absence of vascular risk factors and her young age. A late onset leukoencephalopathy was a relevant consideration; these include metachromatic leukodystrophy (MLD), adrenoleukodystrophy (ALD), Alexander's disease, Krabbe's disease and adult onset leukoencephalopathy with neuroaxonal spheroids (ALSP). Among these conditions, MLD and ALD were unlikely given the negative arylsulphatase and VLCFA tests. The normal lactate was helpful but not definitive evidence against the less commonly encountered mitochondrial disorders at this age, particularly Mitochondrial Encephalopathy with Lactic Acidosis and Stroke Like Syndrome (MELAS). No malignant focus or paraneoplastic antibodies were found in the patient. The MRI and EEG findings were not those typically seen in Creutzfeldt Jakob Disease (CJD). Investigations lacking at this point was testing for the remaining leukodystrophies such as Galactosyl-β-galactosidase for Krabbe's disease and genetic analysis for GFAP mutation seen in Alexander disease.

Follow-up

An assessment approximately 1 year after her initial presentation showed significant further decline in function and personal hygiene. She started to toilet in the sink, had trouble feeding herself and her memory declined further with prominent repetitiveness. A repeat MMSE was 13/30. She had trouble following simple commands and difficulty with language repetition as well. She developed urinary retention, which led to a hospital admission.

The exam this time showed right central facial weakness, right hemiparesis, increased tone in lower extremities, brisk reflexes with bilaterally upgoing toes and clonus. Gait was wide based and spastic with ataxia and postural instability.

Over the next weeks her condition continued to deteriorate. She developed fluctuating level of consciousness and appeared encephalopathic with disorientation to person, place and time. At this point a decision was made, after discussion with the family, to proceed with a brain biopsy.

The biopsy (Fig. 39.2) showed features of a leukoencephalopathic process in combination with dystrophic axonal degeneration characterized by spheroid formation and microglial cell accumulation. There were no findings of vasculitis, granular deposits in vessel smooth muscle, viral inclusions, or a storage disease. The microglial cells were not engaged in active phagocytic stripping of myelin as usually seen in leukodystrophies.

The patient died 3 years after the onset of her symptoms. Prior to death, she developed seizures and was put on anti-epileptics. During her last year of life, she was living in a nursing facility that provided full care. She was unable to swallow and received nutrition through a gatrostomy feeding tube and had an indwelling

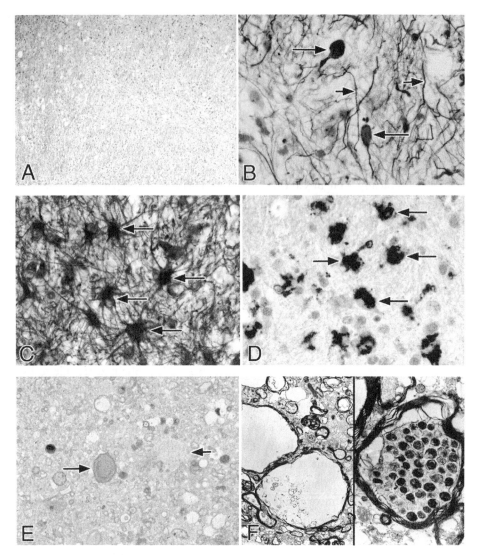

Fig. 39.2. Luxol fast blue/Hematoxlin and eosin (LFB/H&E) stain showing pallor of staining in lower right quadrant as compared to upper left quadrant (A). Bielschowsky showing axonal spheroids (arrows) and axons (truncated arrows) (B). Immunoperoxidase for Vimentin shownig reactive astrocytes (arrows) and background positive processes (C). Immunoperoxidase for CD 68 showing macrophages (arrows) (D). Semithin toluene blue stained upon embedded semithin section showing swollen myelinated axon (short arrow) and macrophage (arrowhead) (E). EM showing swollen axons. Left panel shows two swollen axons with lucent axoplasm and some membranous material; compare with multiple adjacent normally sized axons. Right panel shows a swollen axon with many membrane bound dense bodies (F).

urinary catheter for chronic urinary retention and infections. She was unable to communicate and was described by one of her doctors as being in a persistent vegetative state at the time of her death from urosepsis.

Discussion

Atypical features of dementia in this case include a relatively young age of presentation, a rapid course with early onset rigidity and pyramidal signs, with high signal changes on imaging, and late seizures.

When a dementing illness occurs in the young, an extensive work up is typically conducted to rule out any reversible conditions, which can include infectious, neoplastic and inflammatory disorders. Non-reversible degenerative disorders like AD can still occur in this age group as can Parkinson's disease dementia or dementia with Lewy bodies (Sampson, Warren, & Rossor, 2004). However the imaging findings, the rapid course, and the absence of Parkinson's disease prior to presentation argues against these.

The early presentation with motor features would be atypical for AD or behavioral variant fronto-temporal dementia, even though such findings are more common later in the course of these disorders (Portet, Scarmeas, Cosentino, Helzner, & Stern, 2009). Motor signs are typical manifestations of Lewy Body dementia, or in an atypical parkinsonian disorder such as progressive supra-nuclear gaze palsy or multiple system atrophy. The absence of hallucinations and fluctuations, supranuclear gaze palsy, and autonomic dysfunction, argues against these.

Few of the common dementing disorders present with spasticity or pyramidal signs with the exception of vascular dementia (VaD) (Chui et al., 1992). Patients with VaD do not necessarily have the typically described step-wise deteriorating course as some may manifest with slowly progressing cognitive impairment (Sampson et al., 2004). In addition, patients with VaD can have both pyramidal and extrapyramidal manifestations together, depending on the site of vascular disease (Staekenborg et al., 2008). Vascular risk factors are generally prominent in the history of VaD, and if not, a condition like CADASIL in which one would find a history of migraines and autosomal dominant pattern of inheritance in the family history should be considered (Tournier-Lasserve, Iba-Zizen, Romero, & Bousser, 1991). A hypercoagulable state should also be considered in the absence of vascular risk factors. Some familial cases of Alzheimer disease develop spasticity and seizures, but these occur in the absence of white matter changes (Rudzinski et al., 2008).

A family history is more likely to be revealing when a dementia develops in a young individual (Schott, Fox, & Rossor, 2002). In this scenario the history of the uncle with "behavioral abnormality" was taken as an indicator, among the other red flags, of the atypical nature of the disease process.

While the white matter abnormalities raised the possibility of a vascular cause in the patient, she did not have any vascular risk factors and did not have skin manifestations of CADASIL on biopsy. In adults without a vascular etiology, the degree of white matter disease observed in our patient is atypical. The differential diagnosis of U-fiber sparing white matter disease is broad but includes conditions like ALD, MLD, Krabbe's disease, Alexander's disease, and adult onset leukoencephalopathy with neuroaxonal spheroids (Costello, Eichler, & Eichler, 2009). Other disorders like CJD, MSA, PSP, and Wilson's disease usually have different patterns of signal changes on the MRI and do not involve the subcortical white matter as obviously. CADASIL patients have confluent white mater involvement that extends to the anterior temporal poles and external capsule (O'Sullivan *et al.*, 2001). The changes in PML start posteriorly, usually with visual spatial symptoms (Whiteman *et al.*, 1993).

Typical late onset dementia presents with a slowly progressive course, often with a mild cognitive impairment state prior to the full-blown dementia. Alzheimer disease can present with an amnestic type of MCI (Petersen & Morris, 2005). Degenerative dementias, including Alzheimer disease and dementia with Lewy bodies can sometimes present as a rapidly progressive dementia (Doody *et al.*, 2010; Lopez *et al.*, 2000).

Epilepsy is unusual, though not unheard of, in a setting of dementia. It rarely occurs with AD (Scarmeas *et al.*, 2009) or other degenerative disorders. Its presence should always prompt a search for an atypical process, including adult presentation of a childhood metabolic or storage disorders, such as ceroid lipfuscinosis (Sampson *et al.*, 2004). Our patient had a past history of a single seizure that may have been related to an old brain lesion rather than the current disorder, however seizures re-emerged during the late stages of the disease.

Constitutional symptoms are also important to consider as atypical features of dementia, as it would prompt an investigation for an infectious etiology, particularly HIV with PML as both, together or separately, can cause subcortical white matter disease. Chronic infections like TB, Brucellosis, and Syphilis are also important to exclude and are important to keep in mind in people from endemic areas. Also worth mention is the presence of systematic involvement, for example gastrointestinal symptoms should warrant a search for vitamin B12 or other nutritional deficiencies; weight loss, fever, chills, skin and joint symptoms raise the suspicion of a malignancy or autoimmune process. Weight gain, menstrual changes, and abnormal patterns of hair growth on the other hand would make one suspect an endocrinological disorder like Cushing's or hypothyroidism and both are known to cause cognitive disturbances (Ridha & Josephs, 2006).

This patient had a biopsy proven diagnosis of ALSP, a rare disorder of white matter in adults. It has been described to occur either sporadically or in an autosomal dominant or recessive pattern of inheritance (Wider *et al.*, 2009). The age of onset varies from 22 to 65 years, with hereditary cases occurring in the younger part of the age spectrum, the duration of illness is around 5–9 years and both men and women are affected (Ali, Van Der Voorn, & Powers, 2007; Baba *et al.*, 2006; Freeman *et al.*, 2009; Wider *et al.*, 2009). Behavioral and cognitive manifestations include depression and memory impairment, which are common. A frontal pattern of involvement can occur with apathy or euphoria, disinhibition, and irritability. Apraxia is also described. Other neurological manifestations that are common include pyramidal and/or extrapyramidal signs, gait impairment and epilepsy. Most laboratory investigations including CSF analysis return normal (Ali *et al.*, 2007; Baba *et al.*, 2006; Freeman *et al.*, 2009; Wider *et al.*, 2009). The MRI typically shows abnormal white matter signal that can be confluent or patchy, it is usually of the U-fiber sparing type. There also tends to be predominant frontal involvement and frontal and corpus callosum atrophy (Freeman *et al.*, 2009).

Diagnosis is confirmed by neuropathological examination that demonstrates loss of myelin and axons, presence of gliosis and spheroids. Macrophages that may or may not be pigmented are also present. Hereditary diffuse leukoencephalopathy with axonal spheroids (HDLS) and pigmentary orthochromatic leukodystrophy (POLD), both conditions that can be hereditary or sporadic were previously described as two separate entities, however, a recent review by Wider *et al.* calls to merge them as one entity known as ALSP because the pathology frequently overlaps among them (Wider *et al.*, 2009). The exact pathophysiology of the condition is not yet well known; theories include primary axonal disease, primary myelin disease, oligodendrogliopathy or oxidative stress (Wider *et al.*, 2009). There is of yet no effective treatment for the condition.

In summary, our patient presented at a young age with rapidly progressing dementia, a brain biopsy was able to reveal a leukoencephalopathy known as ALSP as the diagnosis. Unfortunately the patient died after several years from onset with a rapidly progressive course.

Take home messages

- A typical presentations of dementia always deserve a detailed work up to detect potentially reversible causes.
- A leukoencephalopathy should be suspected in adults presenting with various neurologic deficits such as cognitive impairment, pyramidal signs, extrapyramidal signs, ataxia and seizures.

- Brain biopsy may be necessary for diagnosis in dementia, in particular in young individuals with a progressive course.
- ALSP is an increasingly recognized cause of dementia in the young with leukoencephalopathy.

REFERENCES AND SUGGESTED READING

Ali ZS, Van Der Voorn JP, Powers JM (2007). A comparative morphologic analysis of adult onset leukodystrophy with neuroaxonal spheroids and pigmented glia–a role for oxidative damage. *Journal of Neuropathology and Experimental Neurology*, **66**(7), 660–72. doi:10.1097/nen.0b013e3180986247

Baba Y, Ghetti B, Baker MC, Uitti RJ, Hutton ML, Yamaguchi K, Bird T, Lin W, DeLucia MW, Dickson DW, Wszolek ZK (2006). Hereditary diffuse leukoencephalopathy with spheroids: Clinical, pathologic and genetic studies of a new kindred. *Acta Neuropathologica*, **111**(4), 300–11. doi:10.1007/s00401-006-0046-z

Chui HC, Victoroff JI, Margolin D, Jagust W, Shankle R, Katzman R (1992). Criteria for the diagnosis of ischemic vascular dementia proposed by the state of california alzheimer's disease diagnostic and treatment centers. *Neurology*, **42**(3 Pt 1), 473–80.

Costello DJ, Eichler AF, Eichler FS (2009). Leukodystrophies: Classification, diagnosis, and treatment. *The Neurologist*, **15**(6), 319–28. doi:10.1097/NRL.0b013e3181b287c8

Doody RS, Pavlik V, Massman P, Rountree S, Darby E, Chan W (2010). Predicting progression of alzheimer's disease. *Alzheimer's Research & Therapy*, **2**(1), 2. doi:10.1186/alzrt25

Freeman SH, Hyman BT, Sims KB, Hedley-Whyte ET, Vossough A, Frosch MP, Schmahmann JD (2009). Adult onset leukodystrophy with neuroaxonal spheroids: Clinical, neuroimaging and neuropathologic observations. *Brain Pathology (Zurich, Switzerland)*, **19**(1), 39–47. doi:10.1111/j.1750-3639.2008.00163.x

Lopez OL, Wisniewski S, Hamilton RL, Becker JT, Kaufer DI, DeKosky ST (2000). Predictors of progression in patients with AD and lewy bodies. *Neurology*, **54**(9), 1774–9.

O'Sullivan M, Jarosz JM, Martin RJ, Deasy N, Powell JF, Markus HS (2001). MRI hyperintensities of the temporal lobe and external capsule in patients with CADASIL. *Neurology*, **56**(5), 628–34.

Petersen RC, Morris JC (2005). Mild cognitive impairment as a clinical entity and treatment target. *Archives of Neurology*, **62**(7), 1160–3; discussion 1167. doi:10.1001/archneur.62.7.1160

Portet F, Scarmeas N, Cosentino S, Helzner EP, Stern Y (2009). Extrapyramidal signs before and after diagnosis of incident alzheimer disease in a prospective population study. *Archives of Neurology*, **66**(9), 1120–6. doi:10.1001/archneurol.2009.196

Ridha B, Josephs KA (2006). Young-onset dementia: A practical approach to diagnosis. *The Neurologist*, **12**(1), 2–13. doi:10.1097/01.nrl.0000186798.86255.69

Rudzinski LA, Fletcher RM, Dickson DW, Crook R, Hutton ML, Adamson J, Graff-Radford NR (2008). Early onset familial alzheimer disease with spastic paraparesis, dysarthria, and seizures and N135S mutation in PSEN1. *Alzheimer Disease and Associated Disorders*, **22**(3), 299–307. doi:10.1097/WAD.0b013e3181732399

Sampson EL, Warren JD, Rossor MN (2004). Young onset dementia. *Postgraduate Medical Journal*, **80**(941), 125–39.

Scarmeas N, Honig LS, Choi H, Cantero J, Brandt J, Blacker D, Albert M, Amatniek JC, Marder K, Bell K, Hauser WA, Stern Y (2009). Seizures in alzheimer disease: Who, when, and how common? *Archives of Neurology*, **66**(8), 992–7. doi:10.1001/archneurol.2009.130

Schott JM, Fox NC, Rossor MN (2002). Genetics of the dementias. *Journal of Neurology, Neurosurgery, and Psychiatry*, **73** Suppl 2, II27–31.

Staekenborg SS, van der Flier WM, van Straaten EC, Lane R, Barkhof F, Scheltens P (2008). Neurological signs in relation to type of cerebrovascular disease in vascular dementia. *Stroke; a Journal of Cerebral Circulation*, **39**(2), 317–22. doi:10.1161/STROKEAHA.107.493353

Tournier-Lasserve E, Iba-Zizen MT, Romero N, Bousser MG (1991). Autosomal dominant syndrome with strokelike episodes and leukoencephalopathy. *Stroke; a Journal of Cerebral Circulation*, **22**(10), 1297–302.

Whiteman ML, Post MJ, Berger JR, Tate LG, Bell MD, Limonte LP (1993). Progressive multi-focal leukoencephalopathy in 47 HIV-seropositive patients: Neuroimaging with clinical and pathologic correlation. *Radiology*, **187**(1), 233–40.

Wider C, Van Gerpen JA, DeArmond S, Shuster EA, Dickson DW, Wszolek ZK (2009). Leukoencephalopathy with spheroids (HDLS) and pigmentary leukodystrophy (POLD): A single entity? *Neurology*, **72**(22), 1953–59. doi:10.1212/WNL.0b013e3181a826c0

Index

Lightning Source UK Ltd.
Milton Keynes UK
UKOW06f0709161013

219146UK00002B/4/P